Myofaction

Myofascial manipulation

Second Edition

by

Rowland Benjamin D.O.

Copyright © 2002
First Edition June 2002
Second Edition December 2022

Published by R Benjamin

Myofaction - Myofascial manipulation

ISBN 978-0-9581119-4-2

Table of contents

Preface to the Second Edition

Myofaction - Myofascial manipulation was written over twenty years ago, before the age of print-on demand and online publishing. I obtained an ISBN for the book in 2002 and printed one hundred spiral bound copies. I sold about thirty copies to medical libraries around the world and the rest to manual therapists.

There were few outlets available for the book in 2002 and this resulted in the limited sale of the first edition. Now with the arrival of numerous online companies supplying bookshops and individuals around the world, the book will have much greater availability and it is anticipated that the second edition of Myofaction will have a wider distribution.

Over the twenty years since writing Myofaction I have used the technique to treat patients in my various osteopathic clinics. I wanted to run some controlled trials into the effectiveness of the technique but never found the time. I can however report significantly good results with the treatment of my patients, which I credit to the use of myofaction. The twenty years between first writing Myofaction and publishing it today have given me the time to fine tune the technique and it has enabled me to appreciate how effective the technique is in clinical practice.

Myofaction provides health professionals with a unique system of manipulation for each muscle or group of muscles in the body. The book explains massage scientifically and comprehensively. There are three fundamental elements in remedial massage technique, the primary force of compression or transverse pressure, the secondary force of torsion or leverage and the longitudinal or stretch force. These are combined with isometric muscle contraction and focused breathing to produce the myofaction technique.

Myofaction is a highly effective clinical intervention. Although it may be unusual to go into theoretical ideas in the preface, I feel it is necessary to clearly outline why the technique is so effective. Myofaction works because it uses the best elements of remedial massage - cross-fibre kneading, tortional kneading and passive stretching and combines them with isometric contraction and focused breathing. It uses both tension and relaxation. The tension is produced externally with the kneading and stretching actions of the hand and internally with the isometric muscle contraction. This internal tension of the isometric contraction adds another important tension level to the technique, which is absent in the kneading techniques of regular massage.

Myofaction works because the technique acts directly on the muscle to challenge the muscle fibres. Direct action is arguably more effective than indirect action because direct muscle manipulation actually changes the muscle. The application of force on the muscle increases the length of the muscle fibres and stimulates the movement of fluid within and around them. Longer muscle fibres are stronger, more flexible and less tense. Greater fluid movement facilitates the availability of nutrients and oxygen to the muscle and the removal of waste.

Myofaction also works well because the first part of the breathing cycle raises muscle tension to an optimum level and the second part allows time for the muscle to relax. The three types of direct pressure by the hands are maintained against the muscle throughout both the tension phase and the relaxation phase of the technique. They are only released at the end of the one to three repeated breath cycles, depending on how many the therapist wants to use before moving their hand to another part of the muscle.

Increased muscle tension occurs at the end of the inhalation phase of the breathing cycle and while the breath is held in. Relaxation or a decrease in muscle tension occurs at the end of the exhalation phase of breathing and this is assisted by a voluntary letting go of the muscle by the patient. Relaxation is also facilitated by the isometric muscle contraction because the increase in tension generated by the contraction is always followed by post-isometric muscle relaxation.

Another positive aspect of myofaction is that it involves the patient in the treatment. Instead of just being a passive body being treated, the patient connects with the therapist and engages with the treatment, and this provides psychological reinforcement and a better outcome.

The name myofaction is a derivative of muscle (myo) and fascia (fa) and isometric muscle contraction (action). Although the technique mainly treats muscles, fascia surrounds muscles and connects them, and so is an in integrated part of the muscle.

The book is an instruction manual and a reference book on anatomy and myofascial technique. It is written for professional therapists such as for osteopaths, physiotherapists, chiropractors, doctors and advanced masseurs.

The principles of wholism and self-healing which underpin the practice of 'myofaction' are explained in the introduction. There are several useful tables found at the beginning and end of the book including keys for the arrows and applicators. The techniques and anatomical terms used in the book, are defined. To save time, a questionnaire may be given to the patient to support the case history. A brief explanation of the physical examination and a list of muscles and their ranges of movement are provided. In addition to the standard methods of evaluation the 'somafeedback' system is included to assess and correct overuse patterns.

Myofaction - Myofascial manipulation briefly looks at evaluation of the patient in the introduction, the emphasis of the book however is on treatment. The book covers the soft tissues of the human body in a superior to inferior direction. It starts at the head, then works through the cervical spine to the thoracic spine, ribs and lumbar spine. It then follows the upper limb from the shoulder muscles down to the elbow, forearm and hand. The lower limb is covered in a similar way starting with the muscles, which attach on the pelvis and spine and then working through the thigh, leg and feet. Finally, the book looks at the lymphatics system, which is responsible for the drainage of the myofascia.

Each chapter follows a similar approach using bullets and headings. Easy to follow statements describe in chronological order a step by step method of applying the technique. First the anatomy of the region is explained, and a handy anatomical diagram of the area is provided. Then the technique is defined, the position of the patient is described and supporting statements are made. The position of the therapist is described and supporting statements are made, then the applicator is defined (this is the part of the therapist's body which is applied to the patient), the tissue tensions (lock ups) are described, and also the type of technique.

The myofaction technique (also called the active component), kneading, friction and inhibition techniques are illustrated with computer manipulated images showing the therapist performing the technique on the patient. Throughout this book the text, photographs and diagrams always refer to the right side of the body.

The book explains one hundred and forty two different techniques, using two hundred illustrations, one hundred and ninety photographs and eighty six anatomical diagrams. These visual aids help the reader to easily understand the written description of the technique. The arrows in each illustration give an appreciation of the direction of the muscle fibres, the appropriate direction of the applicator and the direction of the isometric muscle contraction. A small mini-key for the arrows is placed below each illustration to remind the reader of the meaning of the different arrows.

This book is a confluence of three skills: clinical skills as an osteopath, lecturing skills in anatomy and soft tissue manipulation, and skills in graphic design. Clinical skills provide the experience, lecturing skill provide the ability to impart knowledge, and the computer skills provide the tools to be able to package the knowledge effectively.

Biography

The author, Rowland Benjamin has worked as an Osteopath for thirty-seven years and in the health and massage field of massage for over forty years. In the late 1970s he established yoga schools in Australia and the U.K and worked with yoga and massage for several years before training as an Osteopath at the N.S.W. College of Natural Therapies and the Pacific College of Osteopathic medicine, Sydney, Australia. He set up his first Osteopathic practice in July 1985 in Sydney, Australia. In 1987 he moved to Liverpool, UK and worked for a year there and used the time for postgraduate studies at The British School of Osteopathy.

Rowland started working as a lecturer in 1987 teaching 'Natural medicine' for Liverpool City Council and 'Natural living' at Burton Manor College, Cheshire, U.K. Since then, he has lectured in Alternative medicine, Natural living, Soft tissue technique, Surface anatomy, Transverse friction, Deep tissue massage, Contemporary health issues, Life skills, Hydrotherapy and Advanced massage at various colleges in Perth, Western Australia.

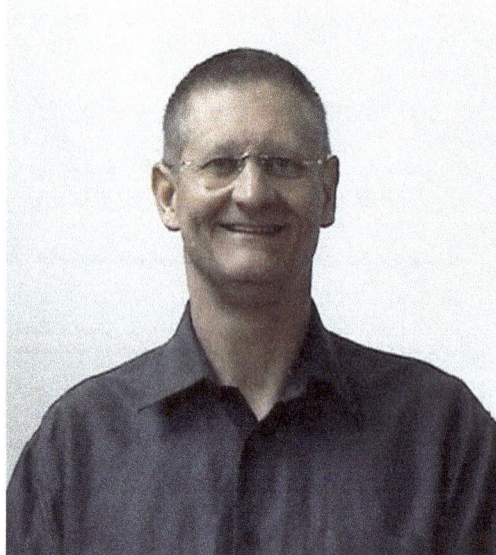

During his career as an Osteopath Rowland has worked in Australia and the UK in private practice and as a locum. In 2015 he published 'Safe Stretch' that looked at individual differences and took them into account when prescribing the right stretches. www.safe-stretch.info. In 2022 he published Massage Yourself, which describes a series of self-massage techniques for muscles, tendons and ligaments www.massage-yourself.com. Rowland also authors environmental books that use cartoons to explain the issues www.ecofreakocartoons.com

Rowland has travelled extensively throughout Australia, New Zealand, Asia, the Middle East, Europe, Africa, North America, Central America and South America and worked as an environmental activist for forty years and runs Information for Action www.informaction.org.

In the 1990s he engaged in a musical career for a few years, writing and performing his song in Australia and the UK. Since 2010 he has been working on the construction of a Permaculture based orchard and nature area in Bridgetown, Western Australia where he resides and practices osteopathy. Progress at Bridgetown Hillside Garden can be viewed at www.bhg.org.au. He continues to practice evidence based and anatomy based manual therapy using self-help systems such as stretching and self-massage to empower his patients.

Acknowledgments

I would like to thank George Stylian D.O., for his influence on my way of approaching soft tissue manipulation. I would like to thank Patrick Sharman, Dragan Mardesic, Blake Casey and Marcus Bryant who were models for the illustrations and David Lehmann, Tristin Apse and Andrew Southern who were models in the photographs and video clips.

I would like to thank Simon Ayles who was a model in the photographs and video clips and who helped with improving the wording of the text. I would like to thank Rachel Handelman who was a model in the photographs and video clips and who helped with filming the video. I would especially like to thank Kim Safety for tracing the photographs. I would also like to thank my partner, Nirada for her support.

Introduction

Myofaction follows the principles of osteopathic medicine. These are the principles of wholism or holism, self-repair or healing, and the interdependence between structure and function.

The concept of wholism has been around since the time of Socrates and Plato, but it was 1928 when J.C. Smuts first coined the term holism. He described it as a philosophy, which looks at whole systems rather than parts. I prefer to use wholism rather than holism because it is accurately spelt this way. Dr Andrew Still, the founder of Osteopathy was one of the first to use wholism in medicine. Although the body is made up of separate tissues and biological systems, it is a unit, but with the parts interdependent on each other. Here are some examples of wholism. A poor mental attitude can lead to physical illness. Conversely prolonged physical illness may lead to mental stress. Ankylosis or loss of movement at a joint such as the ankle can create compensatory stress and inflammation at another joint such as the hip and in time lead to permanent degeneration.

Dr Still observed patients who got better without treatment. In time and under the right conditions some illnesses clear up and symptoms go away. Cuts and bruises, sprains, colds and many types of illnesses respond to their insult by going through an acute phase of repair. These insults may be physical stresses such as cold, injury, a virus, bacteria or psychological stresses. The body has powerful tools for its repair and healing. Dr Still believed that it was better if medicine worked with the healing process. He recommended that the role of the therapist should be to provide the conditions necessary for health, the body's needs and a good environment. He believed that through manipulation and good management of the patient, the body could be made to work better and heal itself more efficiently.

Manipulative treatment should assist the body's natural repair process and other natural functions by influencing the movement of blood and other body fluids and facilitating normal nerve function. Injured tissues cannot be healed directly by manipulation. They only heal if certain repair cells and nutrients can access the damaged tissues through the medium of a good blood supply. Drainage of the damaged area is also essential. Limited drainage of blood, lymph or other body fluids results in the accumulation of waste products, which become irritants to nerves in the immediate tissue. Manipulation facilitates healing by influencing the movement of blood around the repairing tissue. Good circulation is the curative agent.

Structure governs function. From the single cell to the level of whole joints, muscles or organs, the integrity of structures either supports or undermines the healthy running of the body. The converse is also true: function governs structure. So, the rule should be that structure is inter-related with function. Good use or functioning of the body facilitates the stimulation and nourishment of structures that support the body.

Here are a few examples of how impairment in structure affects function: a) an increased thoracic kyphosis impedes diaphragm and rib movement, which is essential for respiration.
b) muscle fibrosis reduces the blood flow necessary for the maintenance of that muscle and tissues near it. c) a joint lesion in the spine decreases movement and reduces local blood flow with resulting nerve irritation. d) a defective vein results in poor drainage and swelling.

Medicine has been in the grip of linear mechanistic thinking for over two hundred years. People are compared with machines; their nervous system is likened to an electrical wiring installation, and their digestive system to a plumbing system. Scientists have tended to break living things down to their parts rather than work with whole systems. Orthodox medicine is still very compartmentalised, with specialists taking an increasingly narrow perspective on the patient's problem and symptoms are treated with little regard for their causes.

The common headache is a good example of linear thinking. Billions of dollars a year are spent worldwide on analgesics to treat headache symptoms. They give relief but often the headaches keep coming back. Many headaches are caused by muscular tension in the neck and shoulders, stress, poor posture, trauma and overuse habits. The muscular tension results in changes in blood flow to the brain. Myofaction would be more appropriate for treating these kinds of 'tension' headaches than analgesics because myofaction addresses the structural changes in the myofascia and the patterns of overuse that are at the cause of the problem. Stress, poor posture and trauma are also causes which may need to be addressed before a satisfactory resolution to the patient's headache can be achieved.

Scientific method splits things into parts so that it can better understand details and processes and communicate them effectively. No living thing, however, ever works as separate parts, and as far as the life sciences are concerned the benefits of fragmentation are clearly limited. The sum of the parts does not make the whole.

Wholistic medicine emphasises a unity between mind and body. This came about as a reaction to the general lack of understanding in medicine of the important role which the mind has in illness. Until the 1960s the body and mind were considered separate entities, and the body was given the focus of attention. The fact that the mind could cause a breakdown in health was largely unrecognised by mainstream medicine. Therefore, a shift from body to mind was necessary to redress the imbalance. The mind and body should not be seen as alternatives but as having varying degrees of involvement in illness. The interplay between mind and body can cause illness and Wholism is concerned with all the factors. In one person's illness the mind may play a major role whereas in another person it may be less significant.

A careful case history is necessary to elicit and evaluate the facts so as to establish the cause of the illness. It is important to make an initial diagnosis. I re-evaluate the diagnosis as the patient and his or her condition changes. The diagnosis is a label, which may change in time. Be aware that a diagnosis can become so firmly entrenched in the mind of a patient as to become a prophecy, a predictive label, a fait accompli.

Nothing in life is static. The longer the duration of any illness the greater the chance of involvement of the mind. Prolonged pain, for example, may lead to psychoemotional changes such as anxiety or depression. These may later develop into physical illnesses such as peptic ulcers or muscular changes. The cause-effect relationship is central to the philosophy of wholistic medicine. If we assume health to be the natural state of human existence and illness an aberration of this state, then for there to be illness there must be a cause. Therefore, it is of primary importance that we remove causes if the patient is to get better.

Wholism is also about considering all the factors which contribute to illness. In one person's illness it may be the mind, in another it may be dietary, occupational, environmental or a combination of several factors. One or several aggravating or causal factors may exist in a single illness. Causal factors include over/under stress, poor nutrition, toxins in our food, water and air, over/under/faulty exercise, occupational problems, trauma, poor posture, medication and unhealthy habits such as smoking and drinking.

It has long been recognised that many of the diseases of Western society are a product of our lifestyles, and therefore under our control.

Genetic factors may lay down the foundations for illness to occur, but it is environmental and use factors over which we have control. Most germs do not cause illness in a healthy person. If they did so there would be no time when we would not be sick because germs exist all around, and within us. Germs particularly proliferate in tissues that are inefficient in removing waste. High levels of toxicity make them more vulnerable to damage.

For some people illnesses such as infections are the only way for them to attract and receive attention and enabling them to take the time to rest in bed and avoid doing something they don't like, such as exams. Illnesses can be straightforward, but peoples' problems frequently are more complex than they appear at first glance. Once again this comes back to the importance of the case history to understand the person one is trying to help.

Health is a positive state of vitality, and not merely the absence of symptoms and signs of illness. To maintain health, humans have to find a balance between their physical, mental, social, emotional and other needs.

If the body is healthy, it must have vitality. Although vitality is not something which can easily be measured scientifically, it does exist and can be deduced even by someone untrained in medicine. A person can be without symptoms of any illness yet lacking in vitality. A sick person, however, will always be lower in vitality because damaged structures will place stresses on different areas of the body. There will be lower energy levels in the body as the body focuses on the process of healing and repair.

Factors which build vitality must be appropriate, qualitatively, quantitatively and timely. Rest is the most valuable means of increasing ones vitality. However, too much rest can be a problem, and so building up the body with an exercise routine of stretching, strengthening, aerobics, stamina and skill development may be required. Too much exercise can devitalise the body and cause injury. Stress can overwhelm the body's coping mechanism, but stress is needed to stimulate and to strengthen the mind and body. Nourishing food is important when hungry. We must be in tune with our natural instincts like thirst and hunger to derive optimal benefit from our food. Overeating results in a diminishing return from our food, a build-up of unwanted fat and the waste products of metabolism in the body and a poor performance by the body generally. Overuse or misuse of the body results in the body using up its reserves of vitality. If vitality is depleted faster than it can be replenished it results in enervation. As well as the obvious fatigue and energy-drain, low vitality also affects digestion and metabolic processes. Waste products of metabolism will not be removed quickly from the body via the blood. The accumulated waste causes toxaemia, which leads to further illness.

Here is a hypothetical look at how vitality is depleted when several illnesses affect the body simultaneously. If the body has 1000 units of vitality to start with and 250 are lost through a back problem, 50 are lost through a toothache and 50 are lost through an emotional problem then only 650 units of vitality will remain. Other health needs which build and support vitality in the body include good hygiene, adequate clothing and housing, a healthy environment, social and sexual relations, play and recreation, a positive mental attitude, a belief system, dignity and self-reliance. The body requires these factors both in health and sickness. Only the proportions differ.

In life, vitality is a constantly changing force, which determines one's resistance to disease. Vitality works as a buffer against stresses acting upon the body. It is when vitality is low that the body is most vulnerable, and its natural defences can be overwhelmed. Disease is the process whereby the body is attempting to restore equilibrium and return to health, and symptoms are the expression of this process brought to conscious awareness. Symptoms are just the tip of a much larger pathological iceberg. The disease process should not be suppressed unless there is danger of irreparable tissue damage, because this is the most significant factor in recovery. Symptoms are signals that something is wrong and obviously must be relieved, but medicine tends to focus on treating the symptoms and misses the big picture. Our bodies are like the environment with its sensitive ecology, and we tamper with it at our cost. The body should be respected, understood and utilised to the greatest advantage.

Wholistic medicine emphasises the patient, not the treatment. In other words, it is not the maximum input of treatment from the maximum number of modalities, but the minimum input of treatment from the optimum number of modalities. Wholistic medicine is also an expression of individual and collective responsibility for health, rather than the will-yourself-well approach, advocated by proponents of rugged individualism.

For a large number of problems treatment may not be necessary, because with sufficient vitality the body heals itself. The most obvious factor for recovery is the removal of causes and providing the body and mind with health needs. As long as the condition is not a medical emergency or there is danger of irreparable damage, treatment should be conservative, safe, effective and health enhancing. No interference is sometimes the best medicine, but it requires experience and sound judgement. Sometimes postural, nutritional or psychoemotional counselling can be utilised to accelerate recovery. The boundaries between therapist and teacher should be diffuse and change to suit the circumstances.

Physical manipulation of the soft tissues and joints can be used to maintain a normal range of movement and enhance better blood-flow and nerve supply to damaged tissues. Hydrotherapy, the use of heat or cold, can be used to increase blood flow and hence tissue repair or reduce pain or unwanted inflammation. Postural, nutritional and basic stress management help may be given. Rest has already been mentioned. It exists as physical rest, mental rest, sensory rest and physiological rest. All may be beneficial at different times.

Working with other practitioners who are skilled in different modalities may be useful at times. All practitioners have limits to their knowledge and skills, and it is important to recognise these limits if we are not to waste the patient's time and money and put them through prolonged discomfort. Maintaining communication with a network of other practitioners is important for effective medicine.

One school of thought in wholistic medicine states that it does not matter what therapy you practice, and it does not matter if the therapy can be proved scientifically. Provided you do no harm and if you have the right attitude, they say, the person you are treating will pick up on the care you are giving them and respond in a positive way.

When a drug with no active ingredient is given to a group of patients in a clinical trial, one third of the group will experience benefit from the drug. It is because they believe in it. This is called the placebo effect. But the placebo effect operates in many situations other than in the clinical trials of drugs. In a Western hospital, symbols such as the doctor's white coat, stethoscope and prescription pad are all placebos which enhance the treatment. In Africa the tribal witch doctor has different symbols and performs different rituals to enhance their treatments, but these are also placebos. In manual therapy, the act of touching the patient can be a placebo, and many popular techniques are placebos. The therapist's body language, their attitude and the phrases they choose to use, combine, to form the bedside manner which is so necessary for recovery. The disdain given to placebo treatment by society is not justified. It is not a trick or the ineffective part of the treatment. Placebos are the health practitioner's best friends. I am not suggesting that we should rely on placebos or use them exclusively to treat physical disease. We should use techniques that have a scientific and anatomical basis supporting them. We should use the best treatment for the problem. But placebos are useful, and if they complement the treatment they should be exploited.

A charismatic physician can utilise the important placebo effect and inspire patients to get better more quickly. This may be called healing, but I believe true healing comes only from within. However useful it may be for the patient to believe in the therapist or symbols of medical power, I believe it is healthier if the patient is encouraged to believe in themselves. Rather than the mystification, which is so common in medical practice, the wholistic approach emphasises empowerment. The therapist should maintain a willingness to give up control over the patient, and the patient, in turn, must be willing to take responsibility for their life. The therapist patient relationship therefore is one based on an attitude of caring and mutual respect.

For health to exist there must be a healthy environment supporting us. The facts indicate that what once was a healthy environment is slowly being eroded away. Environmental disasters like Chernobyl make us dramatically aware of the reality of the global village. Car pollution and deforestation do not have such an immediate impact on our environment and our quality of life, so we often ignore them. We cannot escape from our environment and if we make it unfit to live in then we will surely suffer. Effort is therefore needed on both an individual level and on a social level to manage our environment if we are to maintain or improve our present health.

The wholistic approach is humanistic rather than mechanistic or technology-orientated. This is not to negate the important achievements which have taken place, particularly in the field of surgery and more recently in genetics; they also have their place in wholistic medicine. Wholism is about gaining a perspective on this complex, interrelated and dynamic system of life. It is a bringing together of different health care professions, appropriate to the needs of the patient. It is concerned with fostering self-healing through the process of empowerment and respect. Above all it is caring for the whole person.

Techniques

Treatment is aimed at enabling the body to adapt effectively to acceptable amounts of physical and mental stress placed upon it. It is not an attempt to change a person's posture although this may be possible with long term treatment. Any combination of the techniques can be used. The applicator is that part of the therapist's hand, wrist, elbow or forearm providing the pressure.

Articulation uses repetitive, passive movement, and usually using a lever or fulcrum. The amplitude may be small or large. Sense the feedback from the tissues under your hand. Apply a small bounce at the end of the movement to rapidly produce change and assess tissue reactivity.

Cross fibre kneading uses a slow rhythmical pressure. The amount of force used depends on the depth and the size of the muscle and the thickness of the overlying fascia and other tissues. The patient should cooperate by trying to be as relaxed as possible.

Friction uses firm pressure that is applied over a small surface area. It may be used over ligaments and joint capsules, and between tendons and their sheaths, and for breaking down adhesions at tendon-osseous junctions. Use only for chronic conditions and not when the tissues are inflamed and hence painful. Find the right spot. The therapist's fingers and the patient's skin must move as one. Work across the fibres of the affected structure and systematically cover all the injured area. Apply sufficient pressure to reach deeply enough and make sure the patient's muscles are relaxed. Your posture and the patient's posture should be optimal. Tendons with a sheath must be kept taught.

Pain over a tendon may be due to a strain, either as trauma from a single episode or repetitive actions. Tendonitis is the result. This is characterised by pain and swelling and may be successfully treated using myofascial manipulation. This will increase circulation to the area, help remove scar tissue and with appropriate exercise will restore structural integrity to the damaged tendon. Transverse friction over the tendon and sheath for 3-5 minutes twice a week is required until the condition improves. Rest and strapping may be indicated for the first 48 hours after injury. Ice packs may be applied to the tendon for 15 minutes three times daily.

Inhibition uses firm pressure, held over a small area. Pressure should be increased and decreased gradually and may involve respiratory cooperation. Useful for relaxing spastic muscles, improving local circulation and increasing or decreasing nerve impulses e.g. to the autonomic nervous system

Isometric muscle contraction is a force made by the patient on an unyielding resistance offered by the therapist.

Myofaction is a system of manipulation which corrects structural changes in muscle and fascia (myofascia) that occur as a result of overuse or injury. Isometric muscle contraction is combined with direct pressure on the muscle, usually from a part of the therapists hand, to correct the structural changes. Tissue tension is taken up in three planes. The primary tissue tension is taken up with a combination of compression or transverse/cross-fibre pressure on the muscle. The secondary tissue tension is taken up with pressure on the muscle, usually rotation or torsional force. The longitudinal tissue tension is taken up by taking apart the end attachments of the muscle, like a simple stretch, but not stretched to its full extent.

Muscles are the contractile element in the musculoskeletal system and respond to external and internal stimuli. Initially they respond to physical and psychological insult with temporary changes such as hypertonicity and shortening. These changes are relatively easy to correct with manipulation or self-help systems such as stretching. If however these changes are allowed to persist or not adequately corrected, then they may result in more permanent structural changes such as fibrosis, which involves fibrous infiltrations into the muscle cells. These structural changes are more persistent, and intensive manipulation may be required to correct them.

Fascia is widely distributed throughout the body. It exists between muscle cells and attaches to them. Fascia has a relatively fixed structure and is part of the non-contractile element in the musculoskeletal system. Muscle cells exert a force through the fascia to the tendons. Fascia is slower to respond to overuse but if the muscle element is subjected to long-term insult, then the fascia will become distorted and shortened. Muscle is elastic but fascia is plastic and can be likened to the plastic wrap used on foods. Structural changes in fascia are the most persistent type to treat. More force and a sustained stretch of the fascia is usually required.

Myofaction acts directly to reduce muscle tension, increase blood and lymph circulation, increase muscle length, and increase muscle control, and hence coordination. It also helps to remove overuse habits and reduce involuntary muscle contractions. It works indirectly and generally to increase muscle strength, stamina and efficiency, and also to support the body's ability to heal itself.

Respiratory force is the use of respiration and injunction to induce relaxation. Feel for a release of tension in the muscle during exhalation, and 'take up the slack' by increasing the primary or secondary forces with your applicator or by increasing longitudinal tension. Just before the start of inhalation release your applicator pressure. Reposition your applicator during inhalation.

Stretching uses a slow, purposeful, gradual increase in longitudinal force to separate attachments of muscles, ligaments or fascia. Use a short amplitude for intra articular structures and a longer amplitude for extrinsic structures. It may be rhythmical. The technique should minimise the impact of the stretch reflex. However, an increase in stretch or bounce may be effectively used at the end. Stretching fascia generally requires very slow movement, with medium to heavy pressure.

Anatomical position and terms

Positions may be absolute or relative to other body parts. They assume the anatomical position which is erect with the arms at the side of the body and externally rotated, and the forearms fully supinated. Throughout this text all anatomical terms are related to the patient and not the therapist. Ventral and dorsal are synonyms of anterior and posterior, and these terms apply equally to all quadrupeds. For the superior aspect of the foot refer to dorsum or dorsal surface and for the sole of the foot refer to plantar surface.

Anterior - front of the body or in front of something.
Posterior - back of the body or behind something.

Ventral - front.
Dorsal - back.

Superior - up in a vertical sense.
Inferior - down.

Cephalad - towards the head.
Caudad - towards the feet.

Medial - towards the midline or sagittal plane.
Lateral - away from the midline or sagittal plane.

Deep - away from the surface of the body.
Superficial - towards the surface of the body

Proximal - applies to a limb and refers to something being nearer to the limb root or superior in the anatomical position.

Distal - refers to something being further away from the limb root or inferior in the anatomical position.

Sagittal - the median or midline plane and is named after the sagittal suture.

Coronal - the vertical plane that bisects the front and back halves of the body and is named after the coronal suture.

Transverse or horizontal - the plane which runs across the body horizontally in the anatomical position.

Ipsilateral – on the same side of the body
Contralateral – on the opposite side of the body

Other anatomical and theoretical considerations

All the techniques in this book are based on sound anatomical and scientific knowledge. At the beginning of each chapter a detailed anatomical description of the region is provided which will help the therapist to make a diagnosis of the problem. It is my opinion that referred pain is the exception rather than the rule, and with a good anatomical knowledge, the therapist should be able to name the tissue that is causing the pain and easily come up with a diagnosis.

For convenience physiology tends to look at movements confined to one joint and involving one or only a few muscles. In reality motion is the result of a complex interaction of many joints and muscles (synergists, antagonists, stabilisers) working under the direction of the nervous system.

Muscles function in groups. The principal muscle group or Prime movers are supported, and their direction modified, by Assistant muscles. Neutralisers finely tune motion and counter unwanted movements produced by the prime movers. Antagonists are relaxed by inhibition from the nervous system. This must occur simultaneously with contraction of the prime movers. Stabilisers provide support to the joints which are not being deliberately moved in the manoeuvre, but which may experience some stress in the manoeuvre. Stabilisers support ligamentous function and help maintain apposition (close contact) between joint surfaces during movement.

Movement is necessary for:

1. Locomotion
2. Fluid motion
3. Nerve stimulation
4. Respiration
5. Peristalsis

Loss of movement at a joint may result in:

1. Structural changes to muscles, which results in a) shortness b) atrophy c) weakness
2. Joint degeneration
3. Changes to fascia and other tissues
4. Shortening of ligaments
5. Vascular changes
6. Changes in the neurological feedback

Types of motion restriction include

1. **Contracture** - stiff, inflexible motion with incomplete range of movement. This may be due to shortened muscles and related joint structures.
2. **Spasticity** - stiff inflexible motion with incomplete range of movement. Stretch reflex usually excitable. This is caused by a pyramidal, upper motor neuron lesion.
3. **Spasm** - involuntary muscular contraction. In skeletal muscle the cause is often peripheral nerve irritability.
4. **Rigidity** - stiff and seemingly inflexible with apparently incomplete range of movement, but a slow steady force improves range of movement. This may be caused by tight fascia or an extra pyramidal upper motor neuron lesion.
5. **Flaccidity** - lax motion due to the absence of normal resistance due to muscle tone.
6. **Abrupt** - a sudden jerky motion.

Factors responsible for pathological limitation of joint mobility are

1. **Nerve, blood or muscular interference** due to somatic dysfunction in a related part or segment of the spine, or from causes such as stress or misuse.
2. **Abnormalities or abnormal growths** of tissues or bones in close proximity to the joint. For example, ankylosis, osteophytes or a tumour.
3. **Iatrogenic causes** such as surgical excision or insertion in a muscle or ligament.
4. **Trauma or an injury.** Scars or adhesions after injury must be removed.
5. **Disuse or misuse** resulting in atrophy, or overuse resulting in hypertrophy of muscle.
6. **Psychosomatic factors** with no organic cause.

7. **Biochemical factors** such as prolonged inflammation leading to tissue damage. Inflammation may cause calcium to be deposited in muscle fibres. Diseases such as rheumatoid arthritis or myositis ossificans can cause changes in many types of tissues.
8. **Muscle hypertonicity or fibrosis**. Changes in the nature, density and direction of fibres of intervening tissues; muscle, fascia, fibrocartilage or skin. Normal muscular tone is important for healthy movement. If muscle fibres are hypotonic or hypertonic this will compromise joint stability and function.

Assessment criteria

Myofascial function can be defined according to the following criteria:

1. **What the patient feels** with respect to restriction, pain and other symptoms is noted using a questionnaire or by taking a case history. Although pain can be referred from another site in the body it usually originates at the site of the dysfunction. A good anatomical knowledge is essential in identifying the source of the pain. The psycho-emotional profile of the patient, as determined by the questionnaire and case history, should be taken into account. It is up to the therapist to establish the significance of subjective information. For more detail see the section entitled 'Case history'.

2. **The standing structural analysis** provides information about the position of bony structures when the body is under the influence of gravity. Myofascial dysfunction will often be exaggerated by gravity, and may be more easily seen than when the patient is recumbent. Asymmetry of structure may be due to soft tissue atrophy and hypertrophy, positional change of bony landmarks, or diseases such as osteoarthritis. For more detail see 'Physical examination'.

3. **Palpation** of the myofascia may reveal changes in tissue texture caused by hypertonicity, swelling, hypertrophy, atrophy and spasticity. Change in the skin overlying area of dysfunction may be revealed.

4. **Motion testing** determines the maximum length of the myofascia. This may be a single muscle or group of muscles. This is performed by the therapist who takes the limb or body part to the end of its range of movement, while the patient is relaxed. The range of joint movement can be measured with a goniometer or simple plastic angle ruler. This will provide the absolute measurement which will vary with the age and body type of the patient. In addition, movement of the limb or body part can be compared with the other limb or side. Comparing symmetry provides a relative range of movement. Testing active and passive movement helps differentiate whether a restriction is caused by a shortening of the myofascia or the joint capsule. While range of movement may be reduced, the range may also be exceeded, as in the case of hypermobility, partial or complete dislocation.

5. **Strength testing** determines the ability of a muscle to contract or resist the force from an external object. It is the opinion of the author that in most clinical situations, changes in muscle strength are so small that manual methods of measuring them are unreliable and inaccurate. Strength or weakness is best evaluated by using a calibrated mechanical device that will record a numerical measurement.

6. **Use testing** assesses the patient's ability to relax a single muscle or a group of muscles. Misuse or overuse patterns can be identified using simple feedback techniques. The therapist moves the body part and determines if the patient is able to voluntarily let go. For more detail see 'Somafeedback' Chapter 54.

Questionnaire

PLEASE COMPLETE ALL BLANKS IN CAPITAL LETTERS.
TICK APPLICABLE BOXES.

SURNAME	TITLE Mr ☐ Ms ☐ Mrs ☐ Miss ☐ Other (Please State)	PREVIOUS TREATMENT Osteopathic ☐ Chiropractic ☐ Physiotherapy ☐ Naturopathic ☐ Medical ☐ Other(Please state)
FIRST NAME		
ADDRESS		
TELEPHONE NUMBER Work Home Mobile	IS YOUR WORK? Sitting ☐ Standing ☐ Active ☐ Physically demanding ☐ Mentally demanding ☐	EXERCISE (performed on a regular basis) Stretching ☐ Light weights ☐ Gym aerobics ☐ Walking ☐ Running ☐ Swimming ☐ Yoga ☐ Sports ☐ Other(Please state)
DATE OF BIRTH		
PLACE OF BIRTH		
OCCUPATION	How do you rate your stress levels? Low ☐ Medium ☐ High ☐	
REFERRED BY		
HEALTH FUND		
CHIEF COMPLAINT	How do you cope with stress? Poorly ☐ Moderately ☐ Well ☐	DIAGNOSED DISEASES Osteoarthritis ☐ Osteoporosis ☐ Rheumatism ☐ Malignancy ☐ Infection ☐ Blood vessel disorders ☐ High blood pressure ☐ Other(Please state)
OTHER COMPLAINTS		
FALLS OR ACCIDENTS	How do you rate your energy levels? Low ☐ Medium ☐ High ☐	
PREVIOUS SURGERY		
NAME OF YOUR DOCTOR		
ADDRESS OF YOUR DOCTOR	HOBBIES AND ACTIVITIES	
MEDICATION Past Present		

Case history

Observe the patient entering the room. Notice their gait and attitude. Detailed assessment of gait may be required. Observe the patient's posture, face, speech, body language and manner and actions during the case history for defects, pigmentations, anaemia, jaundice, fidgeting and nervous behaviour.

Basic information Get their full name, address, telephone number, date of birth/age (prone to different types of pathologies), status (single, married, de facto, other), occupation (body use, financial, stressors), ethnic origin (different cultures express illness in different ways), referred by (may need feedback or polite thank you).

Main symptom/complaint Determine the site (specific or general), character (pain, dizziness, pins and needles), severity (numb, ache, sharp pain), and duration (when did it start? is it acute, sub-acute or chronic?). Ask how did it start? (quickly or gradually?), Are there any aggravating factors (is it worse morning/evening, after exercise, rest, when sitting/standing/lying down?), relieving factors (rest, heat/cold, self-help), other signs and symptoms (are they associated with the main symptom, local or referred. How are the patient's energy levels? Do not just get a disease label given by someone else.

Past history of main complaint, other major illnesses, infections, surgery, falls, fractures, accidents, allergies, and previous treatments. Accident history - when, where and how, treatment given. Direction and speed of force, awareness (un/conscious), position and response. By now you should be aware of the patient's attitude to their illness. Family history (brother's, sister's and parent's health/cause of death). Congenital/inherited factors such as cervical ribs, extra or missing vertebrae or muscle attachments, hip deformities. Personal and social history - background of family life and social interests if appropriate. Work - hours, stress/stimulation, dangers, posture, active/sedentary, and economic circumstances. Environmental - home (heating, ventilation, garden), holidays or frequency of breaks.

Psychoemotional Determine their level of stress (too much/little, is source internal/worry or external, management skills), personality (cheerful, anxious, depressed), relationships, history of mental illness (behavioural or organic).

Medication Ask about the name of any past or present medication. Find out their side effects or compound effect from the patient and a reliable pharmaceutical directory.

Present diet Breakfast, Lunch, Dinner, Snacks, idiosyncrasies, allergies. Does diet fulfil the patient's needs for energy, protein (structure), nutrients (vitamins and minerals) and fibre (bulk). Consider the quality of the food, the quantity eaten and the time of day it is eaten. Is the patient able to assimilate, digest, transport, metabolise their food and eliminate their waste? How is the patient's appetite?

Postural Ask how long does the patient spend each day standing, sitting, reclining, and working in unusual positions, or on one weight bearing side? Consider their furniture, mattress, sleeping positions, bad habits.

Exercise/activities Optimally we require a balanced programme of stretching, strengthening, aerobics and skill-development. Find out what the patient enjoys and if possible, use it.

Habits Ask if and how much tea, coffee, sugar, alcohol, tobacco, other drugs, sleep, supplements, medication ie laxatives or sedatives.

Enquire as to their general health, skin, frequency of colds or influenza, bowel action, urine frequency, weight gain/loss.

Record a general evaluation of health - poor, moderate, good, excellent.

Physical examination

Look! You need good lighting. Palpate. Compare symmetry. Check their vital signs. Blood pressure (120/80), weight, height, pulse rate (70-80 beats per minute), respiratory rate (15 breaths per minute), temperature (36.9 deg C).

In the examination we need to consider the interrelations between the various structures (including mind and body), identify and remove the cause of the problem and screen out serious conditions which need referral. The wholistic approach should be adopted but we should be cautious to exercise discrimination, if we are not to be side tracked examining irrelevant tissues, and waste the patient's time and money.

Always examine the area of localised pain or symptom and examine other areas if the problem is referred, compensatory or chronic.

The structural analysis

Posterior view - note symmetry of:
head carriage,
shoulder heights,
scapula bony landmarks
arm distance from side
rotoscoliosis
muscle atrophy and hypertrophy
skin folds at the waist
pelvic bony landmarks
skin folds at the buttocks
skin folds at the knees
valgus or varus of knees
valgus or varus of ankles

Lateral view - note:
head carriage
scapula - is there winging?
anterior-posterior distribution of body
kyphosis
visceroptosis
lordosis
increased lumbosacral angle
pelvic tilt
knee hyperextension

Anterior view - note symmetry of:
face
head carriage
shoulder heights
clavicles
arm distance from side
muscle atrophy and hypertrophy
ribs
sideshifting of trunk
skin folds at the waist
pelvis
patella/ valgus or varus of knees
placement of feet
arches of feet

Gait

The two phases of walking are:

1. **Stance** (60%) includes   a. heel strike   b. flat foot   c. midstance   d. push off

2. **Swing** (40%) includes   a. acceleration   b. midswing   c. deceleration

Ask yourself 'In which phase does the problem occur'? Most occur in the weight bearing stance phase. If there is pain and pathology determine the time spent on the weight bearing leg and the how much the patient's stride decreases.

Painful or antalgic gait may be caused by:

1. a foot problem such as a heel spur, anterior talofibular ligament strain, fallen arches or a metatarsal stress fracture.
2. problems in other joints such as a torn meniscus or ligament damage in the knee or osteoarthritis in the hips or knees.
3. a shoe problem. Look for corns on the dorsum of their toes. Check for rough areas inside the shoe.

Painful calluses may develop over the metatarsal heads as a result of fallen transverse arches. Check if the patient wears down the soles and heels of their shoes excessively or unevenly.

Movement should be smooth and involving the whole body. Does the patient lurch from side to side or walk with their feet wide apart? Osteoarthritis or a fused metatarsophalangeal joint (hallux rigidus) makes hyperextension of the great toe difficult or impossible. Gout may cause pain. Push off may be forced to occur on the side of the foot. Patients whose ankles, knees or hip joints have fused as a result of disease or surgery may have difficulties in all phases of gait, will develop compensations and walk with considerably less energy efficiency.

Myofaction variables

1. Cross fibre force/ Compression
2. Longitudinal force/ Stretch
3. Secondary force/ Torsion
4. Internal force/ Tension
5. Respiratory force/ Breathing

Hypothetical tissue lockup

Compression takes up	20%
Transverse force takes up	20%
Secondary force takes up	20%
Longitudinal force takes up	20%
Contraction force takes up	20%
Total tissue lockup is	100%

The more tension taken up by one, the less tension is available for another.

Throughout this book the text, photographs and diagrams consistently refer to the right side of the body.

Arrows

White arrow

The muscle.

The general direction of the muscle fibres and the place of where the muscle attaches.

Blue arrow

The primary direction of tissue lockup.

This is a transverse force, at right angles to the direction of the muscle fibre and always involving some compression. The amount of compression required depends on how deep the tissue is, the amount of initial tissue slack and how much tension is taken up by the secondary and longitudinal forces.

Green arrow

The secondary direction of tissue lockup.

The force may be in any direction other than the primary direction of tissue lockup, but it is usually a torsional (rotational) force. The secondary force may use a bone as a lever. The lever acts in a counter direction to the primary force to amplify that force.

Red arrow

The stretch direction of tissue lockup.

This is usually along the line of contraction of the muscle and in the same direction as the muscle fibre. This is a longitudinal force. It is also the direction for assessing the ability of the muscle to relax and for correcting the passive component.

Yellow arrow

The contraction tissue lockup.

This is along the line of the muscle fibres. It is a force produced by the muscle and acting on it from within it.

Applicators

Use body weight.

1. One fingertip
   (Small to Medium pressure/ Small surface area).

2. The heads of two or three distal phalanges (a row of fingertips).
   (Medium pressure/ Small to Medium surface area)

3. The heads of interdigitating fingers of both hands.
   (Medium pressure/ Medium surface area)

4. The lateral side of the thumb.
   (Medium pressure/ Medium surface area)

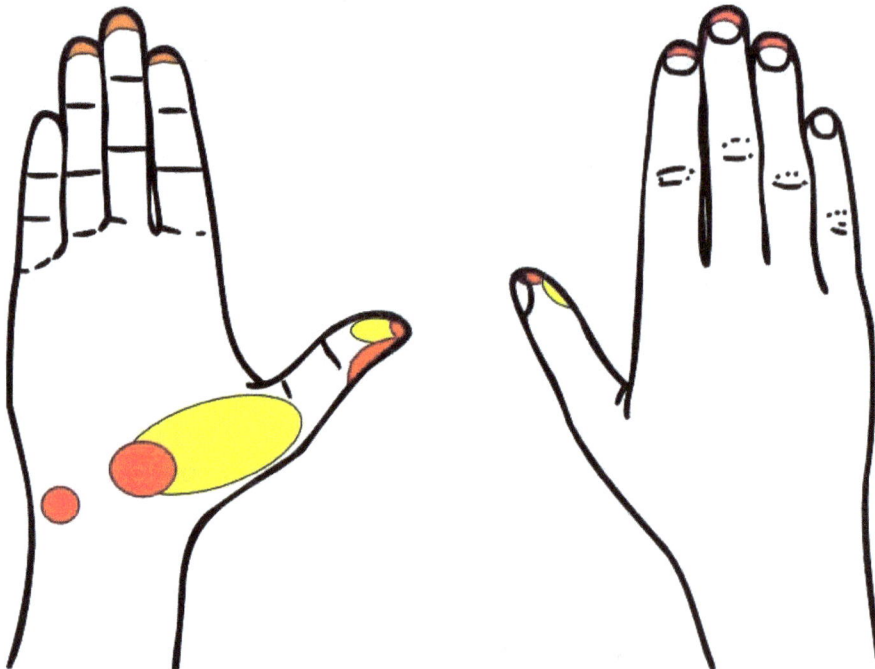

5. The thenar eminence
   (Medium pressure/ Large surface area)

6. Opposition of fingers and thumb to grasp tissue and pull towards therapist.
   (Medium pressure/ Medium surface area)

7. The articular surface of the proximal row of interphalangeal joints (one knuckle or a row of knuckles of the clenched fist).
   (Medium to Large pressure/ Small to Medium surface area)

8. The pad of the thumb.
   (Medium to Large pressure/ Medium surface area)

9. The tip of the thumb.
   (Large pressure/ Small surface area)

10. The tip of the olecranon process
    (Large pressure/ Small surface area)

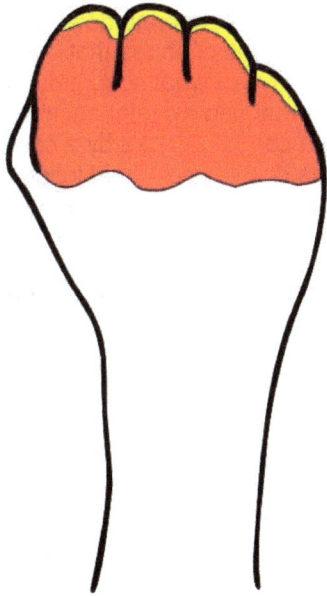

11. The pisiform bone.
   (Large pressure/ Small surface area).

12. The tubercle of the scaphoid and the tubercle of the trapezium (heel of hand).
   (Large pressure/ Medium surface area).

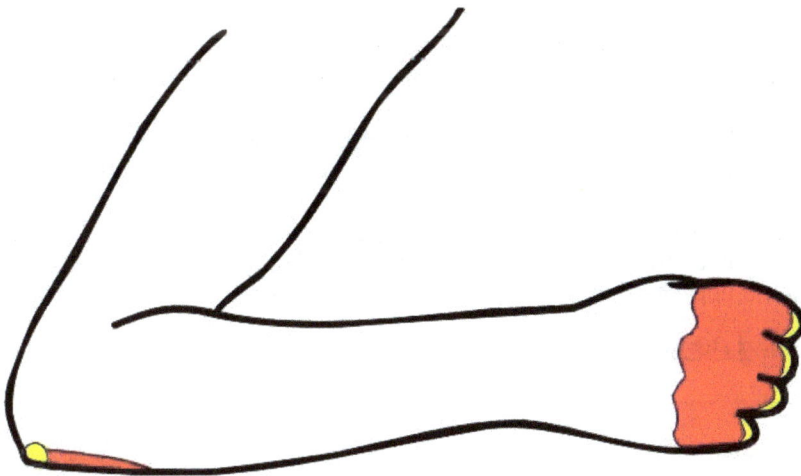

13. The proximal border of the shaft of the ulnar from the olecranon process.
   (Large pressure/ Medium to Large surface area)

14. The dorsal surface of the four proximal phalanges of fingers. (flat part on back of fingers of fist)
   (Large pressure/ Large surface area)

The myofascial manipulation cycles

The graphs A and B are not based on any actual physiological measurements of how muscles respond to manipulation. The total length of the cycle and the breakdown of the time intervals in the cycle are an approximation. The values given to the changes that occur to the muscle in the cycle are also an approximation and representative of what occurs during kneading and myofaction. The shaded area represents the breathing cycle of an inhalation and an exhalation, the dark line represents the pressure that can be exerted by a combination of compression, transverse force, torsion and the longitudinal force. The actual length of the cycle will depend on the patient - their age, gender, level of fitness and lung capacity. Inhalation is given as 80%. This is not maximum inhalation. This is a full but comfortable inhalation and it is assumed that with greater effort the patient could take in a further 20% of air but that this would require a lot of strain. This would defeat the purpose of using breathing in the technique, which is to facilitate relaxation.

A. The kneading cycle

The shaded area shows the breathing cycle over a period of 8 seconds. The inhalation phase is given as 2 seconds and the exhalation phase is given as 6 seconds.

1. The therapist makes applicator contact with the patient at the start of the inhalation phase of the kneading cycle. This is at 0 seconds. (a)
2. The patient takes in a deep inhalation over a period of approximately 2 seconds.
3. For the first 0.5 seconds the therapist's applicator exerts no significant pressure on the muscle. The therapist allows the patient to get use to their touch. (a to b)
4. For the next 1.5 seconds the therapists takes up the skin slack and increases applicator pressure with all of the available compression and some of the longitudinal force (b to c).
5. At the point of full inhalation (x) the applicator pressure is approximately 50%.
6. As the patient exhales the therapist maintains compression and increases applicator pressure by adding a transverse force. The therapist continues to increase the longitudinal force.
7. At about 4 seconds into the breathing cycle the therapist introduces the secondary force. This is usually torsion/rotation but the force may be in any direction other than transverse and it may involve leverage. (d to e)
8. At about 5 seconds into the breathing cycle or 3 seconds into the exhalation phase, the combined compression, torsion, transverse and longitudinal forces are at a maximum. The more use there is of one force, the less there is available for the others.
9. The combination of forces is sustained for about 2.5 seconds. (e to f)
10. At about 7.5 seconds into the breathing cycle or 0.5 seconds before full exhalation, the therapist reduces the applicator pressure and withdraws the applicator contact. (f to g)

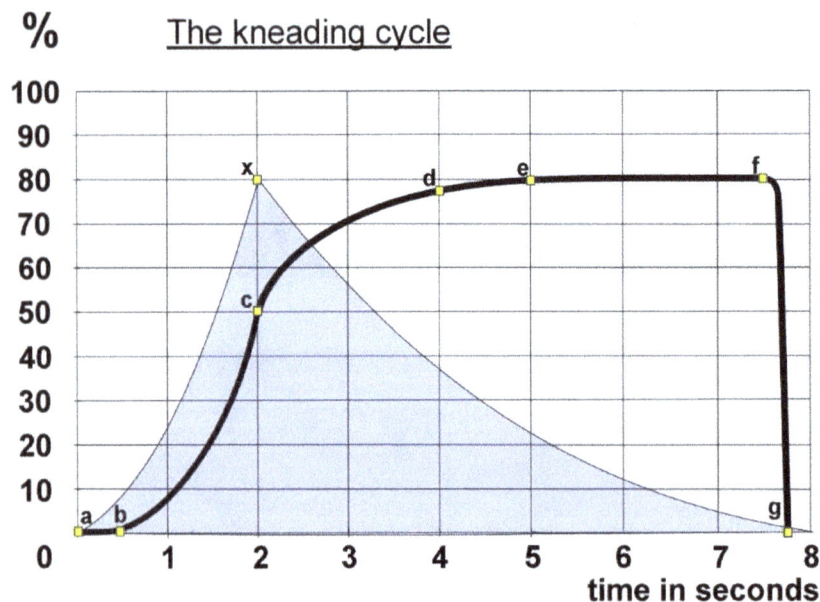

The kneading cycle

B. The myofaction cycle

The shaded area shows the breathing cycle over a period of 12 seconds. The inhalation phase is 2 seconds and the exhalation phase is 6 seconds. In addition, the patient is required to hold their inhalation in for 4 seconds.

1. The therapist makes applicator contact with the patient at the start of the inhalation phase of the myofaction cycle. This is at 0 seconds. (a)
2. The patient is asked to takes in a deep inhalation and hold it in. This takes approximately 2 seconds.
3. For the first 0.5 seconds the therapist's applicator exerts no significant pressure on the muscle. The therapist simply allows the patient to get use to their touch. (a to b)
4. For the next 1.5 seconds the therapists takes up the skin slack and increases applicator pressure with most of the available compression and some of longitudinal force (b to c).
5. At the point of full inhalation (x) the applicator pressure is approximately 40%.
6. At about 2.5 seconds into the breathing cycle the patient is asked to apply a 10% muscle contraction in a given direction. (d)
7. The therapist resists the patient's effort in two ways. Firstly by maintaining their applicator pressure on the muscle directly and secondly by not permitting any movement at the joint.
8. The combination of inhalation, compression and contraction has the effect of increasing tension in the muscle and this is maintained for approximately 3.5 seconds..
9. The patient's muscle contraction should be approximately 10% of full contraction. The applicator will be pushed backwards slightly by the force of the contracting muscle and there will be an increase in the pressure as shown in the graph. (d)
10. If the muscle contraction overwhelms the applicator then this 10% contraction may need to be reduced.
11. At about 6 seconds into the breathing cycle the patient is asked to exhale and relax. (e)
12. As the muscle contraction and the muscle tension subside the therapist increases their applicator pressure. The therapist takes up the post isometric contraction slack in the muscle with a transverse force and an increase in the longitudinal force. (e to g)
13. At about 8 seconds into the breathing cycle the therapist introduces the secondary force. This is usually torsion/rotation but it may be in any direction other than transverse and may involve leverage. (f)
14. At about 9 seconds into the breathing cycle and 3 seconds into the exhalation phase the combined compression, transverse force, longitudinal force and torsion are at a maximum. (g)
15. The combination of forces is sustained for about 2.5 seconds. (g to h)

At about 11.5 seconds into the breathing cycle or 0.5 seconds before full exhalation, the therapist reduces the applicator pressure and withdraws the applicator contact. (h to i)

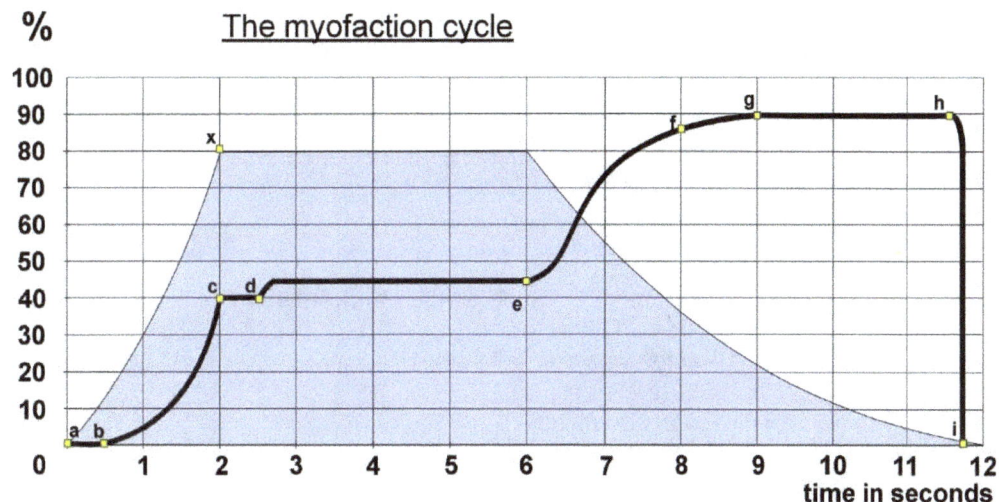

The myofaction cycle

Muscles and ranges of movement (in degrees°)

Isolate motion at the joint being evaluated by stabilising the proximal body part. While the range of joint mobility may be limited or reduced, the range may also be exceeded as in the case of hypermobility, partial or complete dislocations. Range of movement decreases with age, particularly in the spine. Body type, gender, disease and other factors influence the range of movement. The figures below should therefore only be taken as a generalisation.

The Shoulder is a complex of joints working in anatomical cooperation.

Flexion 150 -180°	Extension 40 - 60°
Adduction 30 - 60°	Abduction 180°
Internal Rotation 70 - 95°	External Rotation 80°

With arm abducted 90 °

Internal Rotation 70°	External Rotation 90°
Horizontal Flexion 140°	Horizontal Extension 30°

Other movements include Scapula tilt which is about 60°
Elevation / Depression. The superior to inferior movement of the scapula is about 11 cm
Protraction / Retraction. The medial to lateral movement of the scapula is about 15 cm

Muscles involved

Flexion	Anterior Deltoid (especially after 90°)
	Pectoralis major (clavicular portion)
	Assistants: Biceps and Coracobrachialis
Extension	Latissimus dorsi
	Teres major
	Posterior Deltoid
	Pectoralis major (sternal portion)
	Assistant: Triceps
Adduction	Pectoralis major (sternal)
	Latissimus dorsi
	Teres major
	Assistants: Posterior Deltoid, Biceps and Triceps
Abduction	First phase (0 - 90°)
	Supraspinatus then Middle Deltoid.
	Second phase (90 - 150°)
	Trapezius and Serratus anterior.
	Third phase (150 - 180°)
	Erector spinae muscles and Pectoralis minor
External Rotation	Teres minor
	Infraspinatus
	Assistant: Posterior Deltoid
Internal Rotation	Latissimus dorsi
	Teres major
	Subscapularis
	Pectoralis major
	Assistants: Coracobrachialis and Anterior Deltoid
Horizontal Flexion	Anterior Deltoid
	Pectoralis major (all fibres)
	Subscapularis
	Coracobrachialis.
	Assistant: Biceps
Horizontal Extension	Posterior and Middle Deltoid
	Latissimus dorsi
	Teres major
	Infraspinatus
	Teres minor

18

Scapula Elevation	Levator scapulae
	Upper Trapezius
	Rhomboids
Abduction/Protraction	Serratus Anterior
	Pectoralis Minor
Adduction/Retraction	Rhomboids
	Middle Trapezius

The Elbow includes the humeroulnar joint, humeroradial joint and proximal radioulnar joint.

| Flexion 150° | Extension 0-5° (10°) |
| Supination 80-90° | Pronation 75-85° |

Muscles involved

Flexion	Biceps
	Brachialis
	Brachioradialis
	Assistants: Pronator teres
Extension	Triceps
	Assistant: Anconeus
Pronation	Pronator Teres
	Pronator Quadratus
Supination	Supinator
	Biceps

The Wrist includes the proximal and distal carpal joints and the distal radioulnar joint.

| Abduction 15° | Adduction 30-45° |
| Flexion 80-85° | Extension 70-85° |

Muscles involved

Flexion	Flexor carpi radialis
	Flexor carpi ulnaris
	Palmaris longus.
	Assistants: The finger flexors
	Flexor digitorum profundus and Flexor digitorum superficialis
Extension	Extensor carpi radialis longus
	Extensor carpi radialis brevis
	Extensor carpi ulnaris
	Assistants: The finger extensors
	Extensor digitorum and Extensor pollicis longus
Abduction or Radial deviation	Extensor carpi radialis longus
	Extensor carpi radialis brevis
	Assistants: Flexor carpi radialis, Abductor pollicis longus
	Extensor pollicis longus and brevis
Adduction or Ulnar deviation	Extensor carpi ulnaris
	Flexor carpi ulnaris

The Hand

The thumb

Carpometacarpal joint
  Flexion 15°
  Abduction 70°
  Extension 20°

Metacarpophalangeal joint
  Flexion 90° for the index finger and increasing progressively to the little finger.
  Extension (active) 30 - 40°

Interphalangeal joint
  Flexion 80°
  Extension 15°
  Opposition - the tip of the thumb touches the base or tip of the little finger.

The fingers

Metacarpophalangeal joint
  Flexion 90°
  Extension 45°
  Abduction - Fingers evenly spread.

Proximal interphalangeal joint
  Flexion 100°

Distal interphalangeal joint
  Flexion 80°
  Extension 10°

The Hip

Flexion 90 or 145°	Hyperextension 5-30°
(depending on the knee position)	
External Rotation 45-60°	Internal Rotation 40-50° (greater prone)
Abduction 45°	Adduction 30°

Muscles involved

Flexion	Iliopsoas
	Sartorius,
	Pectineus
	Tensor fascia lata
	Assistants: Rectus femoris, Gracilis,
	Adductor longus and Adductor brevis
Extension	Hamstrings (Semimembranosus, Semitendinosus, Biceps femoris)
	Gluteus maximus (especially in flexion).
	Assistant: Adductor magnus (especially in flexion)
Adduction	Adductor Longus
	Adductor Brevis
	Adductor Magnus
	Gracilis
	Assistants: Pectineus, Gluteus maximus and Hamstrings
Abduction	Gluteus Medius Gluteus Minimus
	Tensor Fascia Lata (especially in extension)
	Assistant: Gluteus maximus
External Rotation	Piriformis
	Quadratus Femoris
	Obturator Internus
	Obturator externus
	Gemellus superior and inferior
	Gluteus maximus

Internal Rotation   Gluteus medius
           Gluteus minimus
           Assistants: Tensor fascia lata and Adductor magnus

The Knee

Flexion/Extension 120-140° (active) 160° (passive) Passive Hyperextension 5-10°
Axial Lateral rotation (knee flexed at right angles) 40° Axial Medial Rotation 30°
Physiological valgus 170-175° Greater in females and children.

Muscles involved
Flexion   Hamstrings
           Sartorius
           Gracilis
           Assistants: Popliteus and Gastrocnemius

Extension   Quadriceps Femoris (Vastus lateralis, medialis, intermedius
           and Rectus femoris)

Lateral Rotation   Biceps Femoris
           Tensor fascia lata

Medial Rotation   Popliteus
           Semimembranosus
           Semitendinosus
           Assistants: Sartorius and Gracilis

Ankle and Foot

Dorsi Flexion 15-25°   Plantar Flexion 40-50°
Subtalar Inversion 5°   Subtalar Eversion 5°
Forefoot Adduction 20°   Forefoot Abduction 10°
Forefoot Inversion 30-35° Forefoot Eversion 15-20°

Toes

Interphalangeal and metacarpophalangeal joints
Flexion (active) 30-40° (passive) 50°
Extension (active) 50-60° (passive) 90°

Great toe

Interphalangeal joint Flexion 70°
Metacarpophalangeal joint Flexion 30° Extension 50-70°

Muscles involved
Plantar Flexion   Gastrocnemius
           Soleus
           Assistants: Peroneus longus and brevis, Tibialis posterior,
           Flexor digitorum longus and Flexor hallucis longus

Dorsi Flexion   Tibialis anterior
           Extensor digitorum longus
           Extensor hallucis longus
           Peroneus tertius

1. Frontalis and occipitalis (Occipitofrontalis)

Anatomy

Occipitofrontalis covers the dome of the skull and is formed by two thin broad muscles, frontalis and occipitalis connected to an aponeurotic sheet, the galea aponeurotica.

Frontalis is formed by two quadrilateral muscles. Their posterior border attaches to the anterior aponeurosis just in front of the coronal suture. Anteriorly they merge with the muscles of the superior orbit: the procerus, corrugator supercilii and orbicularis oculi. There are no bony attachments.

Occipitalis is formed by two quadrilateral muscles attached to the posterior aponeurosis and to the lateral two thirds of the highest nuchal line of the occiput and to the mastoid of the temporal bone.

Actions: Pulls scalp forwards and backwards, raises brow and wrinkles forehead.
Clinical indications: Headaches, scalp injuries, eye strain.
Nerve supply: The facial nerve.

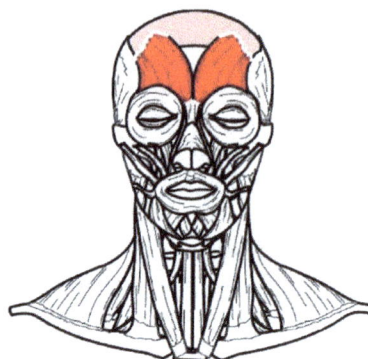

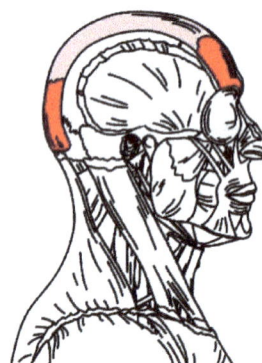

Technique 1.1 Bilateral kneading of frontalis

Patient

- Supine with the head straight and resting on a folded towel or shallow pillow.

Therapist

- Stand or sit at the head of the table.
- Support the patient's head by grasping around the frontal bone and parietal bones with both hands. The fingertips may extend down to the temporal bones.
- Start with both thumbs together either side of the mid-sagittal plane.

Applicator

- The pads of the thumbs of both hands.

Tissue tension

- Take up the longitudinal tension by starting the technique with the forehead relaxed. The eyebrows are therefore depressed.
- Apply compression with pressure from both your thumbs on the middle of the forehead.

Kneading

- Apply a transverse force to the muscle by moving your thumbs apart, sliding them laterally across the muscle.
- Cover the muscle by working along parallel strips.
- Make sure the patient keeps their forehead relaxed.
- Your pressure should be just short of discomfort.

- To relax the muscle, work with the patient's breathing cycle, about 15 breaths per minute.
- To stimulate, increase your speed to about 40 cycles per minute.

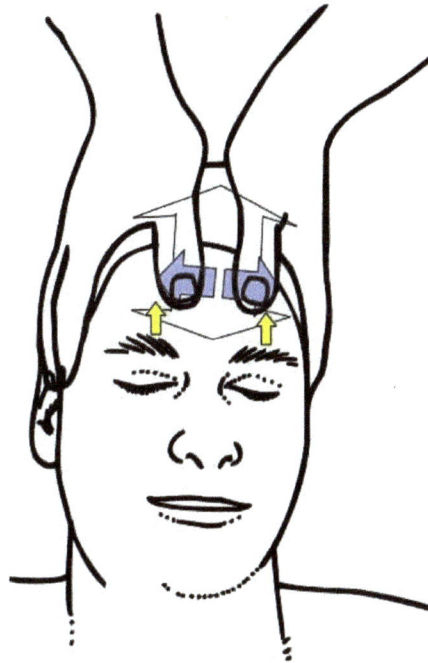

Figure 1.1

Muscle Fibres	⇅	Primary Force	⬇	Secondary Force	↻	Stretch Force	⬇	Contraction Force	⬇

Active component

- Ask the patient to take a deep breath and hold it in.
- Ask the patient to attempt to raise both their eyebrows and thereby contract their frontalis and occipitalis muscles for 3 to 5 seconds using a 10% effort.
- Resist the patient's effort and maintain tissue lockup throughout the technique.
- Ask the patient to exhale and to relax their muscle contraction.
- As soon as you feel that the patient has relaxed their muscles completely (about 1-3 seconds), take up the tissue slack by increasing the lateral pressure on the muscle.
- Take up the slack after each contraction and during exhalation.
- Repeat 2 or 3 times, or as required.

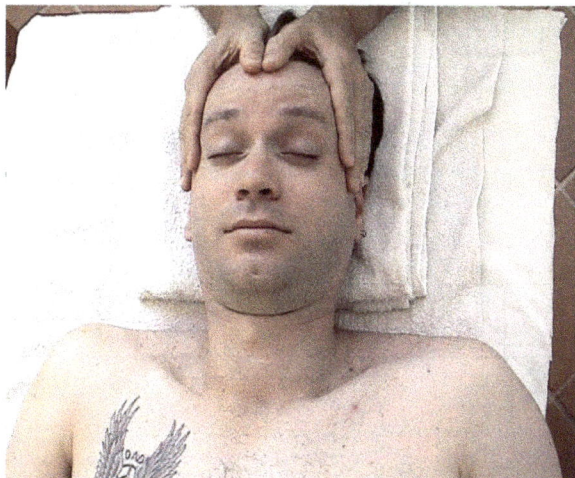

Picture 1.1

Technique 1.2 Unilateral kneading of occipitalis

Patient

- Supine with the head rotated and resting on a folded towel or shallow pillow.

Therapist

- Stand or sit at the head of the table.
- One hand supports the patient's head with a broad hold over the crown. The palm covers both parietal bones and the frontal bone, and the fingers extend towards the occiput.
- The fingers and palm of your other hand add further support by grasping the patient's occiput. The thumb is the applicator, and it rests on the lateral side of occipitalis, which is on the lateral side of the squamous part of the occiput.

Applicator

- The tip or lateral side of the thumb of one hand.

Tissue tension

- Take up the longitudinal tension by pulling the galea aponeurotica anteriorly with your fingertips.
- Apply compression with pressure from your thumb on the side and back of the occiput.

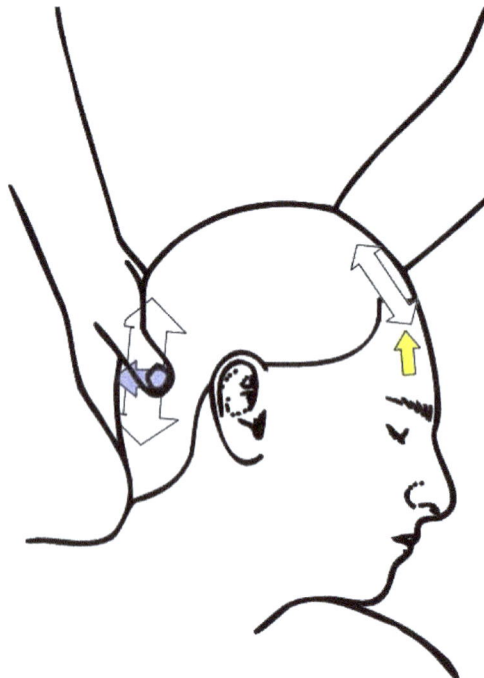

Figure 1.2

Muscle Fibres	⇕	Primary Force	⬇	Secondary Force	↻	Stretch Force	⬇	Contraction Force	⬇

Kneading

- Apply a transverse force to the muscle by moving your thumb posteriorly and medially across the muscle.
- Cover the muscle by working along parallel strips.

- Make sure the patient keeps their forehead relaxed.
- Your pressure should be just short of discomfort.
- To relax the muscle, work with the patient's breathing cycle, about 15 breaths per minute.
- To stimulate, increase your speed to about 40 cycles per minute.

Active component

- Ask the patient to take a deep breath and hold it in.
- Ask the patient to attempt to raise both their eyebrows and thereby contract their frontalis and occipitalis muscles for 3 to 5 seconds using a 10% effort.
- Resist the patient's effort and maintain tissue lockup throughout the technique.
- Ask the patient to exhale and to relax their muscle contraction.
- As soon as you feel that the patient has relaxed their muscles completely (about 1-3 seconds), take up the tissue slack by increasing compression and transverse pressure on the muscle.
- Take up the slack after each contraction and during exhalation.
- Repeat 2 or 3 times, or as required.

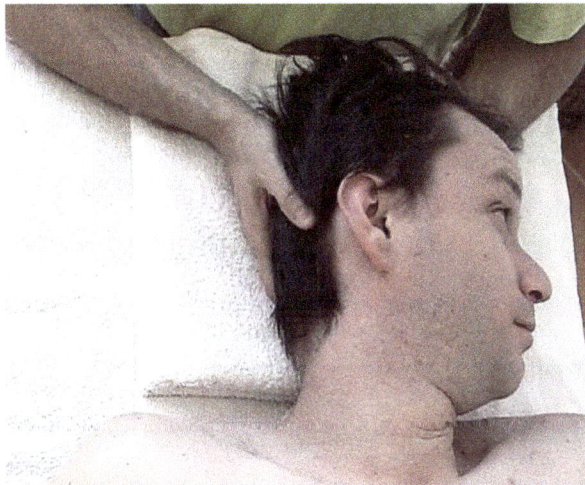

Picture 1.2

2. Muscles of mastication

Anatomy

Temporalis arises from most of the area of the temporal fossa and from the deep surface of temporal fascia. The fibres from this fan-shaped muscle converge on a tendon which passes under the zygomatic arch and then attaches on the coronoid process and the anterior border of the ramus of the mandible. Strong temporal fascia covers the muscle.

Masseter arises on the zygomatic arch and attaches to the lateral ramus and angle of the mandible. The quadrilateral muscle has three layers and is covered by and connected to a layer of fascia, the parotid fascia. Some of the deep fibres also attach on the coronoid process. The strong overlying fascia makes temporalis and masseter difficult to palpate unless they are contracted.
Lateral pterygoid is palpable deep in the buccal cavity. Medial pterygoid not palpable.

Actions: Closes jaw in biting, chewing and speech.
Clinical indications: Dental treatment, malocclusion, neurosis, bruxism and other overuse syndromes.
Nerve supply: Mandibular division of the trigeminal nerve.

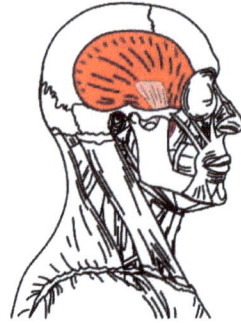

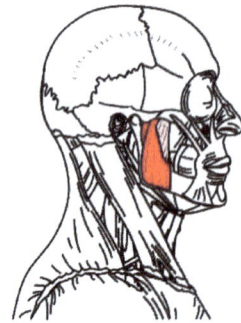

Technique 2.1 Unilateral kneading of temporalis

Patient

- Supine with the head slightly rotated and resting on a folded towel or shallow pillow.

Therapist

- Stand or sit at the head of the table.
- Support the patient's head by grasping the body of the mandible between the fingertips and thumb of one hand. Your palm and forearm add further support by resting against the side of the patient's head.
- The fingers and palm of your other hand add further support by grasping the patient's occiput and the posterior part of the temporal bone.

Applicator

- The tip or lateral side of the thumb of one hand.

Tissue tension

- Take up the longitudinal tension by starting the technique with the jaw depressed and mouth partially open.
- Apply minimal compression with pressure from your thumb. The temple area is sensitive and should be treated with care.
- Add a transverse force to the muscle by flexing your thumb and drawing your thumb across the muscle.
- Remain perpendicular to the muscle by moving in an arc about the muscle attachment on the coranoid process.

26

Kneading

- With the thumb of one hand apply a rhythmical cycle of kneading.
- When the muscle is at an optimal longitudinal tension increase the transverse forces
- Your pressure should be just short of discomfort.
- To relax the muscle, work with the patient's breathing cycle, about 15 breaths per minute.
- To stimulate increase your speed to about 40 cycles per minute.

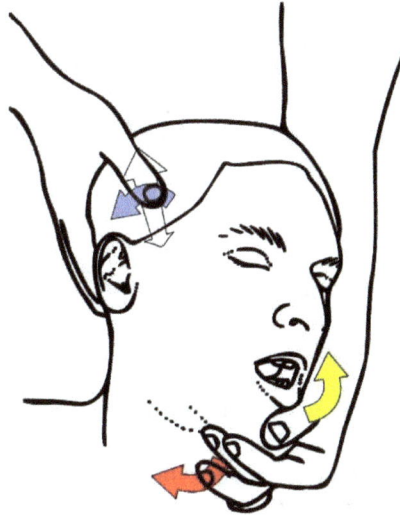

Figure 2.1

Muscle Fibres	⇕	Primary Force	⬇	Secondary Force	↺	Stretch Force	⬇	Contraction Force	⬇

Active component

- Ask the patient to take a deep breath and hold it in.
- Ask the patient to attempt to close their mouth and thereby contract their temporalis muscle for 3 to 5 seconds, using a 10% effort.
- Resist the patient's effort and maintain tissue lockup throughout the technique.
- Ask the patient to exhale and to relax their muscle contraction.
- As soon as you feel that the patient has relaxed their muscles completely (about 1-3 seconds), take up the tissue slack by increasing the primary and longitudinal tension.
- Take up the slack after each contraction and during exhalation.
- Repeat 2 or 3 times, or as required

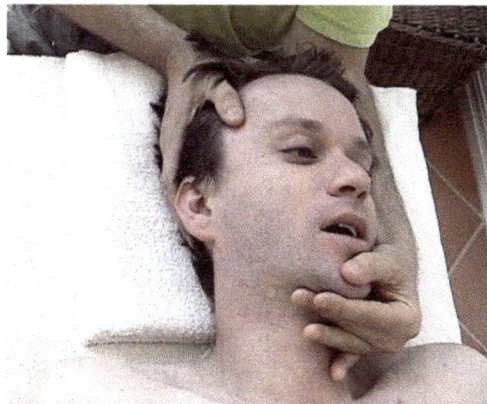

Picture 2.1

Technique 2.2 Unilateral kneading of masseter

Patient

- Supine with the head straight or slightly rotated and resting on a pillow or folded towel.

Therapist

- Stand or sit at the head of the table.
- Support the patient's head by grasping the body of the mandible between the fingertips and thumb of one hand. Your palm and forearm add further support by resting against the side of the patient's head.
- The fingers and palm of your other hand add further support by grasping the patient's occiput and posterior cervical spine.

Applicator

- The tip or lateral side of the thumb of one hand.

Tissue tension

- Take up the longitudinal tension by starting the technique with the jaw depressed and mouth partially open.
- Apply compression with pressure from your thumb.
- Add a transverse force to the muscle by flexing your thumb and drawing your thumb across the muscle.
- Remain perpendicular to the muscle.

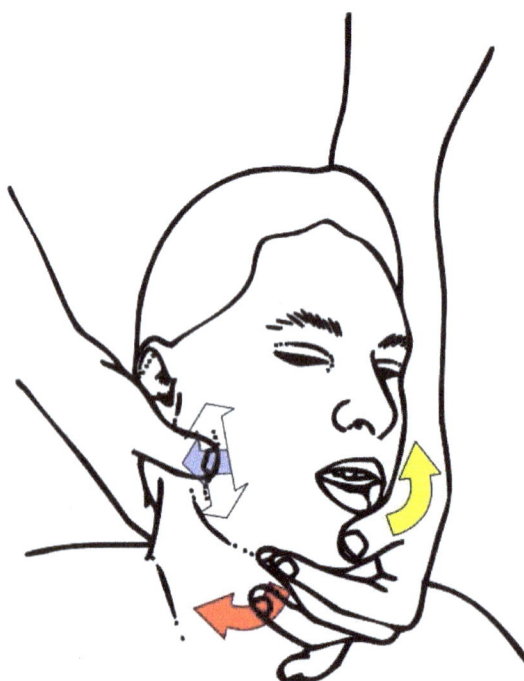

Figure 2.2

Muscle Fibres	⇕	Primary Force	⬇	Secondary Force	↻	Stretch Force	⬇	Contraction Force	⬇

Kneading

- With the thumb of one hand apply a rhythmical cycle of kneading.
- When the muscle is at an optimal longitudinal tension increase the transverse forces
- Your pressure should be just short of discomfort.
- To relax the muscle, work with the patients breathing cycle, about 15 breaths per minute.
- To stimulate increase your speed to about 40 cycles per minute.

Active component

- Ask the patient to take a deep breath and hold it in.
- Ask the patient to attempt to close their mouth and thereby contract their masseter muscle for 3 to 5 seconds, using a 10% effort.
- Resist the patient's effort and maintain tissue lockup throughout the technique.
- Ask the patient to exhale and to relax their muscle contraction.
- As soon as you feel that the patient has relaxed their muscles completely (about 1-3 seconds) take up the tissue slack by increasing the primary and longitudinal tension.
- Take up the slack after each contraction and during exhalation.
- Repeat 2 or 3 times or as required.

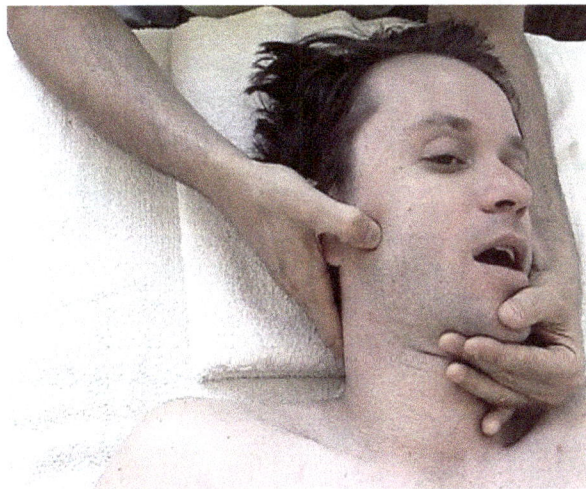

Picture 2.2

Bilateral technique

- Treatment of the temporalis and masseter may be better done bilaterally.
- Ask the patient to take a deep breath in and hold it.
- Take up the tissue slack with compression and transverse pressure.
- Ask the patient to clench his or her jaw.
- Maintain tissue lockup throughout the technique.
- Ask the patient to exhale and to relax their muscle contraction.
- As soon as you feel that the patient has relaxed their muscles completely take up the tissue slack by increasing the compression and transverse tension.

3. Cervical prevertebral muscles

Anatomy

Anterior aspect
The Hyoid bone is U shaped and level with C3. Palpate lateral cornua under the mandible. Thyroid cartilage is level with C4 and C5. It is more prominent in males and easily palpable. The cricoid cartilage is level with C6 and palpable.

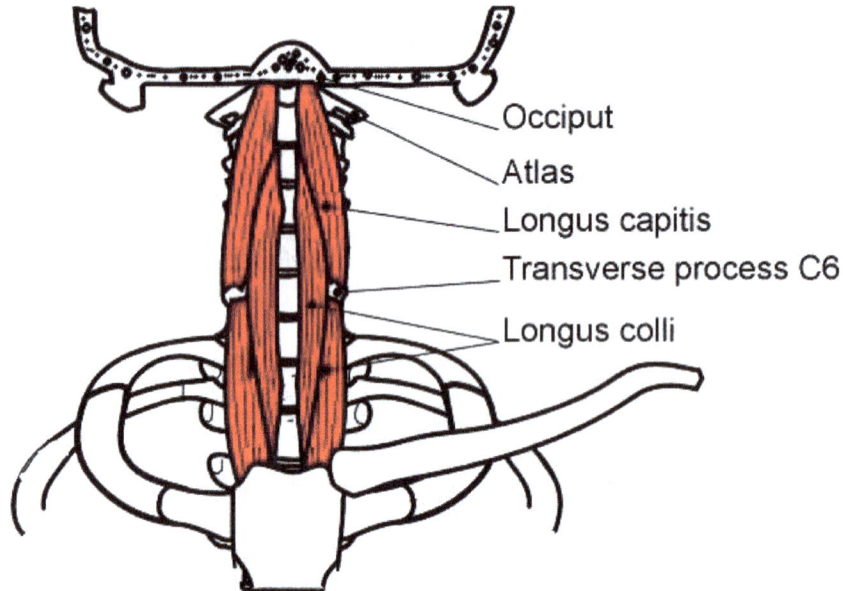

The carotid tubercle is the anterior tubercle of the transverse process of C6. It is a useful landmark and relatively easy to palpate. Palpate unilaterally so as not to occlude the carotid arteries. Trachea rings descend until disappearing under the suprasternal notch

Lateral aspect
The transverse process of C1 is palpable between the mastoid process and the angle of the mandible. The transverse processes of C2 is level with the angle of the jaw.
Except for C1 the cervical transverse processes are not easily palpable. They follow a line from C1 down to the middle of the clavicle.

The **longus capitis** arise on the anterior tubercles of the transverse processes of C3 to C6. The fibres run superiorly and medially over the anterior bodies of the cervical spine and attach onto the basilar part of the occipital bone.

The **longus colli** is in two parts. The inferior oblique fibres arise on the bodies of T1 to T3. The fibres run superiorly and laterally over the anterior bodies of the cervical spine and attach on the anterior tubercles of the transverse processes of C5 and C6. The superior oblique fibres arise on the anterior tubercles of the transverse processes of C3 to C5. The fibres run superiorly and medially over the anterior bodies of the cervical spine and attach on the tubercle of the anterior arch of C1.

The **rectus capitis anterior** arises on the transverse process of C1 and attaches on the basilar occipital bone. The rectus capitis lateralis arises on the transverse process of C1 and attaches on the jugular process of the temporal bone.

The cervical prevertebral muscles are thin and deep to the larynx and not easily palpable. These small anterior suboccipital and prevertebral muscles may be strained when subject to whiplash injuries such as from car accidents.

Technique 3.1 Unilateral kneading of cervical prevertebral muscles from occiput to C7

Patient

- Supine with head straight and resting on a folded towel or shallow pillow.

Therapist

- Stand at the side of the table opposite the patient's head.
- (a) Place the index and middle fingers of your caudad hand onto the ramus of the mandible on the opposite side to which you are standing, and place the thumb of your caudad hand onto the larynx on the same side to which you are standing.
- (b) Alternatively, support the patient's head with a broad hold of the frontal bone with your cephalad hand.
- Place your applicator in the depression between the patients sternocleidomastoid muscle and their larynx and trachea.
- Press down until your fingertips rest against the prevertebral muscles which sit over the bodies of the cervical vertebrae.

Applicator

- The fingertips of one or two fingers. In (a) from your caudad hand, in (b) from your cephalad hand.

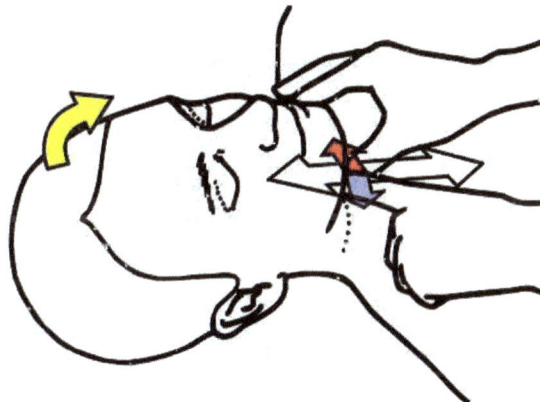

Figure 3.1

Muscle Fibres	⇕	Primary Force	⬇	Secondary Force	↻	Stretch Force	⬇	Contraction Force	⬇

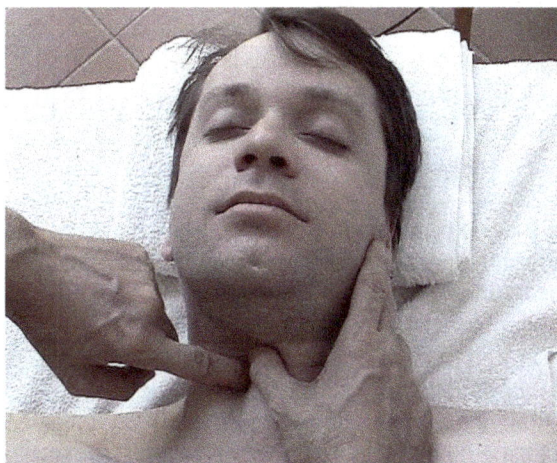

Picture 3.1

Tissue tension

- Gently push the hyoid bone or larynx laterally, away from the spine to facilitate better access for your applicator
- Take up the primary tissue force with minimal compression, by increasing your fingertip pressure, adding a transverse force to the muscle by flexing your finger.
- Your force is perpendicular to the muscle.
- Work across the muscle, from medial to lateral, and then back to medial.
- Longitudinal tension is taken up by starting the technique with the spine in slight extension. A rolled up towel may be placed under the patient's neck to achieve this.

Kneading

- With the fingertips of one hand, apply a rhythmical cycle of transverse pressure.
- Start with a light pressure and build up to a firmer 'friction' pressure.
- Work across the muscle, from medial to lateral, and then back to medial again, by flexing and then extending your finger.
- Ask the patient for feedback. Get them to raise their hand if they feel uncomfortable.
- Your pressure should be just short of discomfort.
- Work over a small surface area at one time.
- Start at the top of the spine and work your way down. Cover the entire area.
- To relax the muscle, work with the patients breathing cycle, about 15 breaths per minute.

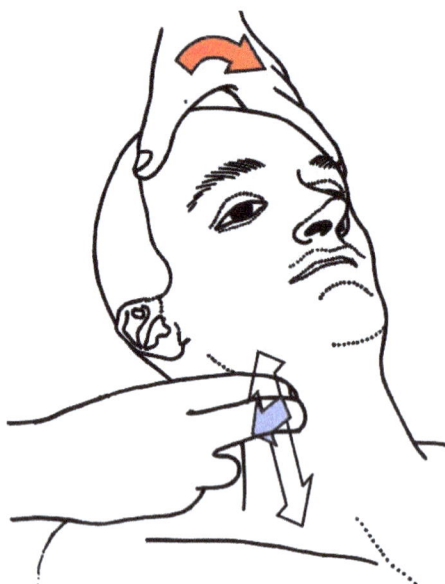

Figure 3.2

Muscle Fibres	⇕	Primary Force	⬇	Secondary Force	↻	Stretch Force	⬇	Contraction Force	⬇

Active component

- Ask the patient to take a deep breath and hold it in.
- Ask the patient to contract their prevertebral muscles by attempting to lift their head off the table, flexing their neck in an arc for 3 to 5 seconds using a 10% effort.
- Alternatively ask the patient to rotate their head and neck.
- Resist the patient's effort and maintain tissue lockup throughout the technique.
- Ask the patient to exhale and to relax their muscle contraction.
- As soon as you feel that the patient has relaxed their muscles completely (about 1-3 seconds), take up the tissue slack by increasing the primary tension.
- Take up the slack after each contraction and during exhalation.
- Repeat 2 or 3 times, or as required.

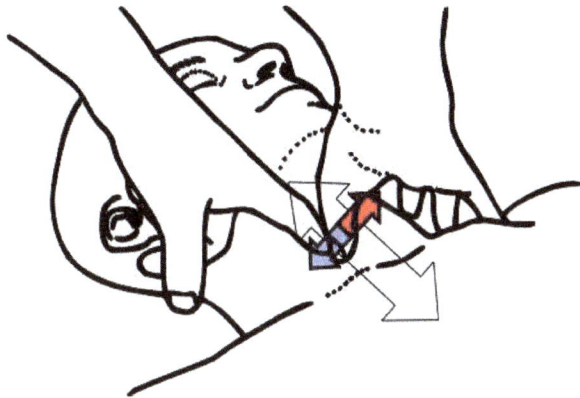

Figure 3.3

Muscle Fibres	↕	Primary Force	⬇	Secondary Force	↻	Stretch Force	⬇	Contraction Force	⬇

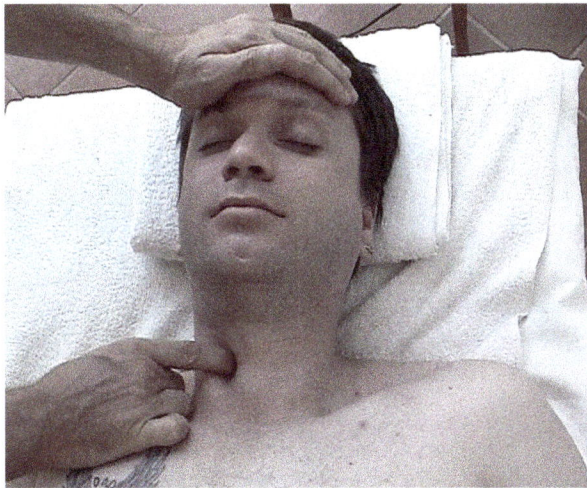

Picture 3.2

4. Superior and inferior hyoid muscles

Anatomy

The **hyoid muscles** arise on the mandible, mastoid process and styloid process, and attach on the clavicle and manubrium via the hyoid. The superior hyoid muscles are palpable in the soft area within the U shape of the mandible, and between the mandible and hyoid. The inferior hyoid muscles are palpable as a thin superficial layer on the anterior of the neck. The hyoid muscles are covered by a layer of deep fascia, the sheet-like platysma muscle and by superficial fascia. The deep fascia invests the vessels, glands and muscles in the region.

Actions: The hyoid muscles are involved in speech, mastication and swallowing. Digastric and mylohyoid depress the mandible or elevate the hyoid. Stylohyoid elevates the hyoid or in combination with other muscles, fixes the hyoid. Omohyoid depresses the hyoid. Thyrohyoid depresses the hyoid or raises the larynx.
Clinical indications: Whiplash, overuse (i.e. singing) and the localised effects of infection.

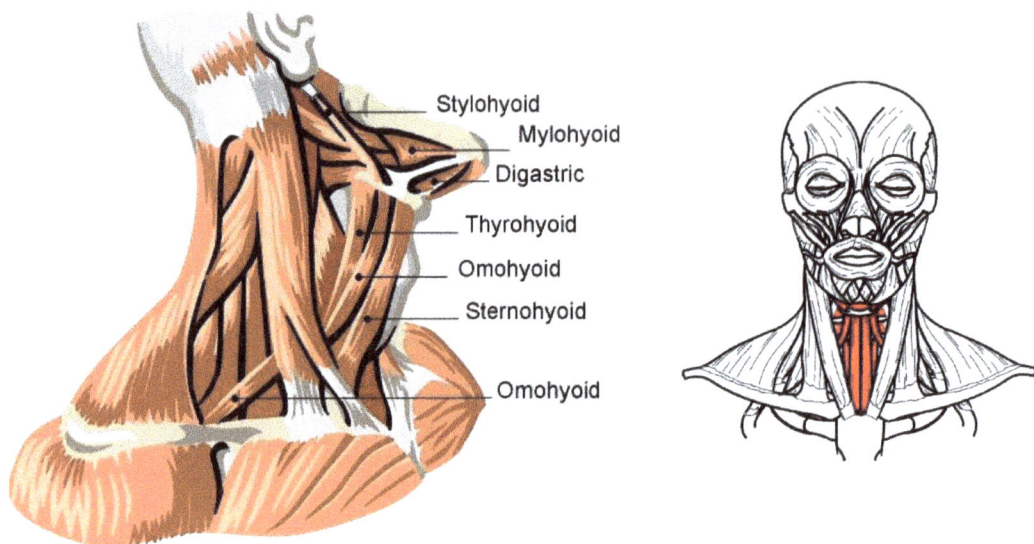

Stylohyoid
Mylohyoid
Digastric
Thyrohyoid
Omohyoid
Sternohyoid

Omohyoid

Technique 4.1 Kneading of superior and inferior hyoid muscles

Patient

- Supine with head in extension.
- A rolled up towel may be placed under the cervical spine to prevent flexion.

Therapist

- Stand at the side of the table, adjacent to the patient's head.
- Place the index and middle fingers of your caudad hand on the ramus of the mandible, on the opposite side to which you are standing.
- Place the thumb of your caudad hand on the hyoid bone, on the same side to which you are standing.
- Rest your thumb on a suitable place on the hyoid to apply longitudinal tension to the muscle you are treating.
- Place your applicator on a superior or inferior hyoid muscle.

Applicator

- The fingertip of the index finger of your cephalad hand.

Tissue tension

- To increase longitudinal tension on the muscles, and to make the muscles more accessible to your applicator, maintain the patient's head in slight extension.
- To take up the longitudinal tension on the superior hyoid muscles, gently push the hyoid bone inferiorly and laterally away from the side you are working.
- Apply compression by increasing your fingertip pressure over the superior hyoid muscles.
- Take up the transverse tissue tension by flexing your finger.
- To take up the longitudinal tension on the inferior hyoid muscles, gently push the hyoid bone superiorly and laterally away from the side you are working.
- For the inferior hyoid muscles, compression is minimal. Only light fingertip pressure is needed to take up the transverse tissue tension.

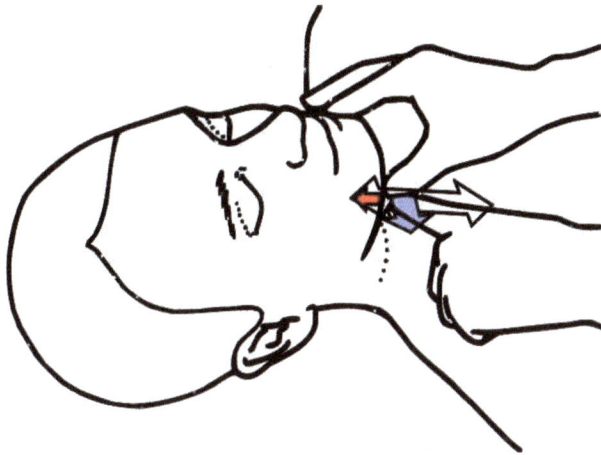

Figure 4.1 Technique for the inferior hyoid muscles

Muscle Fibres	⇕	Primary Force	⬇	Secondary Force	↺	Stretch Force	⬇	Contraction Force	⬇

Kneading

- With the fingertips of one hand, apply a rhythmical cycle of transverse and longitudinal forces.
- The longitudinal tension is produced by pressure on the hyoid with your thumb.
- For your transverse force to remain perpendicular to the superior hyoid muscles, you will need to move the applicator through an arc which runs roughly parallel with, and between, the hyoid and mandible.
- Cover the entire area by following a series of arcs.
- For your force to remain perpendicular to the inferior hyoid muscles, you will need to move the applicator from medial to lateral, or vice versa.
- Cover the entire area by following a series of strips running across the front of the neck, between the hyoid and sternum.
- Ask the patient for feedback. Get them to raise their hand if they feel uncomfortable.
- Your pressure should be just short of discomfort.
- Work over a small surface area at one time.
- Start at the top of the neck and work your way down.
- To relax the muscle, work with the patient's breathing cycle, which is about 15 breaths per minute.

Active component

- Ask the patient to take a deep breath and hold it in.
- Ask the patient to contract their superior or inferior hyoid muscles, by attempting to swallow for 3 to 5 seconds using a 10% effort.

- The patient should not complete the act of swallowing.
- Resist the patient's effort with fingertip pressure on the hyoid bone, maintaining tissue lockup throughout the technique.
- Ask the patient to exhale and to relax their muscle contraction.
- As soon as you feel that the patient has relaxed their muscles completely (about 1-3 seconds), take up the tissue slack by increasing the primary and longitudinal tension.
- Take up the slack after each contraction and during exhalation.
- Repeat 2 or 3 times, or as required.

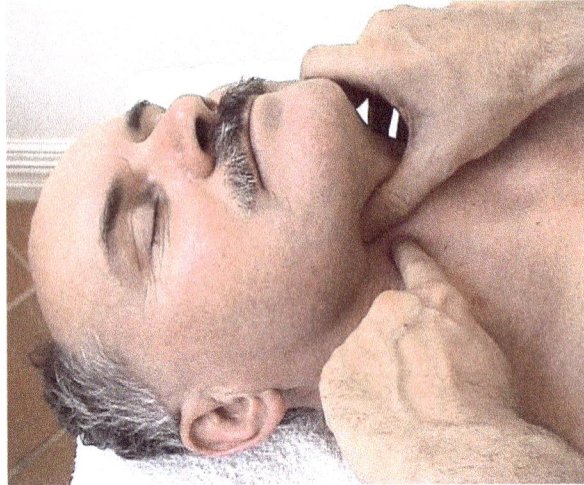

Picture 4.1

Technique 4.2 Kneading the superior and inferior hyoid muscles

Patient

- Supine with head in extension over a rolled up towel.

Therapist

- Stand at the side of the table, opposite the patient's head.
- Support the patient's head with your cephalad hand, maintaining a broad hold of the frontal bone.
- Place your applicator on a superior or inferior hyoid muscle.

Applicator

- The fingertip of the index finger of your caudad hand.

Tissue tension

- To increase longitudinal tension on the muscles and to make the muscles more accessible to your applicator maintain the patient's head in slight extension.
- Rest your index or middle fingertip in a suitable place on the hyoid, to apply longitudinal tension to the muscle you are treating.
- To take up the longitudinal tension on the superior hyoid muscles, gently push the hyoid bone inferiorly and laterally away from the side you are working.
- To take up the longitudinal tension on the inferior hyoid muscles gently push the hyoid bone superiorly and laterally away from the side you are working.
- Apply compression by increasing your fingertip pressure over the hyoid muscles.
- Use light fingertip pressure on the inferior hyoid muscles.
- Take up the transverse tissue tension by flexing your finger.

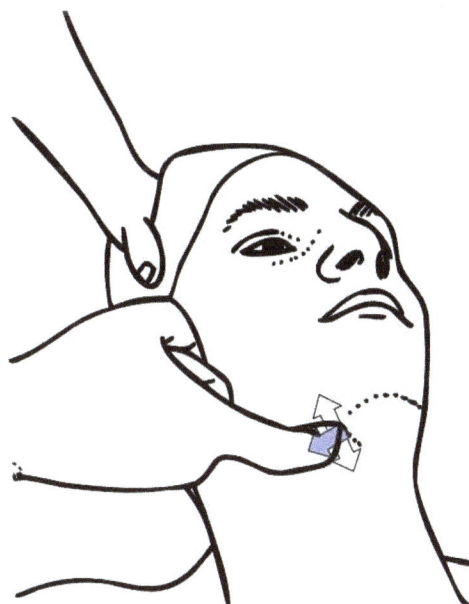

Figure 4.2 Technique for the superior hyoid muscles

Muscle Fibres	⇕	Primary Force	⬇	Secondary Force	↺	Stretch Force	⬇	Contraction Force	⬇

Kneading

- With the fingertips of one hand, apply a rhythmical cycle of transverse and longitudinal forces.
- The longitudinal tension is produced by pressure on the hyoid with your fingertip.
- For your transverse force to remain perpendicular to the superior hyoid muscles, you will need to move the applicator through an arc running roughly parallel with the hyoid and mandible.

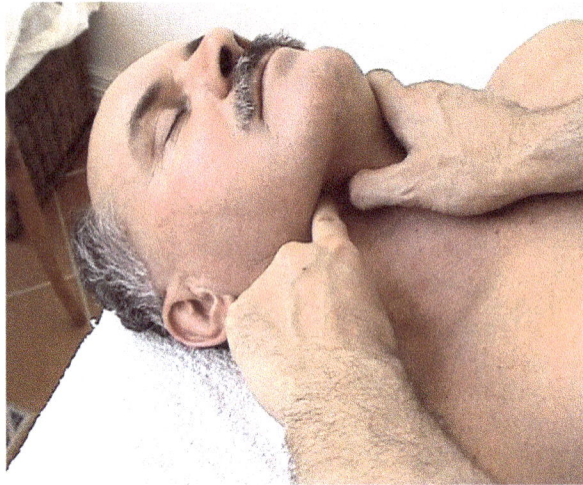

Picture 4.2

- Cover the entire area by following a series of arcs.
- For your force to remain perpendicular to the inferior hyoid muscles you will need to move the applicator from medial to lateral or vice versa.
- Cover the entire area by following a series of strips running across the front of the neck.
- Ask the patient for feedback. Get them to raise their hand if they feel uncomfortable.
- Your pressure should be just short of discomfort.

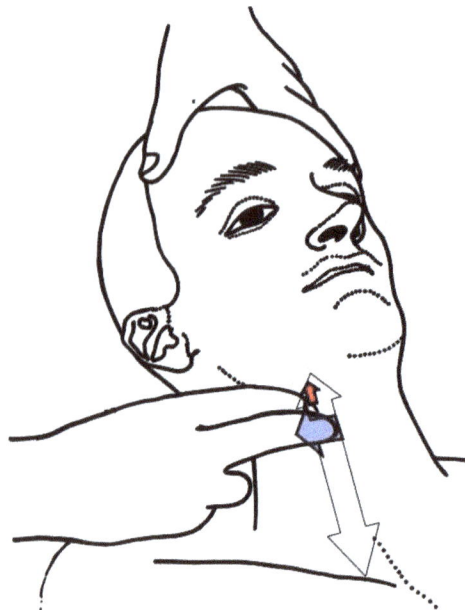

Figure 4.3

Muscle Fibres	⇕	Primary Force	⬇	Secondary Force	↻	Stretch Force	⬇	Contraction Force	⬇

- Work over a small surface area at one time.
- Start at the top of the neck and work your way down.
- To relax the muscle, work with the patient's breathing cycle, which is about 15 breaths per minute.

Active component

- Ask the patient to take a deep breath and hold it in.
- Ask the patient to contract his superior or inferior hyoid muscles by attempting to swallow for 3 to 5 seconds using a 10% effort.
- Resist the patient's effort with fingertip pressure on the hyoid bone and maintain tissue lockup throughout the technique.
- Ask the patient to exhale and to relax their muscle contraction.
- As soon as you feel that the patient has relaxed their muscles completely (about 1-3 seconds), take up the tissue slack by increasing the primary and longitudinal tension.
- Take up the slack after each contraction and during exhalation.
- Repeat 2 or 3 times, or as required.

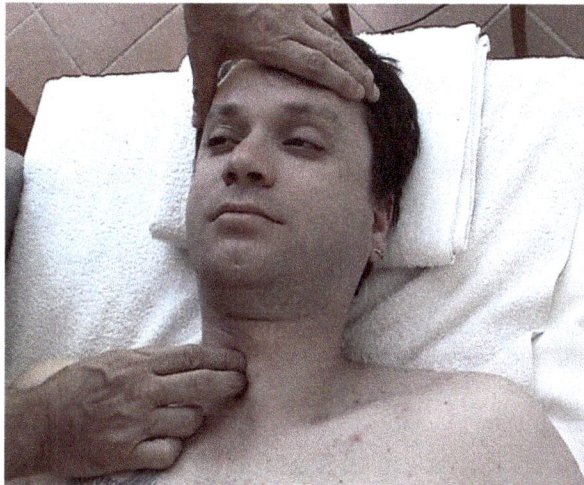

Picture 4.3

5. Sternocleidomastoid

Anatomy

Sternocleidomastoid arises by two heads, one from the sternum and one from the clavicle. Fibres from the two heads spiral and merge but much of the clavicular part attaches on the mastoid process as a strong tendon and much of the sternal part attaches on the lateral half of the superior nuchal line of the occiput as a thin aponeurosis. The platysma and deep cervical fascia cover the muscle.

Action: When both sternocleidomastoid muscles contract they flex the neck when acting with longus colli, and they extend the head and neck when longus colli is relaxed. When one sternocleidomastoid contracts it sidebends the head and neck to the same side and rotates the head to the opposite side. When acting with other muscles, sternocleidomastoid produces level rotation.

Clinical indications: Torticollis and other spasms.

Nerve supply: Accessory nerve and ventral rami of the second, third and sometimes fourth cervical spinal nerves.

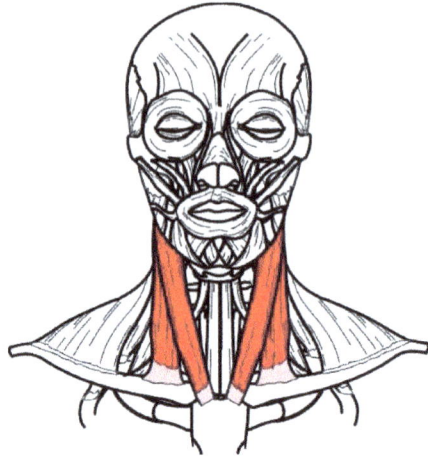

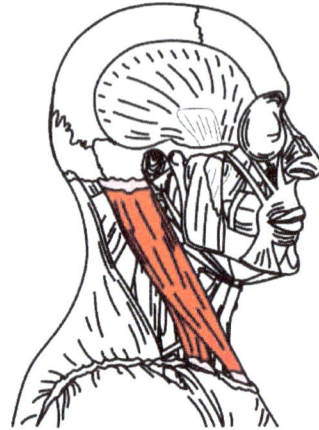

Technique 5.1 Unilateral kneading of sternocleidomastoid

Patient

*   Supine with the head straight and resting on a folded towel or shallow pillow, positioned so as to prevent hyperextension of the head and neck.

Therapist

*   Stand or sit at the side of the table, adjacent to the patient's head.
*   Support the patient's head with a broad hold of the frontal bone with your cephalad hand.
*   Place your index fingertip anterior to the muscle and your thumb posterior to the muscle.
*   Rest the front of your wrist firmly on the table.

Applicator

*   The fingertips and thumb of your caudad hand.

Tissue tension

*   Take up the primary tissue tension on sternocleidomastoid. To take up the compression, grasp the sternocleidomastoid muscle between your index finger and thumb.
*   The transverse tension is taken up by flexing your fingertips.
*   Your force is perpendicular to the muscle and in a posterior direction.
*   Secondary tension is taken up by pushing anteriorly with your thumb, therefore twisting the muscle between your finger and thumb.

- Longitudinal tension is taken up by starting the technique with the head sidebent away and rotated towards you.
- Further secondary tension is taken up when rotating the patient's head away from you.

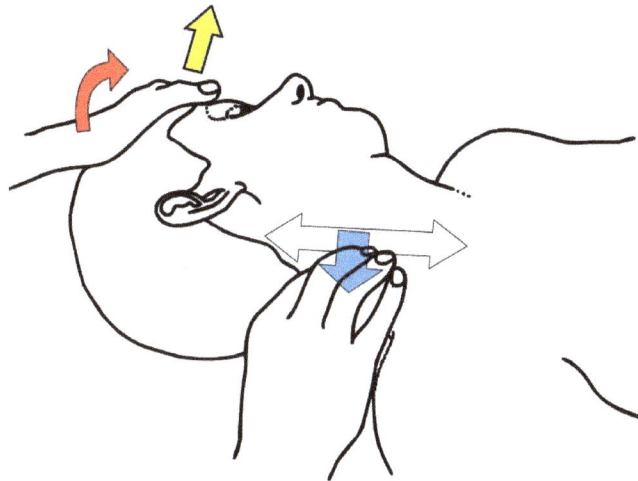

Figure 5.1

Muscle Fibres	↕	Primary Force	⬇	Secondary Force	↻	Stretch Force	⬇	Contraction Force	⬇

Kneading

- With the fingertips and thumb of your caudad hand apply a rhythmical cycle of primary and secondary forces.
- Your hooked fingertips hold back on the muscle as you push the head away.
- Alternatively, by twisting the muscle with your thumb and index fingertip, you can add secondary tension as torsion.
- Your pressure should be just short of discomfort.
- Start at the top of the spine and work your way down.
- To relax the muscle, work with the patient's breathing cycle, which is about 15 breaths per minute.
- To stimulate, increase your speed to about 40 cycles per minute.

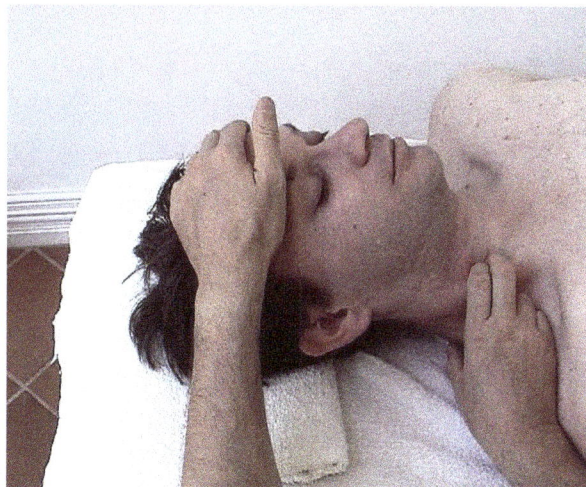

Picture 5.1

Active component

- Ask the patient to take a deep breath and hold it in.
- To activate the sternocleidomastoid muscles, ask the patient to flex their neck for 3 to 5 seconds using a 10% effort.
- Resist the patient's effort and maintain tissue lockup throughout the technique.
- Ask the patient to exhale and to relax their muscle contraction.
- As soon as you feel that the patient has relaxed their muscles completely (about 1-3 seconds), take up the tissue slack by increasing the primary, secondary and longitudinal tension.
- Take up the slack after each contraction and during exhalation.
- Repeat 2 or 3 times or as required.

Technique 5.2 Unilateral kneading of sternocleidomastoid

Patient

- Supine with the head straight and resting on a folded towel or shallow pillow.
- The pillow should be positioned so as to prevent hyperextension of the head and neck.

Therapist

- Stand at the side of the table adjacent to the patient's head.
- Grasp and support the patient's head with your cephalad hand, maintaining a broad hold over the frontal bone.
- Reach across the patient with your caudad hand and hook your fingertips around the sternocleidomastoid on the opposite side to which you are standing.
- Start with your fingertips sitting just behind the muscle and your thumb in front of it.

Applicator

- The fingertips of your caudad hand. Alternatively consider grasping sternocleidomastoid between your fingertips and thumb.

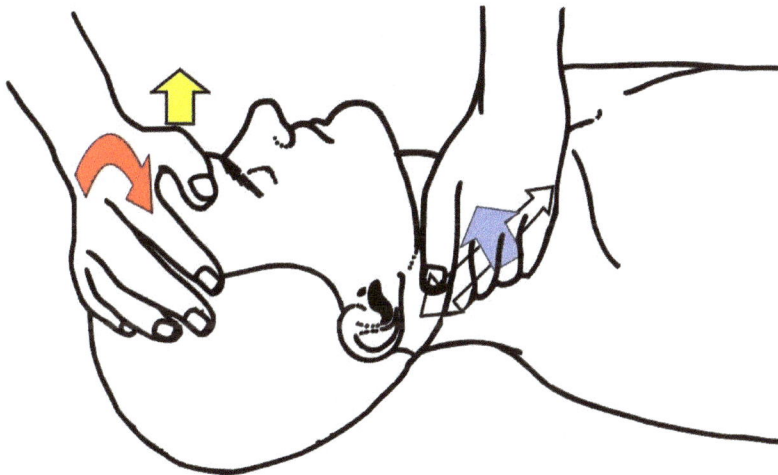

Figure 5.2

Muscle Fibres	⇕	Primary Force	⬇	Secondary Force	↻	Stretch Force	⬇	Contraction Force	⬇

Tissue tension

- Take up the primary tissue tension on sternocleidomastoid. The transverse tension is taken up by flexing your fingertips as you stabilise the patient's head. Gently pull up on the opposite sternocleidomastoid with the fingertips of your caudad hand. Work perpendicular to the muscle and in an anterior direction.
- Alternatively, keep your fingertips in a fixed and flexed position, and rotate the patient's head away from you. Roll their head with your cephalad hand.
- To take up the compression, grasp the sternocleidomastoid muscle between your index finger and thumb. Hold firmly.
- Secondary tension is taken up by twisting the muscle between your finger and thumb.
- Longitudinal tension is taken up by starting the technique with the spine sidebent towards you.
- Further tension is taken up by rotating the patient's head away from you.

Kneading

- With the fingertips of your caudad hand, apply a rhythmical cycle of primary and secondary forces.
- The primary and secondary forces work together to create an optimal tension.
- Work the sternocleidomastoid between finger and thumb.
- Alternatively, hold back on the muscle with hooked fingertips as you push the head away.
- Keep the heel of your hand away from the patient's trachea and larynx.
- Your pressure should be just short of discomfort.
- To relax the muscle, work with the patient's breathing cycle, about 15 breaths per minute.
- To stimulate, increase your speed to about 40 cycles per minute.

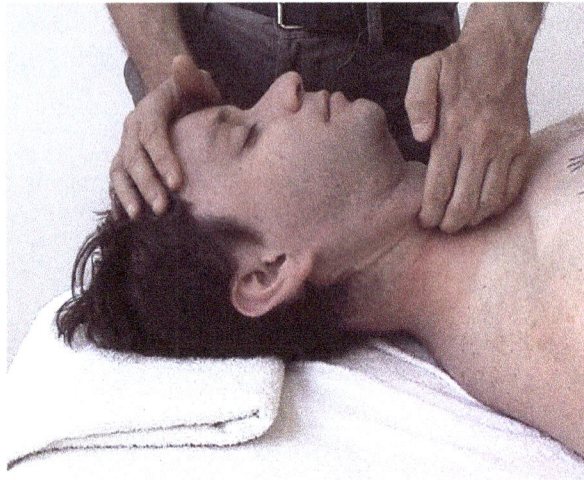

Picture 5.2

Active component

- Ask the patient to take a deep breath in and hold it in.
- Ask the patient to contract their sternocleidomastoid muscles by attempting to lift their head off the table and flex their head and neck.
- Resist the patient's effort and maintain tissue lockup throughout the technique.
- Ask the patient to exhale and to relax their muscle contraction.
- As soon as you feel that the patient has relaxed their muscles completely (about 1-3 seconds), take up the tissue slack by increasing the primary, secondary and longitudinal tension.
- Take up the slack after each contraction and during exhalation.
- Repeat 2 or 3 times or as required.

6. Scalene

Anatomy

The scalene muscles exhibit some variation in the number and levels of cervical vertebrae to which they attach.

Anterior Scalene arises from the anterior tubercles of transverse processes of C3 to 6 and attaches on the scalene tubercle and on a ridge on the upper surface of rib 1. It lies behind sternocleidomastoid and in front of the brachial plexus and subclavian artery.

Middle Scalene arises from the posterior tubercles of transverse processes of C2 to 7 and attaches on the upper surface of rib 1. Sometimes fibres arise from the atlas. The brachial plexus and subclavian artery lie between it and the anterior scalene. The posterior scalene and levator scapulae are posterolateral to it.

Posterior Scalene arises from the posterior tubercles of transverse processes of C5 to 7 and attaches on rib 2.

Action: The scalene raise the upper ribs and sidebend the cervical spine to the same side.
Clinical indications: Chronic respiratory diseases such as asthma or bronchitis. Changes in the muscles may compromise the function of nerves derived from the brachial plexus.
Nerve supply: Cervical nerves from the cervical plexus C1-4 supplies neck muscles and skin.

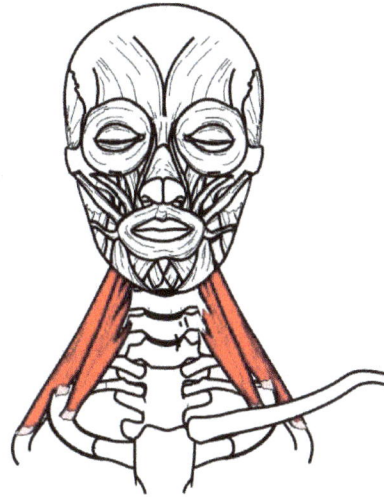

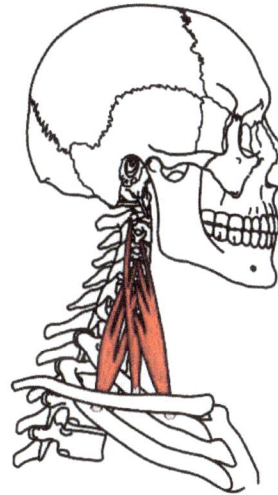

Technique 6.1 Unilateral kneading of anterior, middle and posterior scalene

Patient

- Supine with the head straight and resting on a folded towel or shallow pillow.
- The pillow should be positioned so as to prevent hyperextension of the head and neck.

Therapist

- Stand or sit at the side of the table adjacent to the patient's head.
- Support the patient's head with a broad hold of the frontal bone with your cephalad hand.
- Place your fingertips just anterior to the muscle.
- Rest the front of your wrist firmly on the table.

Applicator

- The fingertips of your caudad hand.

Tissue tension

- Take up the primary tissue tension on the scalene. Due to the close proximity of sensitive neurovascular tissues, compression over the scalene is minimal.
- The transverse tension is taken up by flexing your fingertips as you stabilise the patient's head.
- Alternatively, keep your wrist anchored to the table and your fingertips in a fixed flexed position, and roll the patient's head away from you with your cephalad hand.
- The transverse tension is taken up by flexing your fingertips as you stabilise the patient's head, or by rolling the patient's head away from you.
- Your force is perpendicular to the muscle and in a posterior direction.
- When treating scalene your fingertips should be far enough apart so that they fit between transverse processes of adjacent vertebra. The ease of this technique depends on the size of the therapist's fingers and the size of the patient's neck.
- Secondary tension is taken up when rotating the patient's head away from you.
- Longitudinal tension is taken up by starting the technique with the spine sidebent away from you.

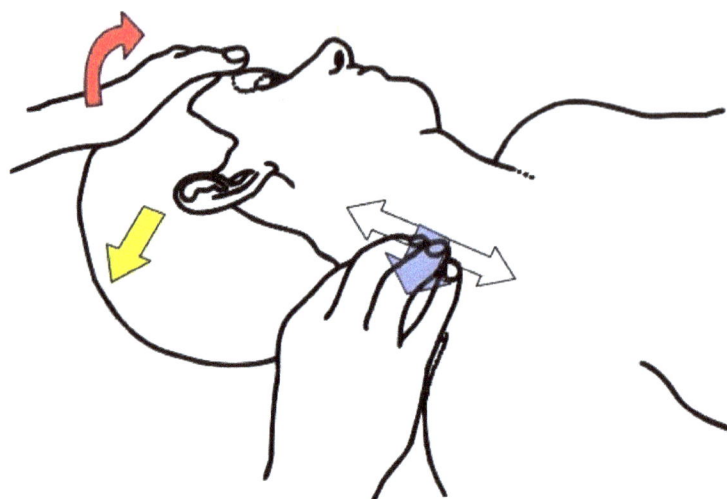

Figure 6.1

Muscle Fibres	↕	Primary Force	⬇	Secondary Force	↻	Stretch Force	⬇	Contraction Force	⬇

Kneading

- With the fingertips of your caudad hand apply a rhythmical cycle of primary and secondary forces.
- Your hooked fingertips hold back on the muscle, or gently pull down on the muscle as you push the head away.
- Your pressure should be just short of discomfort.
- Start at the top of the spine and work your way down.
- To relax the muscle, work with the patients breathing cycle, about 15 breaths per minute.
- To stimulate, increase your speed to about 40 cycles per minute.

Active component

- Ask the patient to take a deep breath and hold it in.
- To activate the scalene muscles, ask the patient to lift their head off the table and sidebend their neck towards you for 3 to 5 seconds using a 10% effort.
- Resist the patient's effort and maintain tissue lockup throughout the technique.
- Ask the patient to exhale and to relax their muscle contraction.

- As soon as you feel that the patient has relaxed their muscles completely (about 1-3 seconds), take up the tissue slack by increasing the primary, secondary and longitudinal tension.
- Take up the slack after each contraction and during exhalation.
- Repeat 2 or 3 times or as required

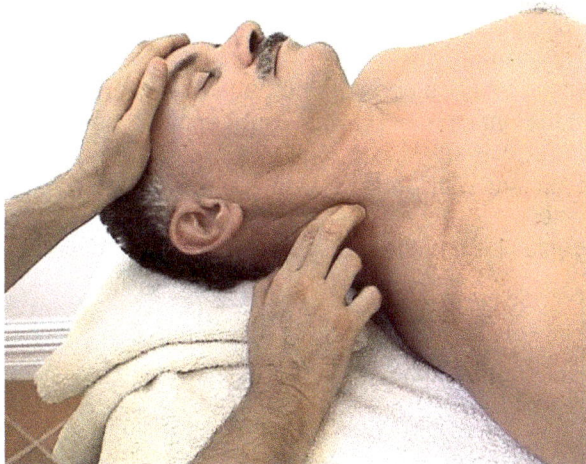

Picture 6.1

Technique 6.2 Unilateral kneading of anterior, middle and posterior scalene

Patient

- Supine with the head straight and resting on a folded towel or shallow pillow. The pillow should be positioned so as to prevent hyperextension of the head and neck.

Therapist

- Stand at the side of the table adjacent to the patient's head.
- Grasp and support the patient's head with your cephalad hand, maintaining a broad hold over the frontal bone.
- Reach across the patient with your caudad hand and hook your fingertips around the opposite side scalene.
- Start with your fingertips behind the transverse process of C1 and the mastoid process.

Applicator

- The fingertips of your caudad hand.

Tissue tension

- Take up the primary tissue tension on the scalene. Due to the close proximity of sensitive neurovascular tissues, compression over the scalene is minimal.
- The transverse tension is taken up by flexing your fingertips as you stabilise the patient's head.
- Gently pull up on the opposite side scalene with the fingertips of your caudad hand.
- Alternatively, keep your fingertips in a fixed and flexed position, and rotate the patient's head away from you. Roll their head with your cephalad hand.
- Work perpendicular to the muscle, in an anterior direction.
- When treating scalene your fingertips should be far enough apart so that they fit between transverse processes of adjacent vertebra. The ease of this technique depends to some degree on the size of the therapist's fingers and the size of the patient's neck.
- Longitudinal tension is taken up by starting the technique with the spine sidebent towards you.
- Further tension is taken up by rotating the patient's head away from you.

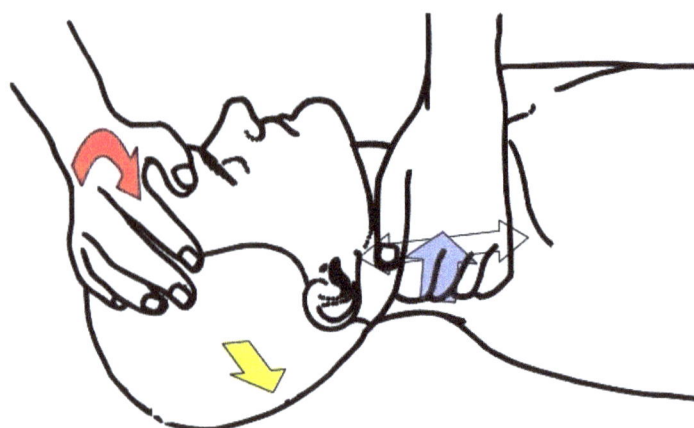

Figure 6.2

Muscle Fibres	⇕	Primary Force	⬇	Secondary Force	↻	Stretch Force	⬇	Contraction Force	⬇

48

Kneading

- With the fingertips of your caudad hand, apply a rhythmical cycle of primary and secondary forces.
- The primary and secondary forces work together to create an optimal tension.
- Use a rake like action with two or three fingertips.
- Alternatively, hold back on the muscle with hooked fingertips as you push the head away.
- Keep the heel of your hand away from the patient's trachea and larynx.
- Your pressure should be just short of discomfort.
- To relax the muscle, work with the patients breathing cycle, about 15 breaths per minute.
- To stimulate, increase your speed to about 40 cycles per minute.

Active component

- Ask the patient to take a deep breath and hold it in.
- Ask the patient to contract their scalene muscles by lifting their head off the table and pushing the head sideways away from you, for 3 to 5 seconds using a 10% effort.
- Resist the patient's effort and maintain tissue lockup throughout the technique.
- Ask the patient to exhale and to relax their muscle contraction.
- As soon as you feel that the patient has relaxed their muscles completely (about 1-3 seconds), take up the tissue slack by increasing the primary, secondary and longitudinal tension.
- Take up the slack after each contraction and during exhalation.
- Repeat 2 or 3 times or as required.

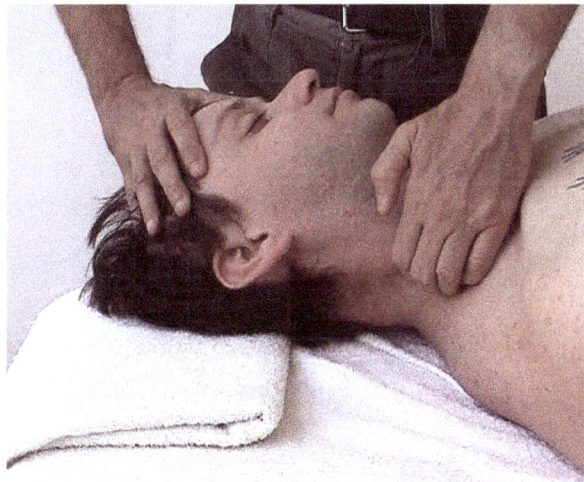

Picture 6.2

Technique 6.3 Unilateral stretching of anterior, middle and posterior scalene

Patient

- Supine with the head straight and resting on a folded towel or shallow pillow.

Therapist

- Stand at the head of the table.
- Grasp and support the patient's head and neck with one hand, maintaining a broad hold over the temporal bone, occipital bone and the upper cervical spine.
- Hook your fingertips around the opposite side of the spinous processes to localise sidebending and for a more effective stretch.
- Reach across the patient's head with your other hand and contact the acromion process.
- Lightly depress the scapula.

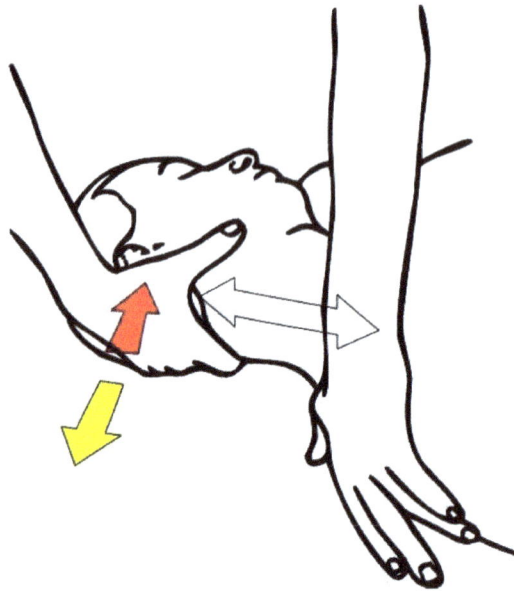

Figure 6.3

Muscle Fibres	⇕	Primary Force	⬇	Secondary Force	↻	Stretch Force	⬇	Contraction Force	⬇

Tissue tension

- Due to the close proximity of sensitive neurovascular tissues, sidebending should be done with care and preferably in combination with mild traction.
- The primary tension is a longitudinal force.

Stretch

- Support the patient's head with your hand and forearm.
- Hold back on the shoulder with your fingers.
- Introduce general and localised sidebending with traction.
- While in sidebending you can introduce variations of rotation, flexion and extension into the technique, to localise the stretch at the appropriate scalene.
- A hand wrap around the sub-occipital area may be necessary to help support the head in a neutral position.
- Care should be taken not to place stress on the sub-occipital muscles.

50

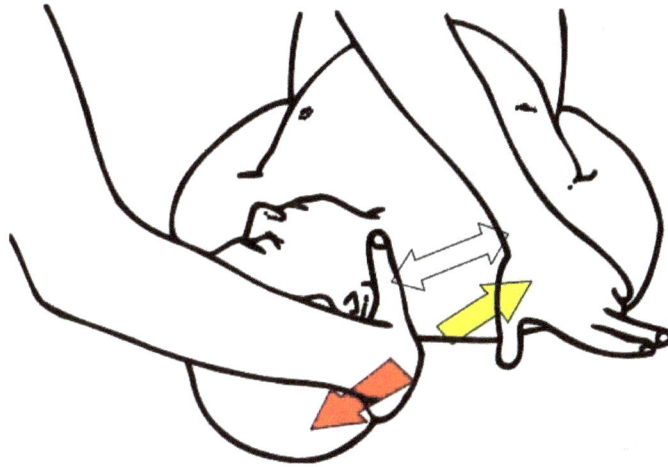

Figure 6.4

Muscle Fibres	⇕	Primary Force	⬇	Secondary Force	↻	Stretch Force	⬇	Contraction Force	⬇

Active component

- Ask the patient to take a deep breath and hold it in.
- Ask the patient to contract their scalene muscles by pushing their head sideways for 3 to 5 seconds using a 10% effort.
- Resist the patient's effort.
- Ask the patient to exhale and to relax their muscle contraction.
- As soon as you feel that the patient has relaxed their muscles completely (about 1-3 seconds), take up the tissue slack by increasing the longitudinal tension.
- Take up the slack after each contraction and during exhalation.
- Repeat 2 or 3 times or as required.

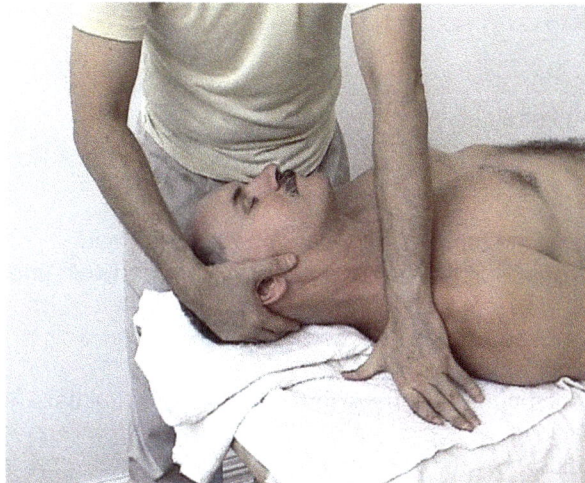

Picture 6.3

7. The suboccipital muscles

Anatomy

The suboccipital muscles are a group of small muscles covered by fascia, dense adipose tissue, the semispinalis capitis medially and the longissimus capitis laterally.

From medial to lateral these consist of:
1. **Rectus capitis posterior minor** running from the inferior nuchal line of the occiput to the tubercle of the posterior arch of the atlas.
2. **Rectus capitis posterior major** running from the inferior nuchal line of the occiput to the spinous process of the axis (C2).
3. **Obliquus capitis inferior** running from the posterior margin of the transverse process of the atlas to the spinous process of the axis.
4. **Obliquus capitis superior** running from the inferior nuchal line of the occiput to posterior margin of the transverse process of the atlas.

Actions: extension, sidebending and rotation of the head, fine-tuning movements and balance of the head on the neck.
Clinical indications: Headaches, whiplash and postural stresses.
Nerve supply: dorsal ramus of the first cervical spinal nerve.

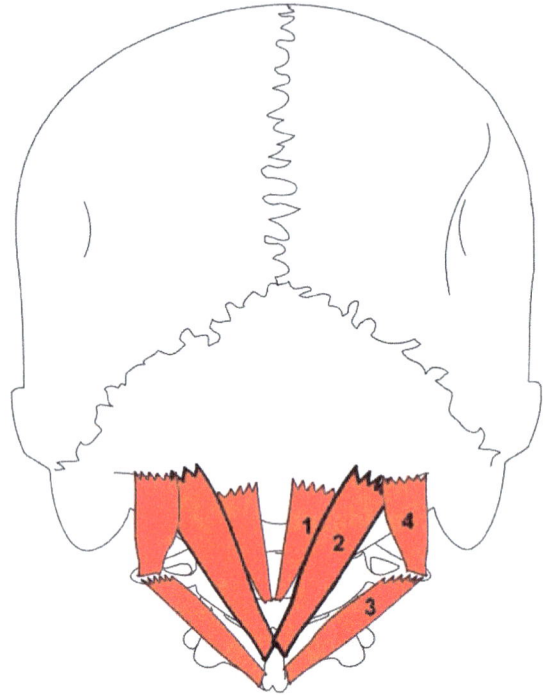

Technique 7.1 Inhibition of the suboccipital muscles

Patient

- Supine with the head straight.

Therapist

- Stand by the corner of the table, adjacent to the patient's head.
- The cephalad hand supports the patient's head with a broad hold under the occiput and the temporal bone.
- Rotate the patient's head until the suboccipital area on one side of the spine is exposed and accessible to your applicator.
- Start with the patient's head and neck in extension and maintain neck extension for the duration of the technique.
- Neck extension helps prevent the superficial neck muscles and fascia from becoming taught and obstructing access to the deeper suboccipital muscles.

Applicator

- The tip of the thumb of your caudad hand or a small T bar.
- Keep your thumb and forearm in a straight line.
- The force is generated along the forearm and the pressure is focused on the tip of the thumb.

Tissue tension

- The applicator is placed on the suboccipital muscle to be treated.
- Take up the primary tissue tension by increasing your thumb pressure with compression on the muscle.
- Apply transverse pressure. Work perpendicular to the muscle.
- Take up the secondary tissue tension with a small amount of thumb rotation.
- Take up the longitudinal tissue tension by flexing the patient's head. Localise movement to the upper cervical spine. Be careful not to induce over tension with too much flexion.

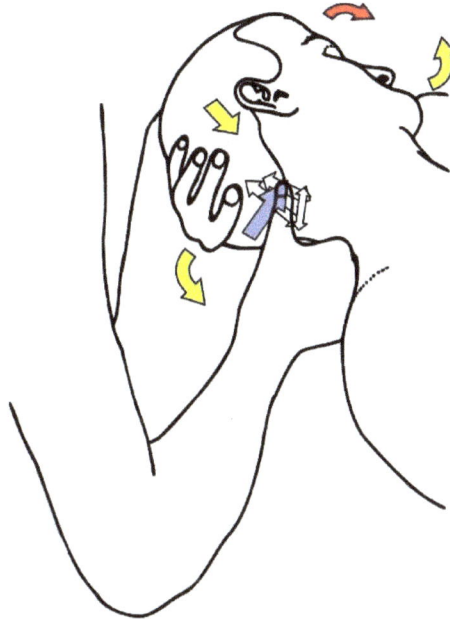

Figure 7.1

Muscle Fibres	⇕	Primary Force	⬇	Secondary Force	↻	Stretch Force	⬇	Contraction Force	⬇

Inhibition

- Apply pressure (compression) on the area of muscle covered by your thumb.
- Start with a light pressure and over about 5 to 10 seconds increase to a firm pressure.
- Your pressure should be just short of discomfort.
- Release slowly.
- To relax the muscle, work with the patients breathing cycle, about 15 breaths per minute.
- Maintain some compression throughout the technique but increase it during exhalation.

Active component

- Ask the patient to take a deep breath and hold it in.
- Ask the patient to push their chin forward and thereby, simultaneously, take their head backwards into extension for 3 to 5 seconds. This involves all four suboccipital muscles.
- Alternatively ask the patient to rotate their head into the table. Contralateral rotation involves the superior oblique.
- Alternatively ask the patient to rotate their head away from the table. Ipsilateral rotation involves the rectus posterior major and inferior oblique.
- Alternatively ask the patient to sidebend their head away from the table. Sidebending involves the rectus posterior major, the superior oblique and the inferior oblique.
- A light pressure is all that is needed, about 10% of full contraction.

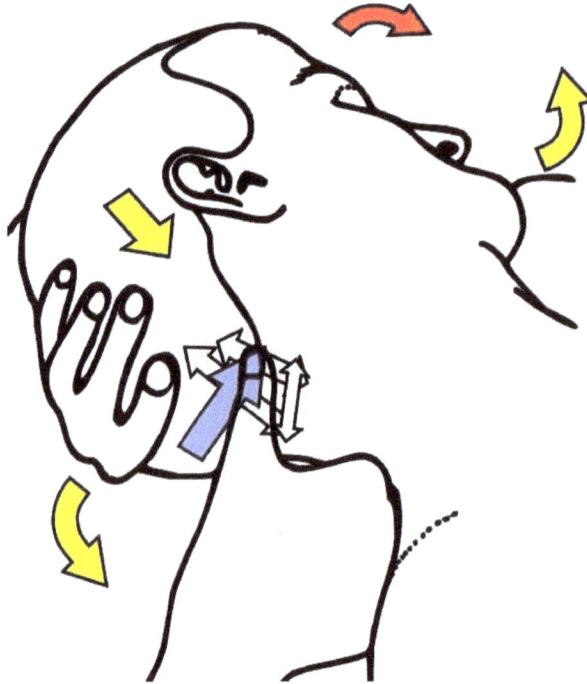

Figure 7.2

Muscle Fibres	↕	Primary Force	⬇	Secondary Force	↻	Stretch Force	⬇	Contraction Force	⬇

- Resist the patient's effort.
- Ask the patient to exhale and relax and then take up the tissue slack presented by increasing your thumb pressure and re-positioning the patient's head in greater degrees of flexion.
- Repeat several times, or as required.

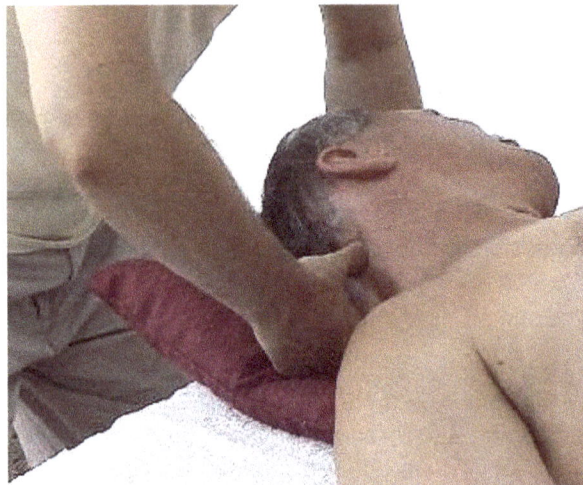

Picture 7.1

54

Technique 7.2 Inhibition and kneading of suboccipital muscles

Patient

- Supine with head straight, resting on a thin pillow or rolled up towel.

Therapist

- Stand or sit at the head of the table.
- Support the patient's occiput in the palm of your left hand.
- Your left hand rests on the table.
- The pads of your fingers rest on the right side of the occiput.
- The fingertip of your index finger rests on a specific sub-occipital muscle, or on several sub-occipital muscles. Accessibility will depend in the size of the therapist's finger and the patient's neck.
- It will be easier to access the muscles if you start with the head and neck in extension.
- Maintain neck extension for the duration of the technique to prevent the superficial neck muscles and fascia from becoming taught and thereby obstructing access to the deeper sub-occipital muscles.
- The thenar and hypothenar areas of your right hand usually sit along the coronal suture, on the left and right sides of the mid-sagittal plane respectively.
- Extremes in the size of the therapist's hand and the patient's head however may require you modifying your point of contact.
- The palm of your hand rests on the patient's frontal bone with fingers facing inferiorly.

Applicator

- The fingertip of the index or forefinger of your left hand for the right sub-occipital muscles.

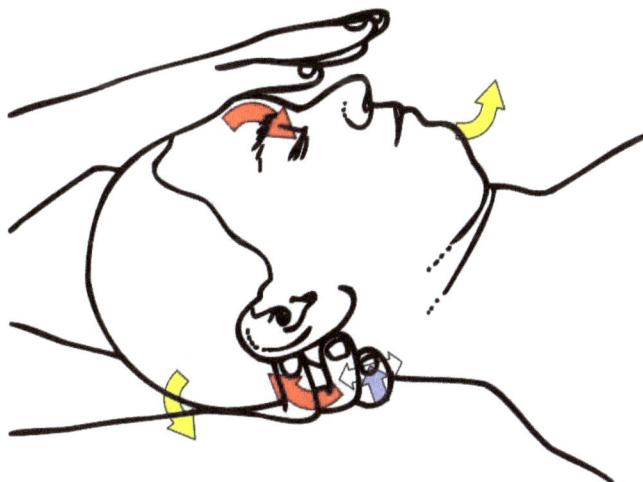

Figure 7.3

Muscle Fibres	⇕	Primary Force	⬇	Secondary Force	↻	Stretch Force	⬇	Contraction Force	⬇

Tissue tension

- Take up the primary tissue tension by increasing your fingertip pressure on the muscle. Flexing the index finger will produce the desired compression and transverse pressure.
- Work perpendicular to the muscle.
- Take up the longitudinal tissue tension by flexing the patient's head.
- Localise movement to the upper cervical spine and to the sub-occipital muscle on the right side.

- This technique requires coordinated movement of both hands and will involve some head rotation (to the right in this case) and sidebending (to the left in this case).

Inhibition

- Apply pressure (compression) on the area of muscle covered by your fingertip.
- Start with a light pressure and over about 5 to 10 seconds increase to a firm pressure.
- Your pressure should be just short of discomfort.
- Release slowly.
- To relax the muscle, work with the patients breathing cycle, about 15 breaths per minute.
- Maintain some compression throughout the technique but increase it during exhalation.

Kneading

- With coordinated movement of both hands and your applicator, apply a rhythmical cycle of primary and longitudinal forces.
- Take care not to pull the patient's hair.
- When the muscle is at an optimal longitudinal tension, increase the primary forces.
- Your pressure should be just short of discomfort.
- To relax the muscle, work with the patients breathing cycle, about 15 breaths per minute.
- To stimulate increase your speed to about 40 cycles per minute.

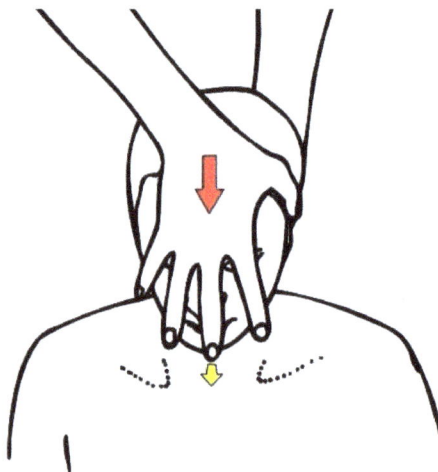 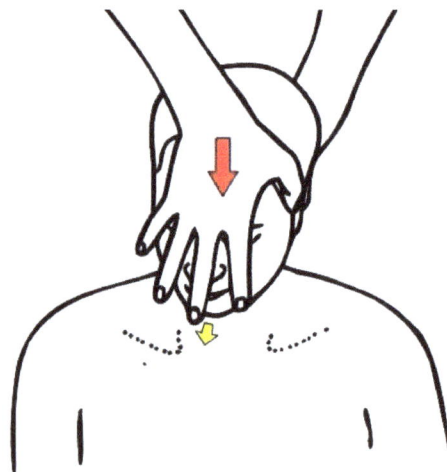

Figure 7.4   Figure 7.5

Muscle Fibres	⇕	Primary Force	⬇	Secondary Force	↻	Stretch Force	⬇	Contraction Force	⬇

Active component

- Ask the patient to take a deep breath and hold it in.
- Ask the patient to push their chin forward and thereby simultaneously take their head backwards into extension for 3 to 5 seconds.
- Alternatively ask the patient to rotate or sidebend their head, depending on which muscle you are treating.
- A light pressure is all that is needed, about 10% of full contraction.
- Resist the patient's effort.
- Ask the patient to exhale and relax, then take up the tissue slack presented by increasing your fingertip pressure (increasing the primary force), and by re-positioning the patient's head in greater degrees of flexion (increasing longitudinal force).
- Repeat several times, or as required.

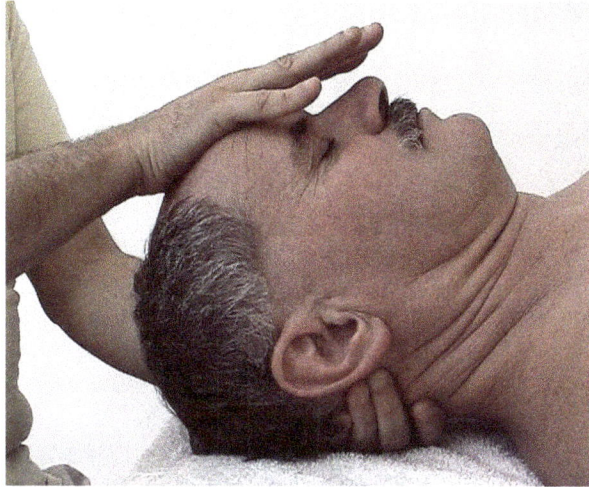

Picture 7.2

Technique 7.3 Inhibition of suboccipital muscles

Patient

- Prone with head rotated away from the therapist.

Therapist

- Stand by the side of the table, near to the patient's head.
- For greatest control grasp a broad area of the crown of the patients head in your cephalad hand. Your spread fingers extend over the frontal bone.
- Grasp the patients neck gently with your caudad hand and place the tip of your thumb on a suboccipital muscle, on the side of the spine nearest the table.

Applicator

- The tip of the thumb of your caudad hand is placed on the suboccipital muscle to be treated.

Tissue tension

- Take up the primary tissue tension by increasing your thumb pressure on the muscle.
- Take up the secondary tissue tension with a small amount of thumb rotation.
- Take up the longitudinal tissue tension by slightly flexing the patient's head.
- To prevent over-tension of the superficial muscles and fascia keep the lower cervical spine in slight extension.

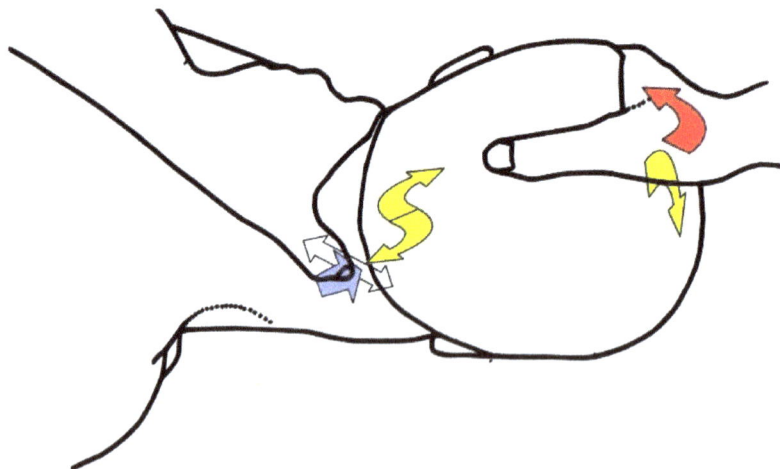

Figure 7.6

Muscle Fibres	⇕	Primary Force	⬇	Secondary Force	↻	Stretch Force	⬇	Contraction Force	⬇

Active component

- Ask the patient to take a deep breath and hold it in.
- Ask the patient to push their chin forward and take their head backwards (head extension) for 3 to 5 seconds. This involves all four suboccipital muscles.
- Alternatively ask the patient to rotate their head into the table. Ipsilateral rotation involves the rectus posterior major and inferior oblique.
- A light pressure is all that is needed, about 10% of maximum contraction.
- Resist their effort.

- Ask the patient to exhale and relax, then take up the tissue slack presented by increasing your thumb pressure, and re-position the patient's head in greater flexion.
- Repeat several times, or as required.

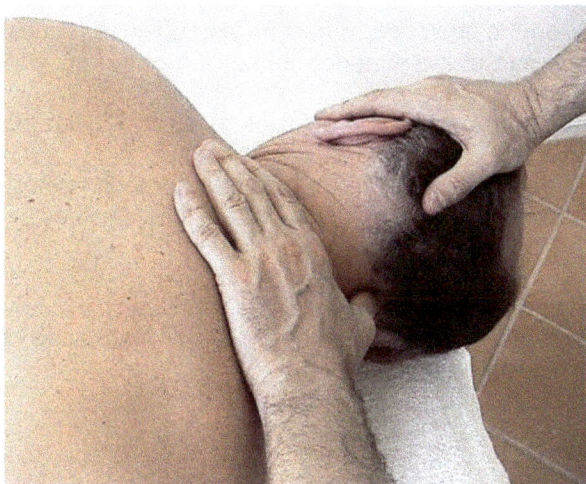

Picture 7.3

8. Posterior cervical muscles

Anatomy

Splenius capitis arises on the ligamentum nuchae and spinous processes of C7 to T3 and attaches under the lateral part of the superior nuchal line of the occiput and on the mastoid process of the temporal bone.

Splenius cervicis arises on the spinous processes of T3 to T6 and attach on the posterior tubercles of the transverse process C1 to T3.

Splenius capitis and splenius cervicis lie deep to sternocleidomastoid, trapezius and the rhomboids and superficial to the segmental muscles, interspinales, intertransversarii and transversospinalis.

Actions: Splenius capitis and splenius cervicis contracting bilaterally extend the head and neck, contracting unilaterally they sidebend and slightly ipsilaterally rotate the head and neck.
Nerve supply: Cervical spinal nerves.

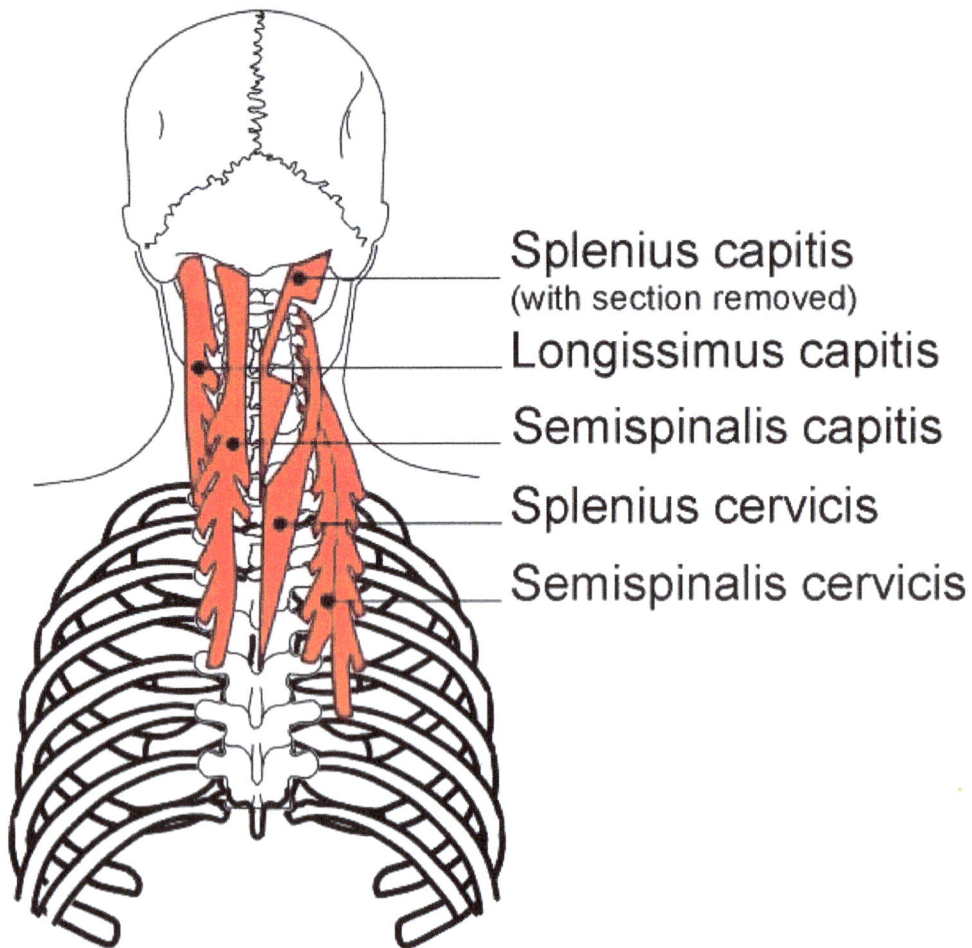

Splenius capitis
(with section removed)
Longissimus capitis
Semispinalis capitis
Splenius cervicis
Semispinalis cervicis

Transversospinalis

Semispinalis thoracis arises on the transverse processes of T6 to T10 and attaches on the spinous processes of C6 to T4. More tendinous in form.

Semispinalis cervicis arises on the transverse processes of T1 to T6 and attaches on the spinous processes of C2 to C5. More muscular especially the fibres that attach on the axis.

Semispinalis capitis arises on the transverse processes of C7 to T6 and the articular processes of C4 to C6 (sometimes C7 & T1) and attaches either side of the mid-sagittal line between the superior and inferior nuchal lines on the occiput.

Action: Extension of the head and cervical spine.
Nerve supply: Dorsal rami of cervical and thoracic nerves.

Multifidus arise on the sacrum (S4), aponeurosis of the erector spinae, posterior superior iliac spine, posterior sacroiliac ligament, mamillary processes of L1 to L5, transverse processes of T1 to T12 and articular processes of C4 to C7. The muscle attaches along the length of a spinous process one to four vertebral segments above.
Nerve supply: Dorsal rami of the spinal nerves.
Rotatores are the deepest muscles. They arise on cervical, thoracic and lumbar transverse processes and attach on the lamina and base of the spinous process of the vertebra above.
Nerve supply: Dorsal rami of the spinal nerves.
Interspinales (Interspinalis) run from one spinous process to the spinous process above. They are present between C2 and T3, and between T11 and L5. They are more distinct in the cervical spine. Sometimes they occur between L5 and the sacrum.
Nerve supply: Dorsal rami of the spinal nerves.
Intertransversarii run from a transverse process to the transverse process above. They are present between C1 and T1, and between T10 and the sacrum. In the cervical and lumbar, pairs of muscles lie either side of the spine.
Nerve supply: Dorsal and ventral rami of the spinal nerves.

Erector spinae
Iliocostalis cervicis arises on the superior border of the angles of ribs 3 to 6 medial to iliocostalis thoracis attachments. It attaches on the posterior tubercles of the transverse process of C4 to C6.
Longissimus cervicis arises on the transverse processes of T1 to T5 medial to longissimus thoracis and to the posterior tubercles of the transverse processes of C2 to C6.
Spinalis cervicis arises on the spinous processes of C7 to T2 and the ligamentum nuchae. It attaches on the spinous processes of C2 to C4. It exhibits variation in its attachments and may be absent.

Cervical spinous processes may be bifid. C2 and C7 (vertebra prominens) are easily palpable. C6 is usually palpable but disappears in extension. Articular pillars and facet joints are at finger-width spacings.

Clinical indications: Whiplash, postural, torticollis, degenerative arthritic changes and congenital defects.

Technique 8.1 Unilateral kneading of cervical muscles from occiput to C7

Patient

- Supine with head straight and resting on a folded towel or shallow pillow.

Therapist

- Stand or sit at the head of the table.
- Support the patient's head with a broad hold over their frontal bone.
- The fingers of your other hand sit in the depression in the middle of the back of neck.
- The pads of your fingertips rest against the medial side of the posterior cervical muscles.
- Your wrists and backs of hands rest on the table or a pillow and act as a fulcrum.

Applicator

- The fingertips of one hand.

Tissue tension

- Take up the primary tissue tension with compression by increasing your fingertip pressure, adding a transverse force to the muscle by simultaneously flexing the fingertips of your hand to pull the muscles away from the middle of the spine.
- Work perpendicular to the muscle, from medial to lateral.
- Take up the secondary tissue tension with a small amount of finger rotation.

- Longitudinal tension is taken up by starting the technique with the spine in slight flexion.
- Try to maintain some flexion for the duration of the technique. A pillow may be placed under the patient's head to prevent hyperextension of the head and neck.

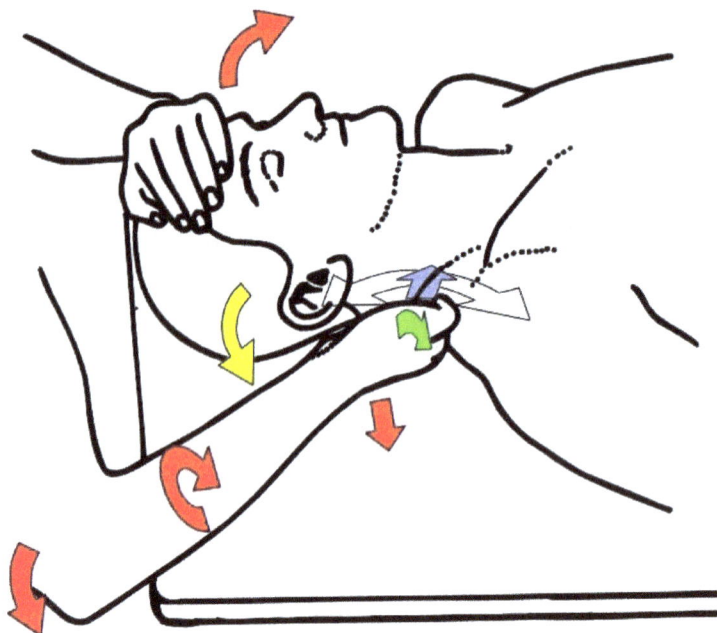

Figure 8.1

Muscle Fibres	↕	Primary Force	⬇	Secondary Force	↺	Stretch Force	⬇	Contraction Force	⬇

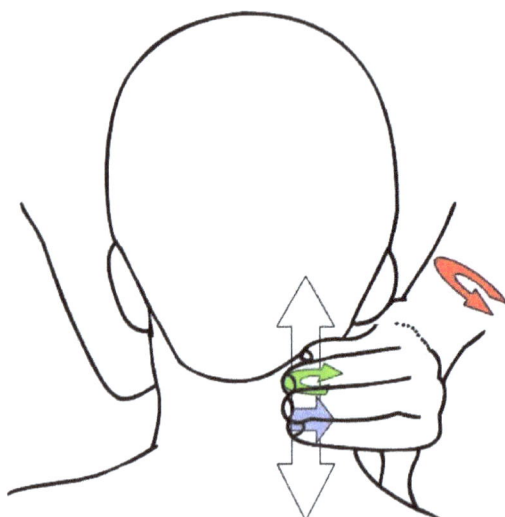

Figure 8.2 View from below

Kneading

- With the fingertips of one hand apply a rhythmical cycle of primary, secondary and longitudinal forces.

- When the muscle is at an optimal longitudinal tension increase the primary and secondary forces
- Your pressure should be just short of discomfort.
- To relax the muscle, work with the patients breathing cycle, about 15 breaths per minute.
- To stimulate, increase your speed to about 40 cycles per minute.

Active component

- Ask the patient to take a deep breath and hold it in.
- Ask the patient to contract his spinal muscles by pushing their head into the table for 3 to 5 seconds using a 10% effort.
- Alternatively ask the patient to rotate their head and neck.
- Resist the patient's effort and maintain tissue lockup throughout the technique.
- Ask the patient to exhale and to relax their muscle contraction.
- As soon as you feel that the patient has relaxed their muscles completely (about 1-3 seconds), take up the tissue slack by increasing the primary, secondary and longitudinal tension.
- Take up the slack after each contraction and during exhalation.
- Repeat 2 or 3 times, or as required.

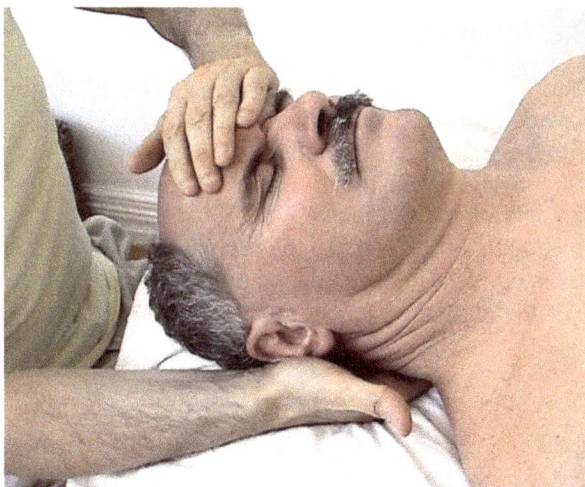

Picture 8.1

Technique 8.2 Bilateral kneading of cervical muscles from occiput to C6

Patient

- Supine with the head straight and resting on a folded towel or shallow pillow.

Therapist

- Stand by the head of the table.
- The fingers of both your hands sit in the depression in the middle of the back of neck.
- The pads of your fingertips rest against the medial side of the posterior cervical muscles.
- Your hypothenar eminences support the patient's head, preventing unwanted extension and rotation.
- Your wrists and backs of both hands rest on the table or a pillow, acting as a fulcrum.

Applicator

- The fingertips of both hands.

Tissue tension

- Take up the primary tissue tension.
- Apply compression by increasing your fingertip pressure.
- Add a transverse force to the muscle by simultaneously flexing the fingertips of your hands to pull the muscles away from the middle of the spine.
- Work perpendicular to the muscle, from medial to lateral.
- Take up the secondary tissue tension with a small amount of wrist abduction and through the fingertips produce torsion to the muscle.
- Longitudinal tension is taken up by starting the technique with the spine in slight flexion.
- Try to maintain some flexion for the duration of the technique. A pillow may be placed under the patient's head to prevent hyperextension of the head and neck.

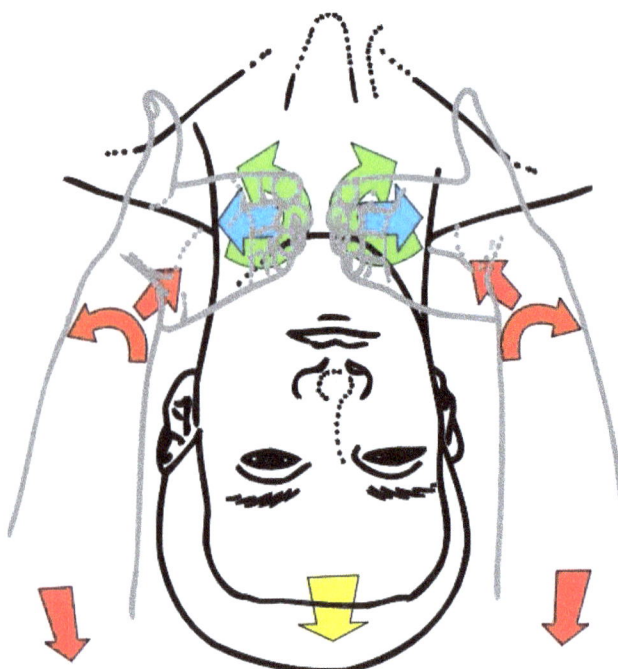

Figure 8.3 View from above

Muscle Fibres	⇕	Primary Force	⬇	Secondary Force	↺	Stretch Force	⬇	Contraction Force	⬇

Kneading

- With the fingertips of one hand apply a rhythmical cycle of primary, secondary and longitudinal forces.
- When the muscle is at an optimal longitudinal tension increase the primary and secondary forces
- Your pressure should be just short of discomfort.
- To relax the muscle, work with the patients breathing cycle, about 15 breaths per minute.
- To stimulate, increase your speed to about 40 cycles per minute.

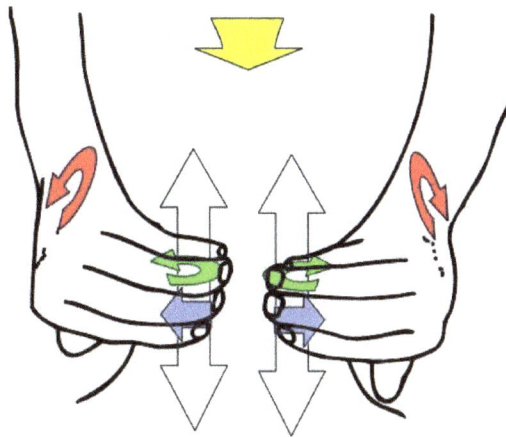

Figure 8.4 View from below

Active component

- Ask the patient to take a deep breath and hold it in.
- Ask the patient to contract their spinal muscles by pushing their head into the table for 3 to 5 seconds using a 10% effort.
- Resist the patient's effort and maintain tissue lockup throughout the technique.
- Ask the patient to exhale and to relax their muscle contraction.
- As soon as you feel that the patient has relaxed their muscles completely (about 1-3 seconds), take up the tissue slack by increasing the primary, secondary and longitudinal tension.
- Take up the slack after each contraction and during exhalation.
- Repeat 2 or 3 times, or as required.

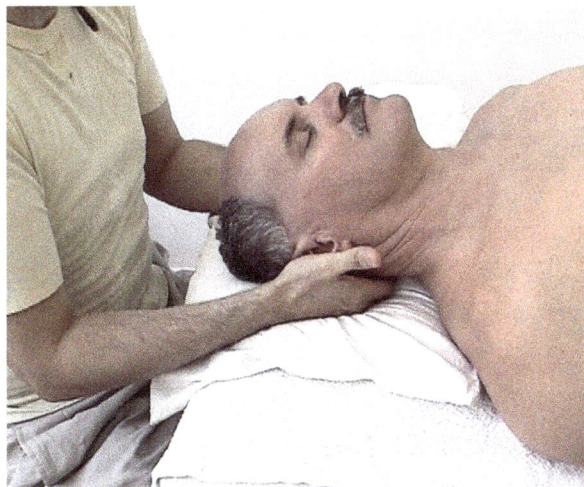

Picture 8.2

Technique 8.3 Inhibition of posterior cervical muscles from C2 to C6

Patient

- Prone with head rotated away from the therapist.

Therapist

- Stand by the side of the couch, adjacent to the patient's head.
- For greatest control, grasp a broad area of the crown of the patient's head in your cephalad hand (optional)
- Grasp the patient's neck gently with your caudad hand, placing the tip of your thumb on a posterior cervical muscle and articular pillar on the side of the spine nearest the table.

Applicator

- The tip of the thumb of your caudad hand.

Tissue tension

- Take up the primary tissue tension by increasing your thumb pressure on the muscle.
- Take up the secondary tissue tension with a small amount of thumb rotation.
- Take up the longitudinal tissue tension by slightly flexing the patient's neck.
- To prevent over-tension of the superficial muscles and fascia, keep the head in slight extension.

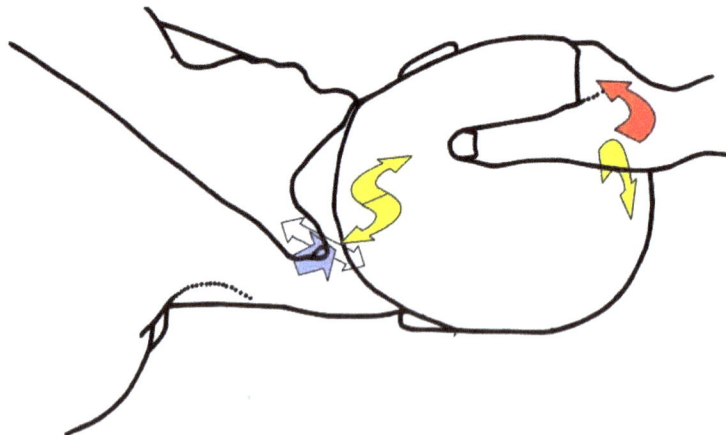

Figure 8.5

Muscle Fibres	⇕	Primary Force	⬇	Secondary Force	↻	Stretch Force	⬇	Contraction Force	⬇

Active component

- Ask the patient to take a deep breath and hold it in.
- Ask the patient to push their neck straight backwards into your applicator (neck extension) for 3 to 5 seconds.
- Alternatively, ask the patient to rotate their head into the table.
- A light pressure is all that is needed, about 10% of maximum contraction.
- Resist their effort with your applicator, not with your cephalad hand.
- Ask the patient to relax and then take up the tissue slack presented by increasing your thumb pressure.
- Re-position the patient's cervical spine in greater flexion.
- Repeat several times, or as required.

66

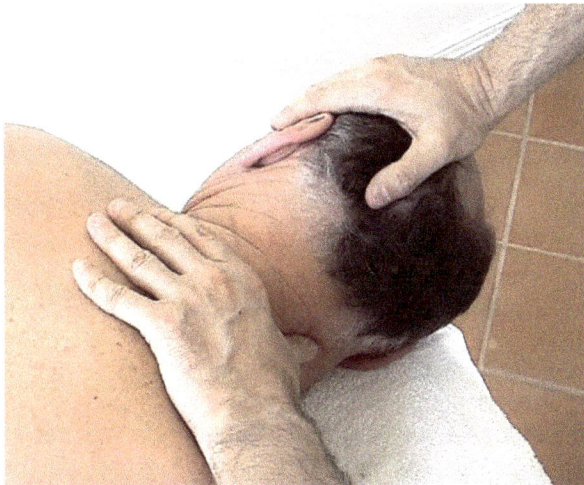

Picture 8.3

Technique 8.4 Unilateral kneading of posterior cervical muscles from the occiput to C7

Patient

- Supine with the head straight and resting on a folded towel or shallow pillow.

Therapist

- Stand at the side of the table adjacent to the patient's head.
- Grasp and support the patient's head with your cephalad hand, maintaining a broad hold over the frontal bone.
- Reach across the patient with your caudad hand and hook your fingertips around the opposite side posterior cervical muscles.
- Your fingertips sit in the depression in the middle of the back of neck.
- The pads of your fingertips rest against the medial side of the posterior cervical muscles.

Applicator

- The fingertips of your caudad hand.

Tissue tension

- Take up the primary tissue tension with compression, by increasing your fingertip pressure, adding a transverse force to the muscle by flexing your fingertips.
- Alternatively, keep your fingertips in a fixed flexed position and your forearm extended and lean back.
- Pull the muscle away from the spine.
- Work perpendicular to the muscle, from medial to lateral.
- Longitudinal tension is taken up by starting the technique with the spine in slight flexion.
- Try to maintain some flexion for the duration of the technique. A pillow may be placed under the patient's head to prevent hyperextension of the head and neck.
- Further tension is taken up by rotating the patient's head away from you.

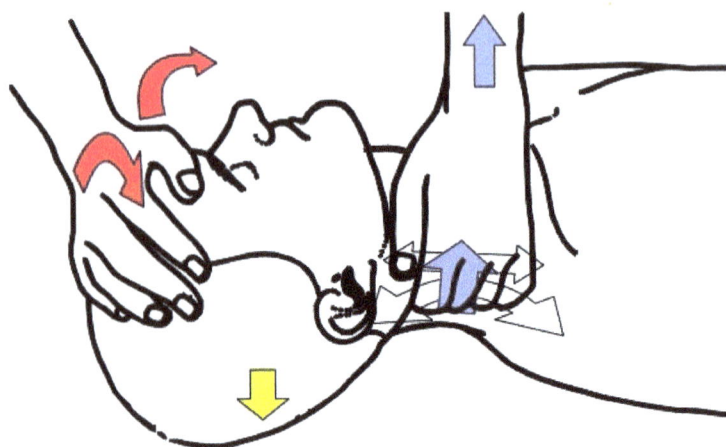

Figure 8.6

Muscle Fibres	⇕	Primary Force	⬇	Secondary Force	↻	Stretch Force	⬇	Contraction Force	⬇

Kneading

- With the fingertips of your caudad hand apply a rhythmical cycle of primary, secondary and longitudinal forces.
- When the muscle is at an optimal longitudinal tension increase the primary forces.

- Use a push-pull action.
- Keep your wrist and the palm of your caudad hand away from the patient's neck. Do not allow your hand to obstruct movement of the cervical spine, or reduce the force going through to your fingertips.
- Your pressure should be just short of discomfort.
- To relax the muscle, work with the patients breathing cycle, about 15 breaths per minute.
- To stimulate, increase your speed to about 40 cycles per minute.

Active component

- Ask the patient to take a deep breath and hold it in.
- Ask the patient to contract their posterior cervical muscles by pushing their head backward into the table for 3 to 5 seconds using a 10% effort.
- Alternatively, ask the patient to rotate their head into your applicator.
- Resist the patient's effort and maintain tissue lockup throughout the technique.
- Ask the patient to exhale and to relax their muscle contraction.
- As soon as you feel that the patient has relaxed their muscles completely (about 1-3 seconds), take up the tissue slack by increasing the primary tension, secondary and longitudinal tension.
- Take up the slack after each contraction and during exhalation.
- Repeat 2 or 3 times, or as required.

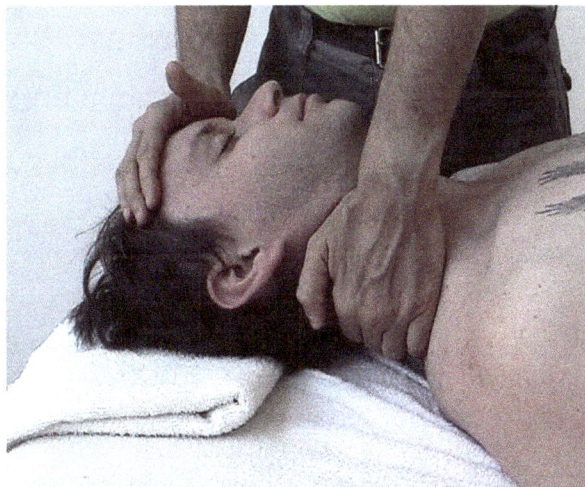

Picture 8.4

9. Erector spinae (Sacrospinalis/Paravertebral muscles)

Anatomy

The erector spinae is made up of muscles of different lengths and attachments. The composition and size of muscle and tendon varies throughout the length of the spine.
It arises on the sacrum as a broad thick tendon, and in the lumbar becomes a thick muscle. In the thoracic it separates into three distinct columns, from lateral to medial they are the iliocostalis, longissimus and spinalis. A paravertebral gutter is formed between the bulk of the muscle mass and lumbar and thoracic vertebral spinous processes.

The erector spinae arises on the spinous processes of T11 and 12 and all lumbar vertebrae and their supraspinous ligaments, the median and lateral sacral crests and a medial area on the iliac crest. Its fibres merge with the sacrotuberous and posterior sacroiliac ligaments and with the gluteus maximus.

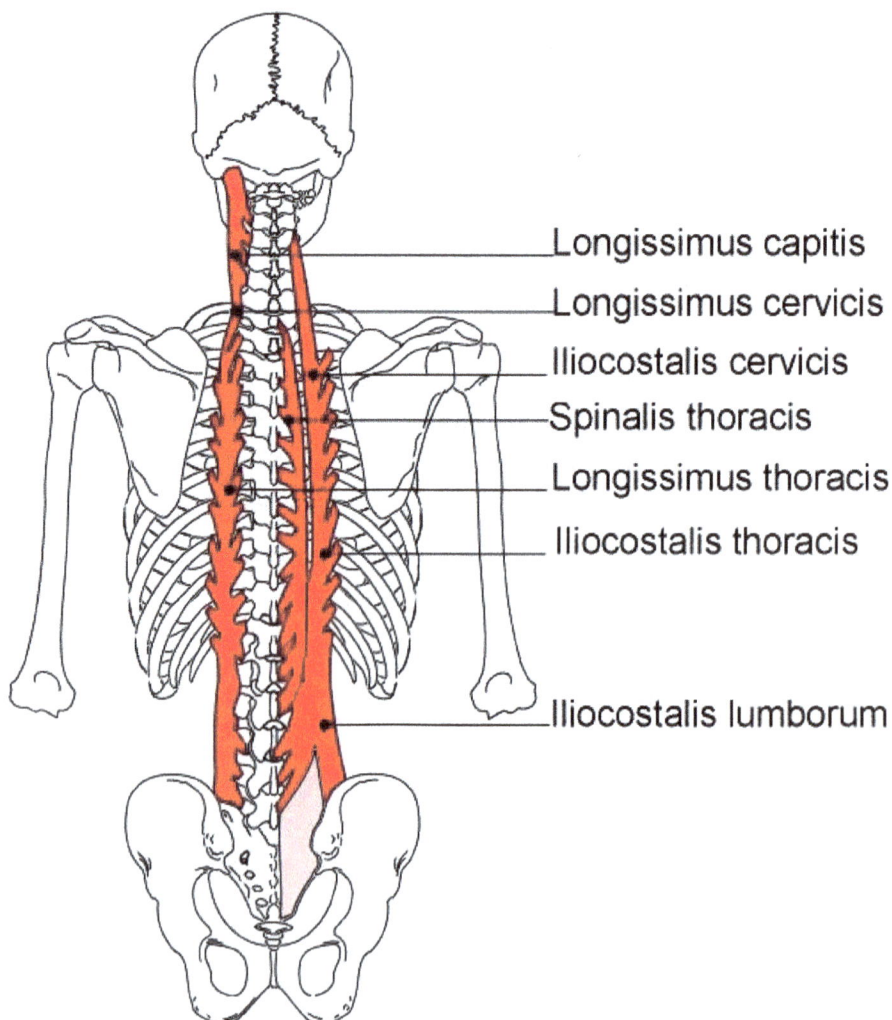

Longissimus capitis
Longissimus cervicis
Iliocostalis cervicis
Spinalis thoracis
Longissimus thoracis
Iliocostalis thoracis

Iliocostalis lumborum

Iliocostalis
Iliocostalis lumborum attaches onto the inferior borders of the angles of ribs 6 to 12.
Iliocostalis thoracis arises on the superior border of the angles of ribs 6 to 12. It attaches onto the superior border of the angles of ribs 1 to 6 and the transverse process of C7.
Iliocostalis cervicis arises on the superior border of the angles of ribs 3 to 6 medial to iliocostalis thoracis attachments. It attaches onto the posterior tubercles of the transverse process of C4 to C6.

70

Longissimus

Longissimus thoracis arises on the iliocostalis lumborum, posterior transverse processes of lumbar vertebrae and the thoracolumbar fascia. It attaches onto the tips of the transverse processes of all thoracic vertebrae and between the tubercles and angles of ribs 3 to 12.

Longissimus cervicis arises on the transverse processes of T1 to T5 medial to longissimus thoracis and to the posterior tubercles of the transverse processes of C2 to C6.

Longissimus capitis arises on the transverse processes of T1 to T5 and the articular processes of C4 to C7. It attaches onto the posterior mastoid process, deep to splenius capitis and sternocleidomastoid.

Spinalis

Spinalis thoracis merges anteriorly with semispinalis thoracis and laterally with longissimus thoracis. It arises on the spinous processes of T11 to L2. The tendons unite into a small muscle and this later separates as distinct tendons, which attach on the spinous processes of T1 to T4-8.

Spinalis cervicis arises on the spinous processes of C7 to T2 and the ligamentum nuchae. It attaches onto the spinous processes of C2 to C4. It exhibits variation in its attachments and may be absent.

Spinalis capitis blends with the semispinalis capitis.

Actions: Bilateral contraction produces extension of the vertebral column and head. Unilateral contraction produces sidebending and rotation.

Nerve supply: Dorsal rami of cervical, thoracic and lumbar spinal nerves.

Transversospinalis

Semispinalis thoracis arises on the transverse processes of T6 to T10 and attaches onto the spinous processes of C6 to T4. More tendinous in form.

Semispinalis cervicis arises on the transverse processes of T1 to T6 and attaches onto the spinous processes of C2 to C5. More muscular, especially the fibres that attach on the axis.

Semispinalis capitis arises on the transverse processes of C7 to T6 and the articular processes of C4 to C6 (sometimes C7 & T1) and attaches either side of the mid-sagittal line, between the superior and inferior nuchal lines on the occiput.

Nerve supply: Dorsal rami of cervical and thoracic nerves.

Action: Extension of the head and cervical spine.

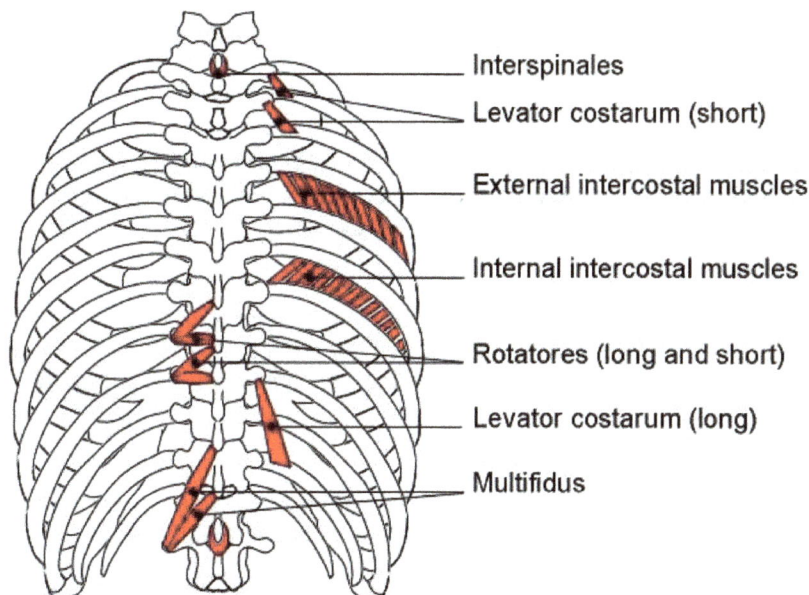

Interspinales
Levator costarum (short)
External intercostal muscles
Internal intercostal muscles
Rotatores (long and short)
Levator costarum (long)
Multifidus

Multifidus arises on the sacrum (S4), aponeurosis of the erector spinae, posterior superior iliac spine, posterior sacroiliac ligament, mamillary processes of L1 to L5, transverse processes of T1 to T12 and articular processes of C4 to C7. The muscle attaches along the length of a spinous process, one to four vertebral segments above.

Nerve supply: Dorsal rami of the spinal nerves.

Rotatores are the deepest muscles. They arise on cervical, thoracic and lumbar transverse processes and attach onto the lamina and base of the spinous process of the vertebra above.
Nerve supply: Dorsal rami of the spinal nerves.

Interspinales (interspinalis) run from a spinous process to the spinous process above. They are present between C2 and T3, and between T11 and L5. They are more distinct in the cervical spine. Sometimes they occur between L5 and the sacrum.
Nerve supply: Dorsal rami of the spinal nerves.

Intertransversarii run from a transverse process to the transverse process above. They are present between C1 and T1, and between T10 and the sacrum. In the cervical and lumbar, pairs of muscles lie either side of the spine.
Nerve supply: Dorsal and ventral rami of the spinal nerves.

Actions: The short muscles of the back show intermittent contractions in the upright position and have a mainly postural function. They work with rectus abdominis muscles and they protect the spine from injury by finetuning the movements of individual vertebrae. They prevent the longer muscles exerting buckling forces on the spine. They produce extension, sidebending and rotation.

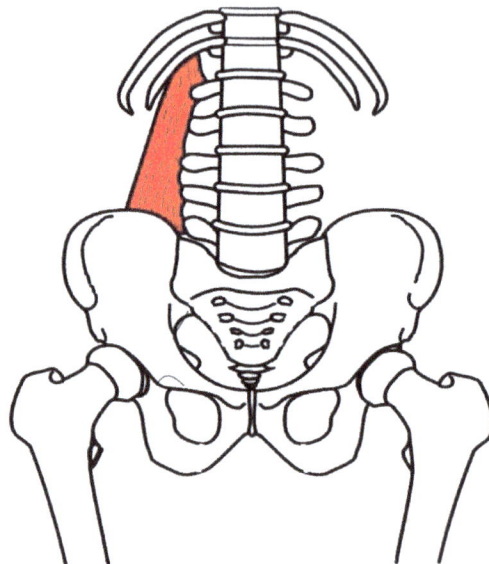

Quadratus lumborum arises on the posterior iliac crest and attaches on rib 12 and the tip of transverse processes of lumbar vertebrae L1 to 4. It lies deep to erector spinae.
Action: It sidebends the spine and fixes the lower ribs.
Nerve supply: T12 to L1.

Serratus posterior superior arises from the ligamentum nuchae, spinous processes and supraspinous ligaments from C7 to T3 and attaches just lateral to the angles of ribs 2 to 5. It covers a layer of fascia and lies deep to the rhomboids. It may be absent or vary the vertebral levels of attachment.
Nerve supply: Intercostal nerves 2 to 5.

Thoracolumbar fascia extends from the ligamentum nuchae to the medial crest of the sacrum. It is continuous with the deep cervical fascia and it extends laterally to the rib angles, abdominal aponeurosis and iliac crest.

In the cervical spine it attaches onto the ligamentum nuchae and cervical transverse processes. In the thoracic it attaches onto the tips of all thoracic spinous processes and supraspinous ligaments, and to the rib angles laterally. It is thin and lies between the erector spinae and the muscles connecting the spine to the upper limb.

In the lumbar it is thick and strong and has three layers. The posterior layer is the most superficial layer and attaches on the spines of lumbar and sacral vertebrae and supraspinous ligaments. The middle layer attaches onto the tips of all lumbar transverse processes and intertransverse ligaments. The anterior layer attaches onto the anterior surface of all lumbar transverse processes (medially), the arcuate ligament (superiorly), iliolumbar ligament and the iliac crest (inferiorly). The thoracolumbar fascia encloses and intermeshes with muscles in the lumbar region. The posterior and middle layers pass behind and in front of erector spinae. The middle and anterior layer passes behind, and in front of, quadratus lumborum. All three layers join laterally and become continuous with the aponeurosis of the transversus abdominis.

Technique 9.1 Strong kneading of thoracic and lumbar erector spinae from T1 to L5

Patient

- Prone with head rotated towards you.

Therapist

- Stand by the side of the table.
- Place your forearm so it sits parallel to the spine and your olecranon process rests against the patient's spinous processes, on the side of the spine nearest you.
- Take up any skin slack by moving your olecranon process over the spinous processes into the paravertebral gutter on the opposite side of the spine to which you are standing.
- For the upper thoracic, the olecranon process should point cephalad and for the lumbar the olecranon process should point caudad.
- Your free hand grasps your forearm and helps control the applicator.

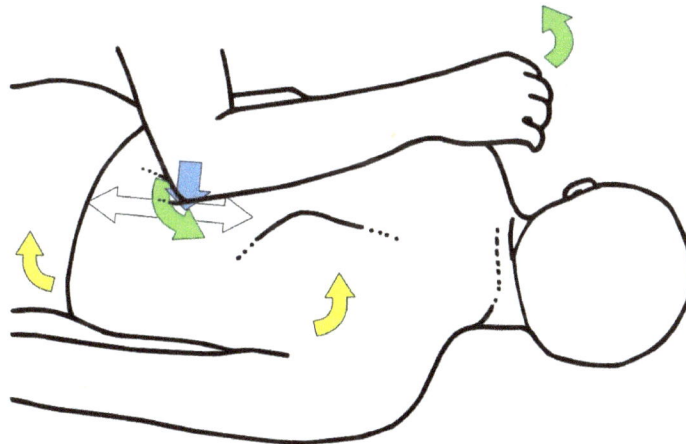

Figure 9.1

Muscle Fibres	⇕	Primary Force	⬇	Secondary Force	↻	Stretch Force	⬇	Contraction Force	⬇

Applicator

- Proximal border of ulnar shaft and olecranon process.

Tissue tension

- Take up the primary tissue tension with compression and a transverse force moving from medial to lateral over the muscles with your applicator.
- Take up the secondary tissue tension (torsion) by applying a rotation force with your applicator.
- Take up the longitudinal tension by starting the technique with the patient's spine sidebent towards you.

- A pillow may be placed under the patient's chest or abdomen if there are areas of the spine that are hyper-extended.

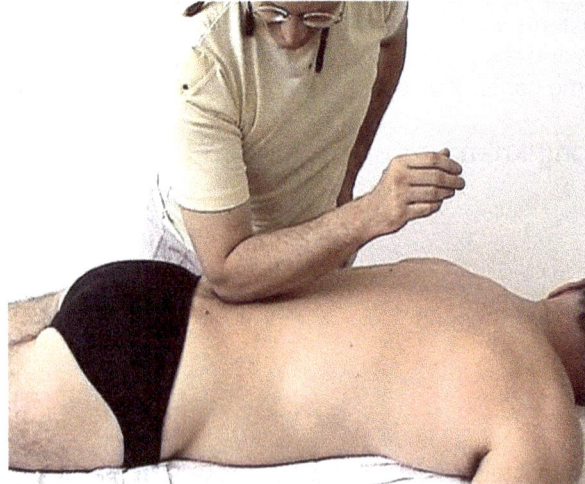

Picture 9.1

Kneading

- Apply a rhythmical cycle of primary and secondary forces.
- Begin with compression, introduce transverse tension and then rotation.
- Your pressure should be just short of discomfort.
- To relax the muscle, work with the patient's breathing cycle, about 15 breaths per minute.

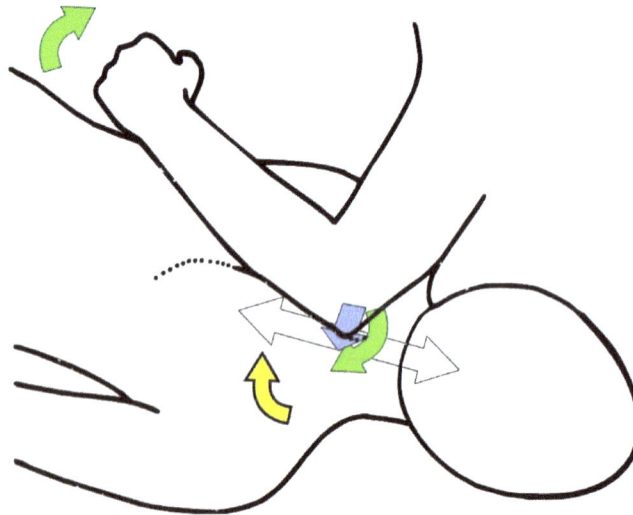

Figure 9.2

Muscle Fibres	⇕	Primary Force	⬇	Secondary Force	↻	Stretch Force	⬇	Contraction Force	⬇

Active component

- Ask the patient to take a deep breath and hold it in.
- Ask the patient to contract their spinal muscles for 3 to 5 seconds using a 10% effort.

    When working on the upper thoracic spine, ask the patient to lift their head upward and backward off the table.

74

When working on the mid-thoracic spine, ask the patient to rotate their spine by lifting the shoulder and rib cage on the opposite side, off the table.

When working on the lumbar, ask the patient to rotate their spine by lifting the pelvis on the opposite side to which you are standing, off the table.
Alternatively, ask the patient to lift the leg on the near side to which you are standing, off the table, less than 1 cm (1/2").

- Resist their effort and maintain tissue lockup throughout the technique.
- Ask the patient to exhale and to relax their muscle contraction.
- As soon as you feel that the patient has relaxed their muscles completely (about 1-3 seconds), take up the tissue slack by increasing the primary and secondary tension.
- Take up the slack after each contraction and during exhalation.
- Repeat 2 or 3 times, or as required.

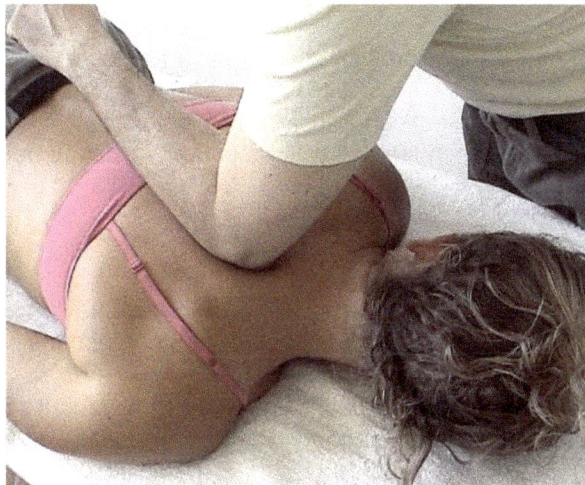

Picture 9.1b

Technique 9.2 Kneading of the upper thoracic erector spinae from T1 to T6

Patient

- Prone with their head rotated towards you.

Therapist

- Stand by the side of the table near to the head end. Your forearms are crossed.
- The heel of your caudad hand sits under the occiput and your fingers cover the occiput.
- Your cephalad hand makes contact with the muscle to be treated.

Applicator

- Pisiform bone, heel of hand or thenar eminence.

Tissue tension

- Take up the primary tissue tension with compression and by applying a transverse force on the muscle.
- Take up the secondary tissue tension with your applicator applying a rotation force.
- Take up the longitudinal/stretch tension with flexion and traction applied by the cephalad hand on the occiput.

Kneading

- Apply a rhythmical cycle of primary, secondary and longitudinal forces.
- When the muscle is at an optimal longitudinal tension, increase the other forces.
- Your pressure should be just short of discomfort.
- To relax the muscle, work with the patient's breathing cycle, about 15 breaths per minute.
- To stimulate, increase your speed to about 40 cycles per minute.

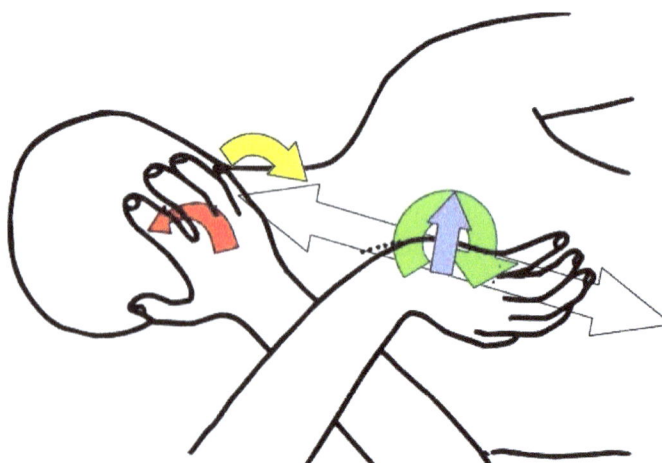

Figure 9.3

Muscle Fibres	⇕	Primary Force	⬇	Secondary Force	↻	Stretch Force	⬇	Contraction Force	⬇

Active component

- Ask the patient to take a deep breath and hold it in.
- Ask the patient to attempt to lift their head and neck upward and backward off the table for 3 to 5 seconds using a 10% effort. The erector spinae muscles of the upper thoracic will contract.

- Resist their effort and maintain tissue lockup throughout inhalation.
- Ask the patient to exhale and to relax their muscle contraction.
- As soon as you feel that the patient has relaxed their upper thoracic muscles completely (about 1-3 seconds), take up the tissue slack by increasing the primary, secondary and longitudinal tension.
- Take up the slack after each contraction and during exhalation. Repeat as required.

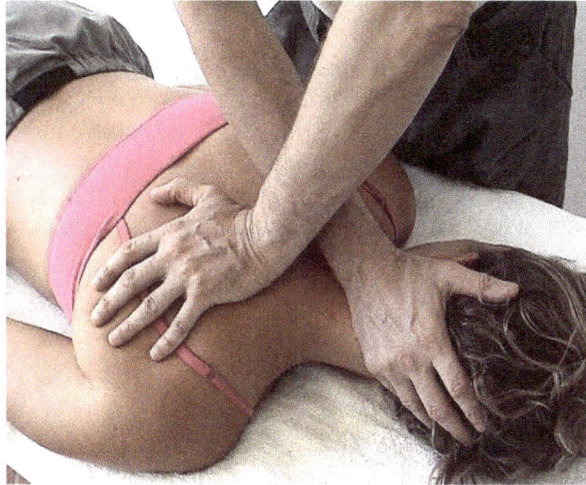

Picture 9.2

Technique 9.3 Kneading of thoracic and lumbar erector spinae from T1 to L5

Patient

- Prone with head rotated towards you.

Therapist

- Stand by the side of the table.
- Your forearms are at right angles and make a T shape.
- The pisiform bone and hypothenar eminence of your caudad hand rest in the nearside paravertebral gutter, the carpal groove rests over the paravertebral muscles, the thenar eminence rests on the lateral side of the rib angle and your fingers point cephalad.
- The applicator of your cephalad hand is placed in the paravertebral gutter on the opposite side of the spine, just medial to the muscle to be treated, and adjacent to the caudad hand.

Applicator

- Pisiform bone, heel of hand and thenar eminence.

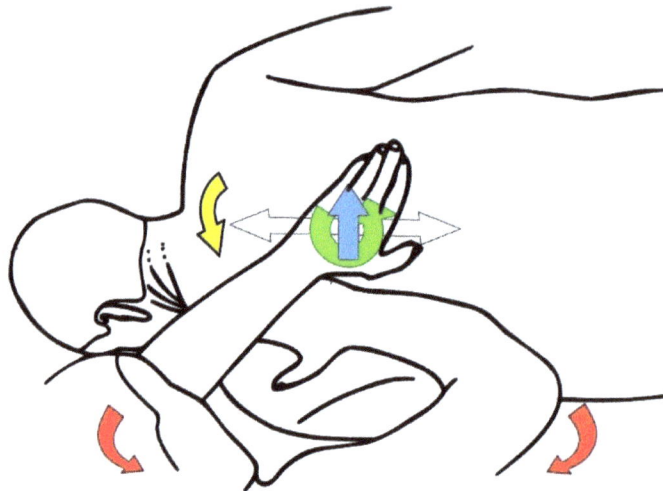

Figure 9.4

Muscle Fibres	⇕	Primary Force	⬇	Secondary Force	↻	Stretch Force	⬇	Contraction Force	⬇

Tissue tension

- Take up the primary tissue tension with your applicator, with compression and a medial to lateral transverse force on the muscles.
- Take up the secondary tissue tension (torsion) with your applicator, by applying a rotation force. Avoid skin stretch by taking some slack into the paravertebral gutter.
- Think of the movement as a twist of both hands in opposite directions. The caudad hand going clockwise and the cephalad hand going anticlockwise.
- Take up the longitudinal tension by starting the technique with the spine sidebent towards you.
- If both hands push down on the transverse processes on either side of the spine with equal pressure, then there will be no rotation.
- Use just enough downward pressure to stabilise the nearside spine, but not too much so that you produce extension in the spine and shortness in the muscles.

- A pillow may be placed under the patient's chest or abdomen, where the spine is hyper-extended.
- The pisiform of your caudad hand can be used to create rotation and sideshifting in the spine and leverage on adjacent vertebra to increase longitudinal tension in muscles.

Kneading

- Apply a rhythmical cycle of primary and secondary forces.
- When the muscle is at an optimal compression and transverse tension, increase the secondary forces.
- Your pressure should be just short of discomfort.
- To relax the muscle, work with the patient's breathing cycle, about 15 breaths per minute.
- To stimulate, increase your speed to about 40 cycles per minute.

Active component

- Ask the patient to take a deep breath and hold it in.
- Ask the patient to contract their spinal muscles for 3 to 5 seconds using a 10% effort.

  When working on the upper thoracic spine ask the patient to lift their head upwards and backwards off the table.

  When working on the mid-thoracic spine ask the patient to rotate their spine by lifting the shoulder and rib cage on the opposite side, off the table.

  When working on the lumbar ask the patient to rotate their spine by lifting the pelvis on the opposite side, off the table or lifting his leg on the near side, no more than 1 cm (1/2") off the table.

- Resist their effort and maintain tissue lockup throughout the technique.
- Ask the patient to exhale and to relax their muscle contraction.
- As soon as you feel that the patient has relaxed their muscles completely (about 1-3 seconds), take up the tissue slack by increasing the primary and secondary tension.
- Take up the slack after each contraction and during exhalation.
- Repeat 2 or 3 times, or as required.

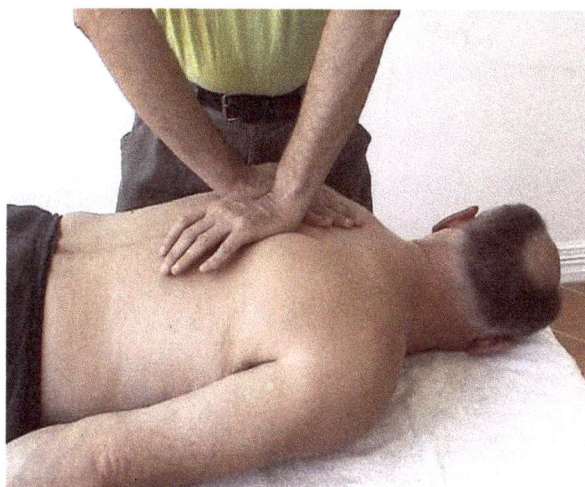

Picture 9.3

Technique 9.4 Kneading of thoracic and lumbar erector spinae from T1 to L5

Patient

- Prone with head rotated towards you.

Therapist

- Stand by the side of the table.
- Place the full length of your thumb against a group of spinous processes on the side of the spine nearest you. (Fig 9.5)
- Place the thenar eminence of your other hand over the dorsum of the proximal phalanx of your thumb.
- The thenar eminence of one hand reinforces the 'passive' thumb of the other hand.
- Take up any skin slack as you slide your thumb over the spinous processes into the paravertebral gutter on the opposite side of the spine (Fig 9.6). Both hands move together.
- To reach the upper thoracic muscles use the thumb of your caudad hand. Your thumb will point cephalad.
- To reach the lower lumbar muscles use the thumb of your cephalad hand. Your thumb will point caudad.

Applicator

- The thumb as a passive tool reinforced by the thenar eminence of the other hand.
- Alternatively, your knuckles or the heel of one hand reinforced by the heel of the other hand.

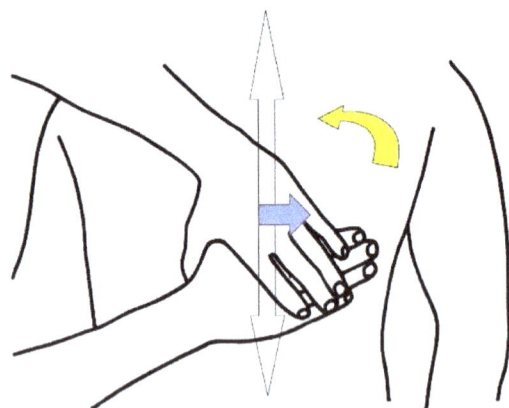

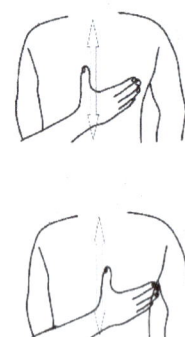

Figure 9.5   Figure 9.6 & Figure 9.7

Muscle Fibres	⇕	Primary Force	⬇	Secondary Force	↻	Stretch Force	⬇	Contraction Force	⬇

Tissue tension

- Take up the primary tissue tension with compression and then increase tissue tension using a transverse force to the muscle. Work from medial to lateral.
- There is no secondary tissue lockup.
- Longitudinal tension is taken up by starting the technique with the spine sidebent towards you.
- A pillow may be placed under the patient's chest or abdomen to minimise hyperextension.
- As the applicator is applied to only one side of the spine there will be a small amount of rotation.

Kneading

- Apply a rhythmical cycle of compression and medial to lateral transverse force.
- Your pressure should be just short of discomfort.
- To relax the muscle, work with the patient's breathing cycle, about 15 breaths per minute.
- To stimulate, increase your speed to about 40 cycles per minute.

Active component

- Ask the patient to take a deep breath in and hold it in.
- Ask the patient to contract their spinal muscles for 3 to 5 seconds using a 10% effort.

  When working on the upper thoracic spine, ask the patient to lift their head upward and backward off the table.

  When working on the mid-thoracic spine, ask the patient to rotate their spine by lifting the shoulder and rib cage on the opposite side to which you are standing, off the table.

  When working on the lumbar, ask the patient to rotate their spine by lifting the pelvis on the opposite side to which you are standing, off the table.
  Alternatively, ask the patient to lift the leg on the near side to which you are standing, off the table less than 1 cm (1/2").

- Resist the patient's effort and maintain tissue lockup throughout the technique.
- Ask the patient to exhale and to relax their muscle contraction.
- As soon as you feel that the patient has relaxed their muscles completely (about 1-3 seconds), take up the tissue slack by increasing the primary tension.
- Take up the slack after each contraction and during exhalation.
- Repeat 2 or 3 times, or as required.

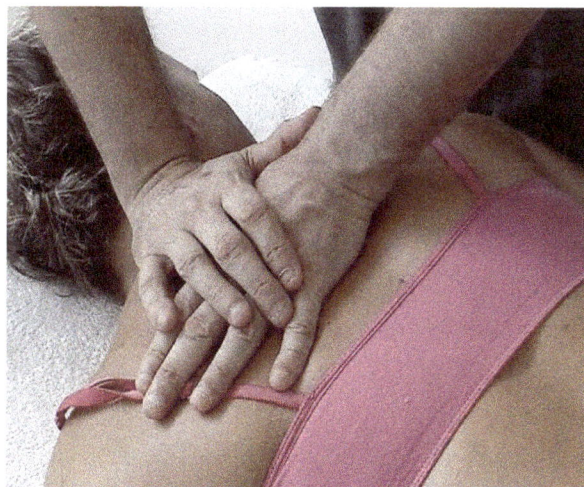

Picture 9.4

<u>Technique 9.5</u> Kneading the thoracic spine from T1 to T12 This technique is most effective from T6 to T12

Patient

- Prone with head straight or rotated towards you.

Therapist

- Stand by the side of the table facing the patient.

Applicator

- The heads of the distal phalanges of a row of interdigitating fingers (fingertips) of one or both hands.
- The heels of your hand.
- Your knuckles.
- Use a broad contact.

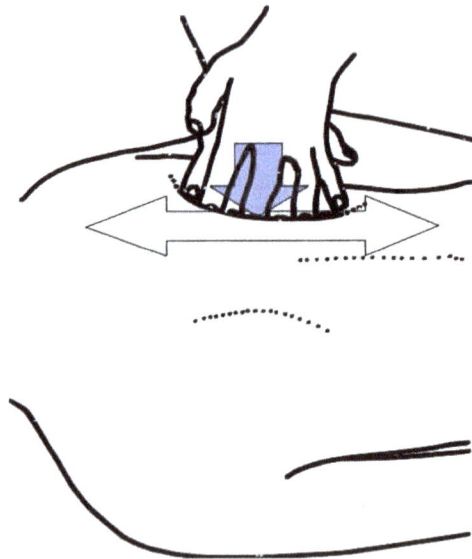

<u>Figure 9.8</u>

Muscle Fibres	⇕	Primary Force	⬇	Secondary Force	↻	Stretch Force	⬇	Contraction Force	⬇

Tissue tension

- Take up the primary tissue tension with your applicator, with compression and a lateral to medial transverse force on the muscles.
- There is no secondary tissue tension lockup.
- Take up the longitudinal tension by starting the technique with the patient's spine sidebent away from you. (optional)
- A pillow may be placed under the patient's chest or abdomen if there are areas in the spine, which are hyper-extended.

Kneading

- Start close to the rib angles and work deeply over iliocostalis and then the remaining paravertebral muscles.
- Apply a rhythmical cycle of lateral to medial force.
- Your pressure should be just short of discomfort.

- To relax the muscles, work with the patient's breathing cycle, which is about 15 breaths per minute.
- To stimulate, increase your speed to about 40 cycles per minute.
- This technique is good for well-built patients.

Active component

- If you use one hand as the applicator, the other hand is available to offer resistance to the patient's effort.
- Ask the patient to take a deep breath and hold it in.
- Ask the patient to contract their spinal muscles for 3 to 5 seconds using a 10% effort.

   When working on the upper thoracic spine, ask the patient to lift their head upward and backward off the table.

   When working on the mid-thoracic spine, ask the patient to sidebend their spine by pushing their shoulder towards you.

- Resist their effort and maintain tissue lockup throughout the technique.
- Ask the patient to exhale and to relax their muscle contraction.
- As soon as you feel that the patient has relaxed their muscles completely (about 1-3 seconds) take up the tissue slack by increasing the primary tension.
- Take up the slack after each contraction and during exhalation.
- Repeat 2 or 3 times or as required.

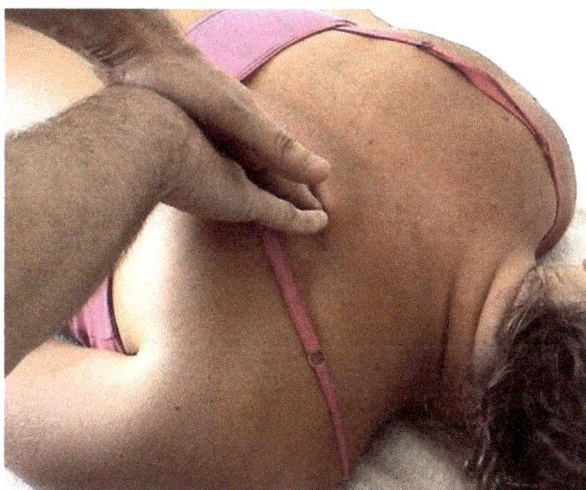

Picture 9.5

Technique 9.6 Stretch for quadratus lumborum, thoracolumbar fascia and erector spinae from T8 to L3

Patient

- Prone with head straight or rotated towards you.

Therapist

- Stand by the side of the table adjacent to the patient's lower lumbar spine.
- With your caudad hand grasp the anterior superior iliac spine of the patient's pelvis, on the opposite side to which you are standing.
- Your cephalad hand makes contact on a rib angle or lower thoracic transverse process, on the opposite side to which you are standing.

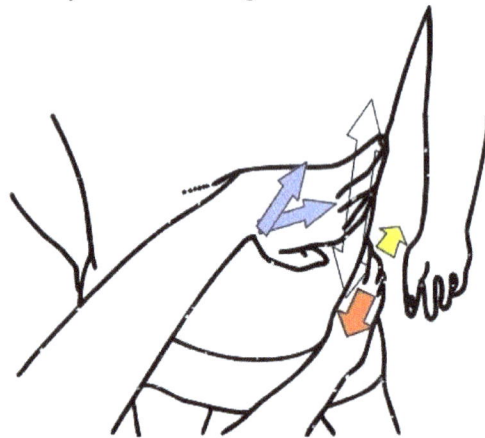

Figure 9.9

Muscle Fibres	⇕	Primary Force	⬇	Secondary Force	↻	Stretch Force	⬇	Contraction Force	⬇

Applicator

- Pisiform bone, heel of hand or thenar eminence.

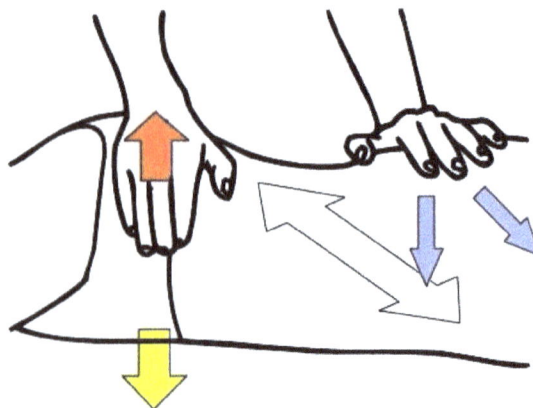

Figure 9.10

Muscle Fibres	⇕	Primary Force	⬇	Secondary Force	↻	Stretch Force	⬇	Contraction Force	⬇

Tissue tension

- Longitudinal tension is greater if you start the technique with the patient sidebent towards you.
- Take up longitudinal tissue tension by applying a transverse or oblique force with your cephalad hand, to a lower thoracic rib angle or transverse process. Your force is in an anterior, superior and lateral direction.
- Add longitudinal tissue tension with your caudad hand, by taking the anterior superior iliac spine in an inferior and posterior direction.

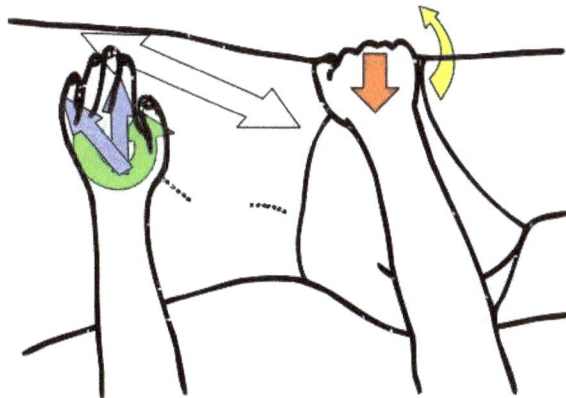

Figure 9.11

Muscle Fibres	⇕	Primary Force	⬇	Secondary Force	↻	Stretch Force	⬇	Contraction Force	⬇

Active component

- Ask the patient to take a deep breath and hold it in.
- Ask the patient to attempt to pull their pelvis down towards the table (anterior) or up to their head (superior) for 3 to 5 seconds using a 10% effort. The abdominal muscles, quadratus lumborum and erector spinae muscles will contract.
- Resist their effort and maintain tissue lockup throughout inhalation.
- Ask the patient to exhale and to relax their muscle contraction.
- As soon as you feel that the patient has relaxed their muscles completely (about 1-3 seconds), take up the tissue slack by increasing the longitudinal tensions.
- Take up the slack after each contraction and during exhalation.
- Repeat 2 or 3 times, or as required.

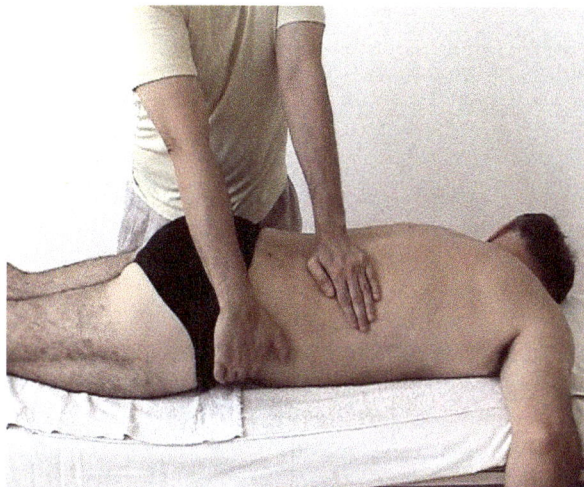

Picture 9.6

<u>Technique 9.7</u> Traction and mild stretch for the thoracolumbar fascia, quadratus lumborum and lumbar erector spinae from L1 to L5

Patient

- Supine with the hips and knees flexed and feet close together.

Therapist

- Sit on the side of the table and on the patient's feet, to fix them to the table.
- Reach around the patient's thighs and grasp one knee with your cephalad hand. Your forearm rests against the superior aspect of the other knee.
- Grasp the end of the table with your caudad hand.

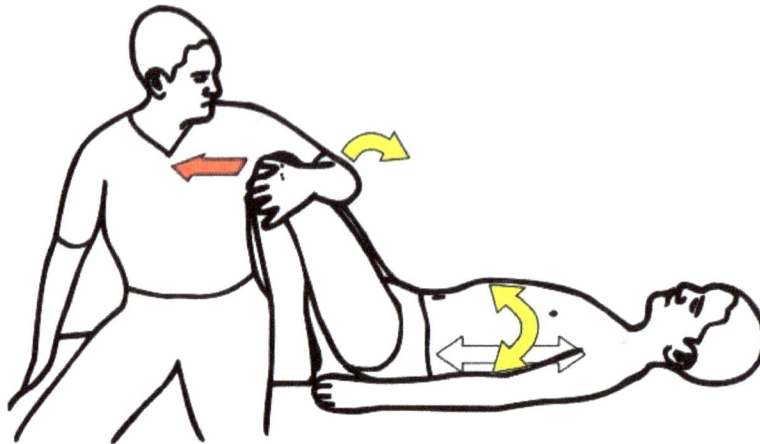

<u>Figure 9.12</u>

Muscle Fibres	↕	Primary Force	⬇	Secondary Force	↻	Stretch Force	⬇	Contraction Force	⬇

Tissue tension

- Take up the longitudinal tension with traction.
- Use your caudad arm as an anchor.
- Lean back and pull on the patient's knees.
- The patient's feet act as a fulcrum and the pull is transmitted through the pelvis to the lumbar spine.
- This produces a longitudinal stretch to the myofascia and traction to the spine.
- Use rotation and traction of the patient's hips to induce subtle forces on the tissues.

Traction and Stretch

- Apply a rhythmical cycle of on-off traction or sustained traction for up to five minutes.
- Work with the patients breathing cycle, about 15 breaths per minute.

Active component

- Ask the patient to take a deep breath and hold it in.
- Ask the patient to either a) attempt to push their feet into the table (extend their hips)
- b) flatten their backs into the table (flex their lumbar spine) c) pull their knees towards their head d) take their knees to one side - for 3 to 5 seconds using a 10% effort.
- Resist their effort and maintain tissue lockup throughout the inhalation.
- Ask the patient to exhale and to relax their muscle contraction.

- As soon as you feel that the patient has relaxed their muscles completely (about 1-3 seconds), take up the tissue slack by increasing traction.
- Take up the slack after each contraction and during exhalation.
- Repeat 2 or 3 times, or as required.

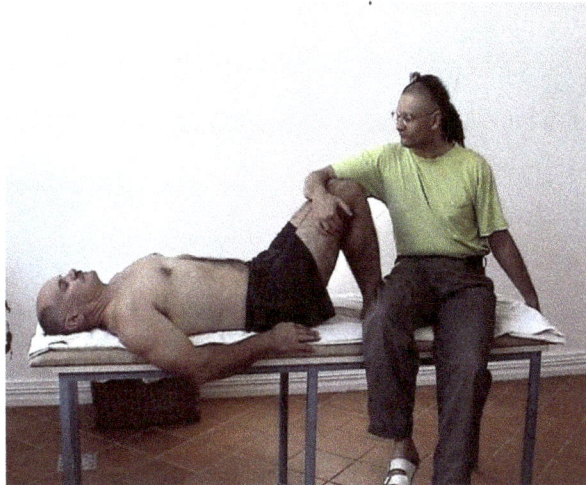

Picture 9.7

Technique 9.8 Inhibition of the upper thoracic erector spinae from T1 to T6

Patient

- Prone with their head rotated or forward in face hole.

Therapist

- Stand at the head of the table.

Applicator

- Pads of thumbs.

Tissue tension

- Take up the tissue tension by gradually increasing your thumb pressure on the muscle.
- Your pressure is directed perpendicular to the muscle.
- Make sure the force goes through your thumbs and not your fingers.

Inhibition

- Apply pressure as compression on the area of muscle covered by pad of your thumb.
- Your pressure should be just short of discomfort.
- To relax the muscle work with the patient's breathing cycle, about 15 breaths per minute.
- Maintain some compression throughout the technique but increase it during exhalation.

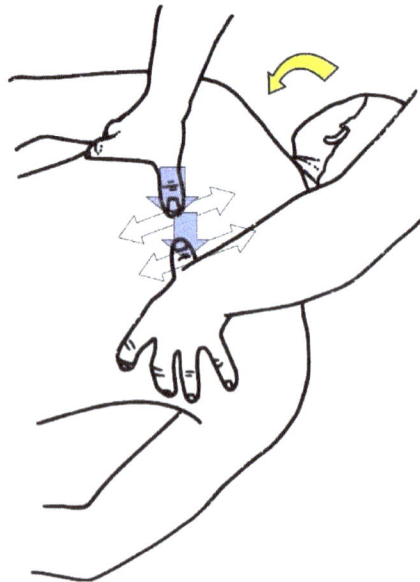

Figure 9.13

Muscle Fibres	⇕	Primary Force	⬇	Secondary Force	↺	Stretch Force	⬇	Contraction Force	⬇

Active component

- Ask the patient to take a deep breath and hold it in.
- Ask the patient to attempt to lift their head and neck upward and backward off the table for 3 to 5 seconds using a 10% effort. The upper thoracic muscles will contract.
- Maintain tissue compression.

- Ask the patient to exhale and to relax their muscle contraction. As soon as you feel that the patient has relaxed their upper thoracic muscles completely (about 1-3 seconds), take up the tissue slack by increasing the compression.
- Take up the slack after each contraction and during exhalation.
- Repeat 2 or 3 times, or as required.

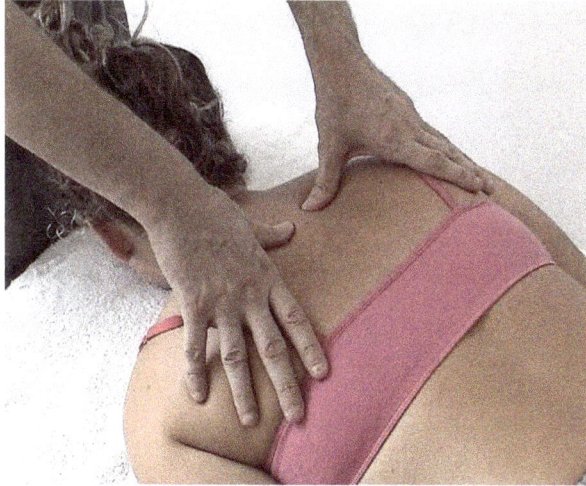

Picture 9.8

Technique 9.9 Kneading the upper thoracic from T1 to T6 (sometimes to T9)

Patient

- Sidelying near to the edge of the table closest to the therapist and facing the therapist.
- The trunk should remain perpendicular to the table.
- The forearm of the arm, on which the patient is lying, is flexed at the elbow and rests against the front of their chest.

Therapist

- Stand by the side of the table, adjacent to the patient's rib cage and facing the patient.
- Lean over the patient's rib cage and shoulder.
- Abduct the patient's arm and drape it over your cephalad arm.
- Grasp the paravertebral muscles with the fingertips of one or both hands.

Applicator

- All fingertips of one or both hands.

Tissue tension

- Take up the primary tissue tension with compression, adding a medial to lateral transverse force by pulling up on the paravertebral muscles with your fingertips.
- Take up the secondary tissue tension by increasing abduction and extension of the patient's arm with your cephalad shoulder.
- To increase longitudinal tension a pillow can be placed under the patient's rib cage to sidebend their spine towards the table.

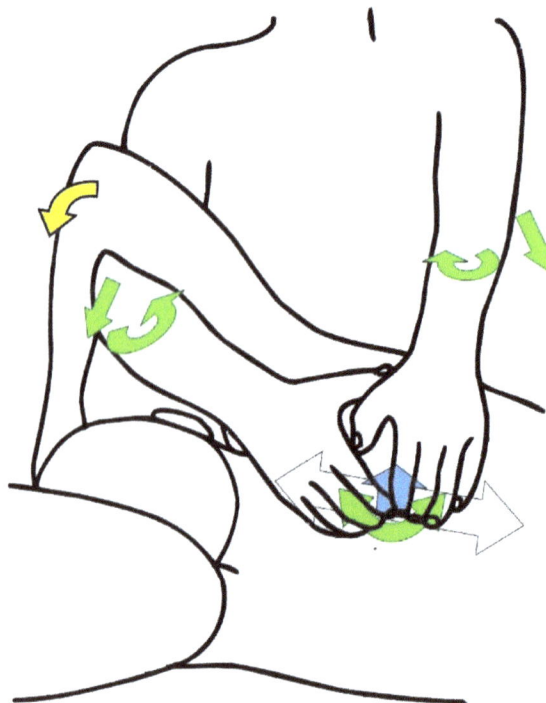

Figure 9.14

Muscle Fibres	⇕	Primary Force	⬇	Secondary Force	↺	Stretch Force	⬇	Contraction Force	⬇

90

Kneading

- Apply a rhythmical cycle of primary and secondary forces.
- When the muscle is at an optimal level of secondary tension add compression and increase the transverse pressure.
- Your pressure should be just short of discomfort.
- To relax the muscle, work with the patients breathing cycle, about 15 breaths per minute.
- To stimulate, increase your speed to about 40 cycles per minute.

Active component

- Ask the patient to take a deep breath and hold it in.
- Ask the patient to try to bring their arm back and towards the table and so further extend and abduct their shoulder for 3 to 5 seconds using a 20% effort. The spinal muscles will contract.
- Resist their effort and maintain tissue lockup throughout the technique.
- Ask the patient to exhale and to relax their muscle contraction.
- As soon as you feel that the patient has relaxed their spinal muscles completely (about 1-3 seconds), take up the tissue slack by increasing the primary and secondary tension.
- Take up the slack after each contraction and during exhalation.
- Repeat 2 or 3 times, or as required.

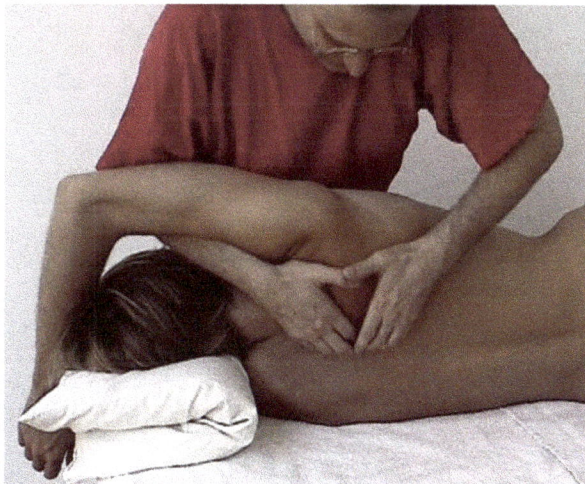

Picture 9.9

Technique 9.10 Mild stretch for quadratus lumborum, lumbar fascia and lumbar erector spinae from T12 to L5

Patient

- Prone with head rotated towards you.
- A large pillow may be placed under the abdomen.
- An arm can be abducted to add tension to the lumbar fascia.
- The patient can be positioned in sidebending.

Therapist

- Stand by the side of the table, adjacent to the patient's lumbar spine.
- Your forearms are crossed.
- The heel of your caudad hand sits under a rib angle on the side of the spine nearest you (as in Figure 9.15), or under a rib angle on the side of the spine furthest away from you.
- Place the applicator of your cephalad hand on the medial border of the lumbar erector spinae muscles (paravertebral gutter) or on the ilium on the opposite side of the spine.

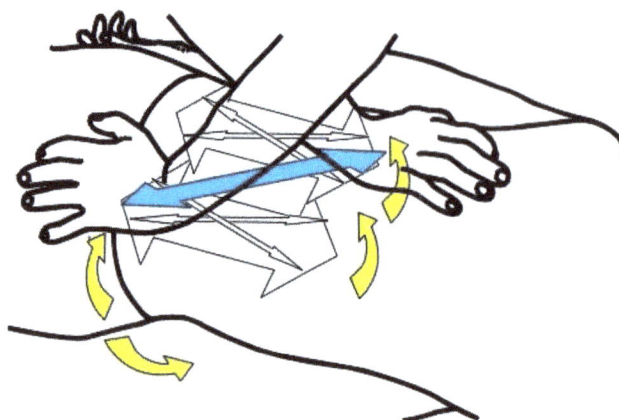

Figure 9.15

Muscle Fibres	⇕	Primary Force	⬇	Secondary Force	↻	Stretch Force	⬇	Contraction Force	⬇

Applicator

- Pisiform bone, heel of hand or thenar eminence of both hands.

Tissue tension

- Take up the longitudinal tension by applying an inferior force to the ilium with the cephalad hand and a superior force to a lower rib angle with the caudad hand.
- Combinations of medial and lateral pressure (transverse force) are applied.
- Any secondary tissue tension applied to the muscle is a rotation (torsion).
- Compare the right and left sides of the body for the relative amount of resistance that is encountered.

Stretch

- Your crossed arms induce an opposing force along one side of the lumbar, or diagonally across both sides of the lumbar.
- Push anteriorly, inferiorly and transversely (medially or laterally) on the ilium with your cephalad hand.

- Push anteriorly, superiorly and transversely (medially or laterally) on the rib angle with your caudad hand.
- Increased pressure is applied and sustained when resistance is encountered.
- Work with the patients breathing cycle, about 15 breaths per minute.

Active component

- Ask the patient to take a deep breath and hold it in.
- Ask the patient to attempt to either a) lift their pelvis up towards their head (superior) b) lift their pelvis off the table (posterior) c) lift one side of their rib cage off the table d) lift both sides of their rib cage off the table (posterior) - for 3 to 5 seconds using a 10% effort.
- The erector spinae muscles of the lumbar will contract.
- Resist their effort and maintain tissue lockup throughout inhalation.
- Ask the patient to exhale and to relax their muscle contraction.
- As soon as you feel that the patient has relaxed their lumbar muscles completely (about 1-3 seconds), take up the tissue slack by increasing the longitudinal tension.
- Take up the slack after each contraction and during exhalation.
- Repeat 2 or 3 times, or as required.

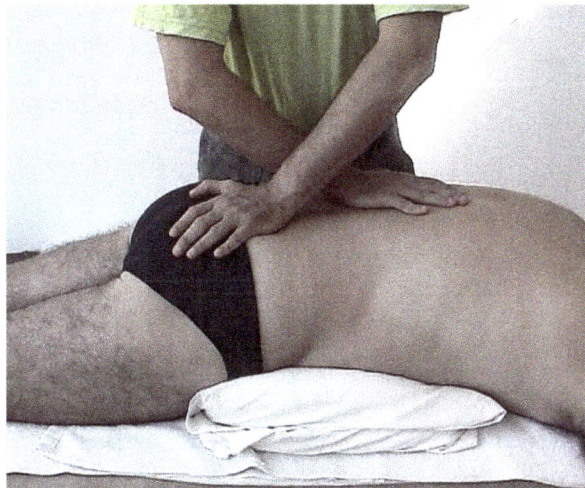

Picture 9.10

<u>Technique 9.11</u> Inhibition of lumbar fascia, quadratus lumborum and lumbar erector spinae from L1 to L5

Patient

- Prone with head rotated towards you.
- A pillow may be placed under the abdomen.

Applicator

- Olecranon process of either forearm.

Therapist

- Stand by the side of the table adjacent to the patient's lumbar spine.
- Place your olecranon process in the paravertebral gutter, on the same side of the spine that you are standing.
- Slide your applicator over a spinous process and into the paravertebral gutter on the opposite side of the spine, so it sits against the medial border of the erector spinae.

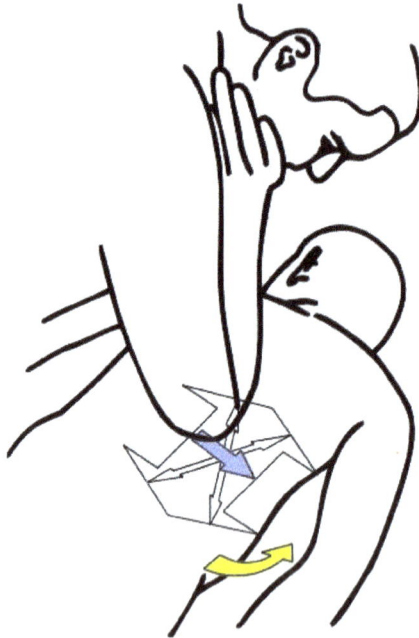

<u>Figure 9.16</u>

Muscle Fibres	⇕	Primary Force	⬇	Secondary Force	↻	Stretch Force	⬇	Contraction Force	⬇

Tissue tension

- Take up the primary tissue tension with your applicator. Apply compression and then increase tissue tension using a transverse force.
- Work from medial to lateral and along parallel strips.
- There is no secondary tissue lockup.
- Longitudinal (stretch) tension is taken up by starting the technique with the spine sidebent towards you.
- A pillow may be placed under the patient's chest or abdomen to minimise hyperextension.

Inhibition

- Press downwards towards the table with a medium to heavy pressure.

- Maintain compression as you slowly push away with a medial to lateral force.
- Increase your pressure when you encounter areas of tight, thick lumbar fascia and hypertonic muscle.
- Your pressure should be just short of discomfort.
- Work with the patients breathing cycle which is about 15 breaths per minute.

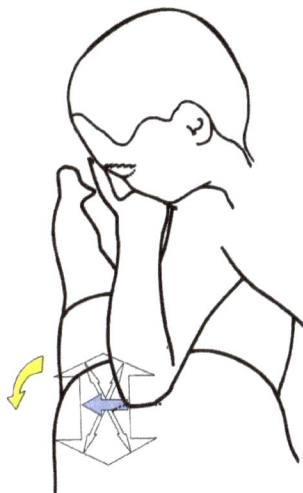

Figure 9.17

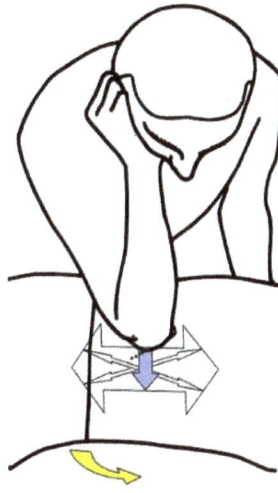

Figure 9.18

Muscle Fibres	⇕	Primary Force	⬇	Secondary Force	↻	Stretch Force	⬇	Contraction Force	⬇

Active component

- Ask the patient to take a deep inhalation and hold it in.
- Ask the patient to contract their spinal muscles for 3 to 5 seconds using a 10% effort.
- Ask the patient to rotate their spine away from you by lifting their rib cage off the table.
- Alternatively, ask the patient to rotate his spine by lifting the pelvis on the opposite side, up and off the table or up towards their head
- Alternatively, ask the patient to lift their leg on the near side, up and off the table.
- Resist the patient's effort with your applicator or with assistance from your free hand and maintain tissue lockup throughout the technique.
- Ask the patient to exhale and to relax their muscle contraction.
- As soon as you feel that the patient has relaxed their muscles completely (about 1-3 seconds), take up the tissue slack by increasing the primary tension.
- Take up the slack after each contraction and during exhalation.
- Repeat 2 or 3 times or as required.

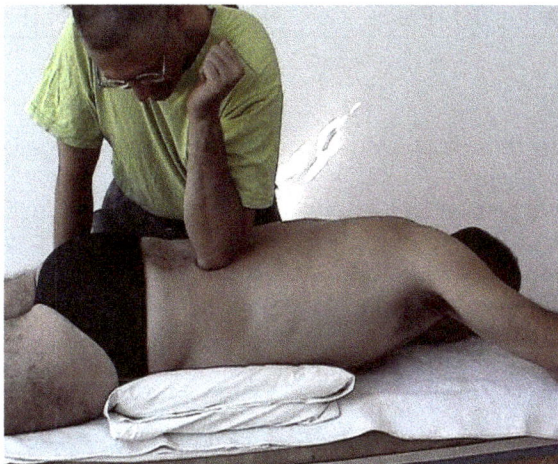

Picture 9.11

Technique 9.12 Stretch for quadratus lumborum, thoracolumbar fascia and erector spinae from T8 to L5

Patient

- Prone with head rotated towards you.
- The patient's arm on the opposite side to which you are standing, is internally rotated and at their side when you are stretching quadratus lumborum and erector spinae.
- The arm is fully abducted and externally rotated when stretching the thoracolumbar fascia.

Therapist

- Stand by the side of the table, adjacent to the patient's lower lumbar spine.
- Grasp the patient's opposite side thigh just above the knee with your caudad hand.
- Extend the patient's thigh.
- Reach under their thigh and fix your fist on the couch beside the other thigh.
- Take care not to put pressure on the patella.
- Your cephalad hand makes contact on the opposite side rib angle or lower thoracic transverse process.

Applicator

- Pisiform bone, heel of hand or thenar eminence.

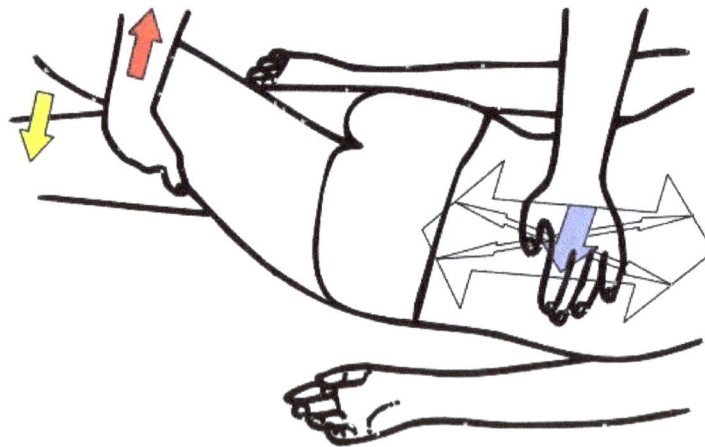

Figure 9.19

Muscle Fibres	⇕	Primary Force	⬇	Secondary Force	↻	Stretch Force	⬇	Contraction Force	⬇

Tissue tension

- Take up the longitudinal tension by starting the technique with the patient's lumbar sidebent towards you.
- Take up the longitudinal tension by further extending and then adducting the patient's thigh with your caudad hand. This is best done by extending the elbow of your caudad arm and moving the leg over your fist which acts as a fulcrum.
- Take up the tissue tension with your cephalad hand by applying compression and a transverse or oblique force with your applicator on the rib or Tp.
- Secondary tissue tension may be taken up with your applicator by applying a rotation force (torsion).

Active component

- Ask the patient to take a deep breath and hold it in.
- Ask the patient to attempt to take their thigh to the side away from you for 3 to 5 seconds using a 20% effort. The quadratus lumborum and erector spinae muscles will contract to stabilise the pelvis when the hip abductors contract.
- Resist their effort and maintain tissue lockup throughout inhalation.
- Ask the patient to exhale and to relax their muscle contraction.
- As soon as you feel that the patient has relaxed their muscles completely (about 1-3 seconds), take up the tissue slack by increasing the primary, secondary, longitudinal and other tensions.
- Take up the slack after each contraction and during exhalation.
- Repeat 2 or 3 times, or as required.

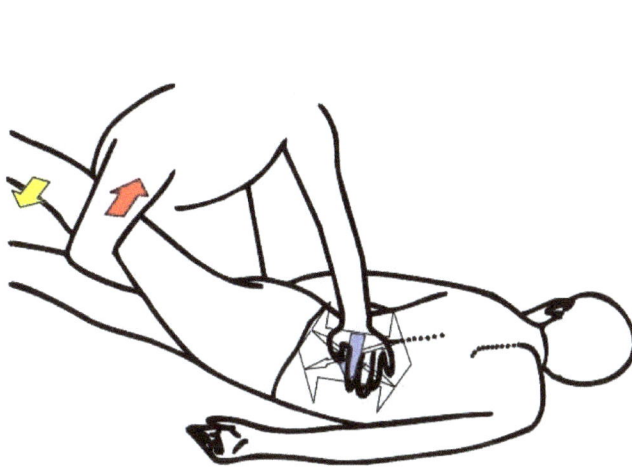

Figure 9.20

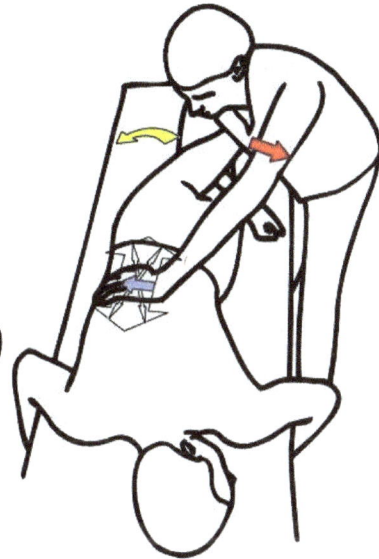

Figure 9.21

Muscle Fibres	⇕	Primary Force	🔽	Secondary Force	🔄	Stretch Force	🔽	Contraction Force	🔽

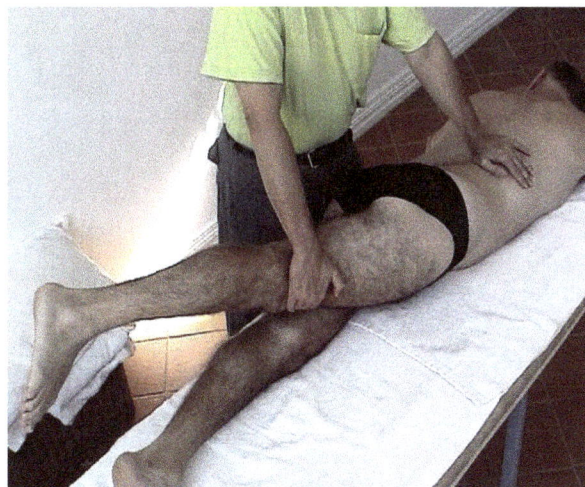

Picture 9.12

97

Technique 9.13 Kneading or inhibition of quadratus lumborum, thoracolumbar fascia, lower thoracic and lumbar erector spinae from T8 to L5 using leverage

Patient

- Supine with the hips and knees flexed and thighs crossed.
- Take care not to compress the testes in males!

Therapist

- Stand by the side of the table near to the patient's pelvis.
- Reach under both legs and grasp the patient's top knee with your caudad hand.
- The popliteal fossa of the patient's bottom leg rests on your deltoid muscle.
- You should now have a secure hold on the patient's lower limbs, which are locked in a fixed position; through the lower limbs you should be able to easily control the patient's pelvis and lumbar spine.
- Rotate the patient's legs away from you to expose the area to be treated. This should be on the side of the spine nearest you.
- Make contact on the tissue with your applicator.

Applicator

- Flexed or extended fingertips, pisiform, heel of hand, thenar eminence or dorsum of clenched fists (MCP joints).

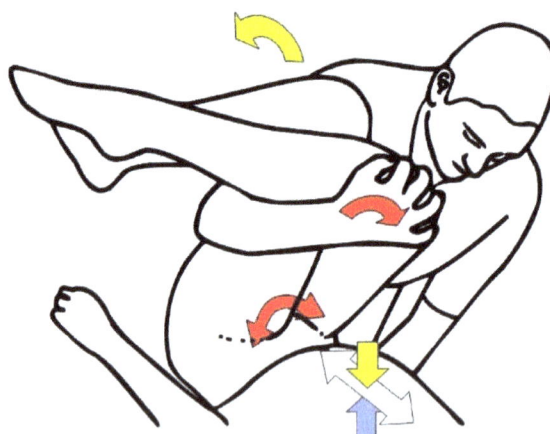

Figure 9.22

Muscle Fibres	⇕	Primary Force	⬇	Secondary Force	↻	Stretch Force	⬇	Contraction Force	⬇

Tissue tension

- Take up the longitudinal tension with flexion and rotation of the patient's hips. This force is produces flexion and sidebending in the lumbar spine. The patient's feet should point away from you as you execute the manoeuvre.
- The primary tissue tension is compression, which is achieved by flexing the patient's hips and bringing the patient's knees towards you, thereby taking more of their body weight over your applicator.
- Use combinations of increased flexion, rotation of the pelvis toward you and sidebending of the pelvis away.

Kneading or Inhibition

- Apply a rhythmical cycle of compression and longitudinal forces.
- Circumduct the hips to knead the muscles. Roll the patient's lumbar over your applicator.

- Your applicator can be used passively or actively push against the lumbar tissues.
- The forces generated by leverage can be massive so care should be taken not to damage your fingers.
- Use a sustained hold to inhibit the muscles.
- Your pressure should be just short of discomfort.
- To relax the muscle work with the patient's breathing cycle, about 15 breaths per minute.

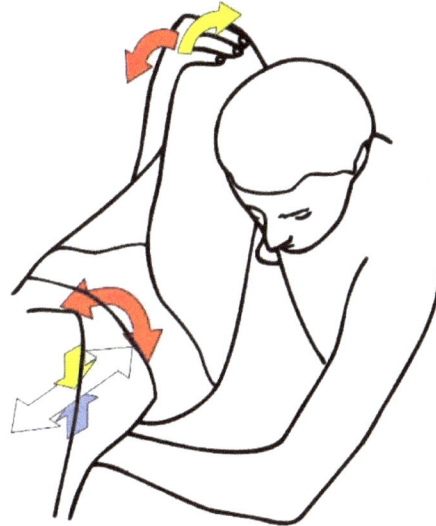

Figure 9.23

Muscle Fibres	⇕	Primary Force	⬇	Secondary Force	↺	Stretch Force	⬇	Contraction Force	⬇

Active component

- Ask the patient to take a deep breath and hold it in.
- Ask the patient to attempt to push their legs back to the table (extend their hips and spine) or rotate their hips so their feet point towards you (sidebend their spine) for 3 to 5 seconds using a 20% effort.
- Resist their effort and maintain tissue lockup throughout inhalation.
- Ask the patient to exhale and to relax their muscle contraction.
- As soon as you feel that the patient has relaxed their muscles completely (about 1-3 seconds), take up the tissue slack by increasing flexion.
- Take up the slack after each contraction and during exhalation.
- Repeat 2 or 3 times, or as required.

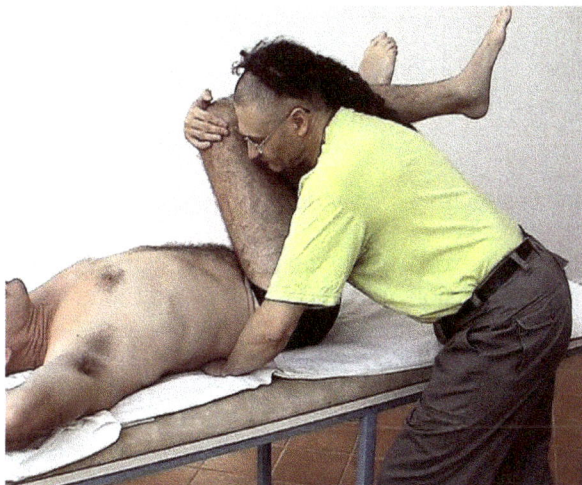

Picture 9.13

Technique 9.14 Kneading of thoracic erector spinae from T4 to T12

Patient

- Seated with legs hanging over the side of the table.
- Their forehead is resting on their folded forearms.
- Their knees are together.

Therapist

- Stand by the side of the table facing the patient.
- Place one knee against the patient's knees to provide support and counter any forward slide of the patient when you execute the manoeuvre.
- The patient rests one arm on your shoulder. Support their weight.
- Be mindful that the patient's face does not get pushed into your armpit.
- Reach around either side of the patient's rib cage with both hands.
- Place your applicators in the paravertebral gutters either side of the spine. Your fingertips rest just medial to the muscles.

Applicator

- Fingertips of both hands.

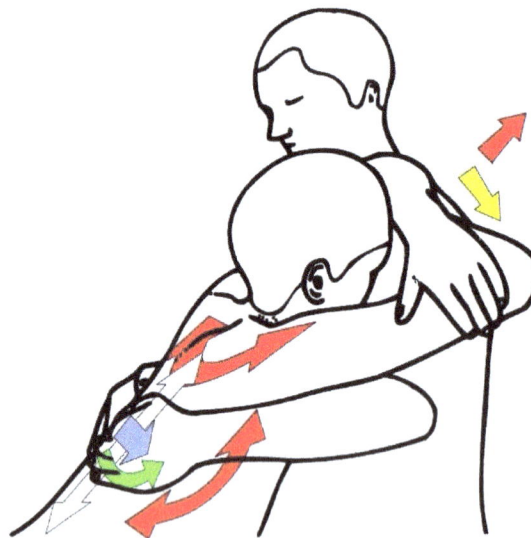

Figure 9.24

Muscle Fibres	⇕	Primary Force	⬇	Secondary Force	↺	Stretch Force	⬇	Contraction Force	⬇

Tissue tension

- Take up the primary tissue tension by applying compression and a medial to lateral transverse force on the muscle.
- Take up the secondary tissue tension by applying a rotation force (torsion).
- Take up the longitudinal tension with sideshifting (sidebending) and traction, applied through the patient's shoulders to the spine.

Kneading

- Apply a rhythmical cycle of primary, secondary and longitudinal forces.
- When the muscle is at an optimal longitudinal tension, increase the primary and secondary forces.
- Your pressure should be just short of discomfort.

- To relax the muscle work with the patient's breathing cycle, about 15 breaths per minute.

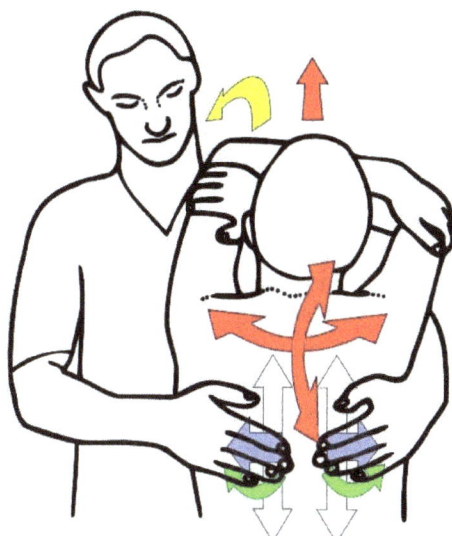

Figure 9.25

Muscle Fibres	↕	Primary Force	⬇	Secondary Force	↻	Stretch Force	⬇	Contraction Force	⬇

Active component

- Ask the patient to take a deep breath and hold it in.
- Ask the patient to attempt to either a) push their head into their forearms (head and neck flexion), b) push their forearms into your shoulders (shoulder extension), or c) push their elbow sideways against your shoulders (sidebending of the spine), for 3 to 5 seconds using a 20% effort. Various muscles of the trunk will contract depending on the direction of force.
- Resist their effort and maintain tissue lockup throughout inhalation.
- Ask the patient to exhale and to relax their muscle contraction.
- As soon as you feel that the patient has relaxed their muscles completely (about 1-3 seconds), take up the tissue slack by increasing the primary, secondary and longitudinal tension.
- Take up the slack after each contraction, during exhalation.
- Repeat 2 or 3 times, or as required.

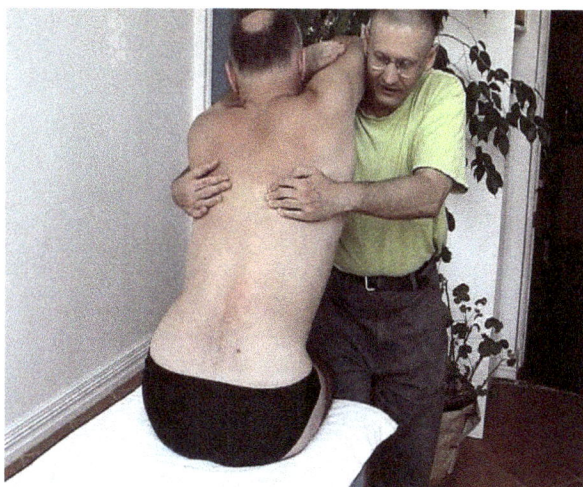

Picture 9.14

Technique 9.15 Kneading of thoracic erector spinae from T3 to T12

Patient

- Seated with legs hanging over the side of the table.
- Ask the patient to be relaxed but sit up straight. Do not allow them to slouch forward.
- Initially their forearms are folded and arms flexed about 90 degrees.

Therapist

- Stand at the side of the table, behind and to one side of the patient.
- Reach over the patient's shoulder and feed your hand through the patient's folded arms.
- Reach under the patient's arm and grasp a group of ribs high up in the axilla.
- Ask the patient to drop their arms and relax. Their forearms should remain folded.
- Your axilla rests on the patient's shoulder and should merge with it.
- Support the weight of the patient's shoulder.
- Place your applicators in the paravertebral gutters just medial to the erector spinae.
- When treating the upper thoracic, sideshift the patient.
- A translation of your forces goes through the spine and ribs in a horizontal plane.
- When treating the lower thoracic, sidebend the patient more.
- Do this by pushing down obliquely on the patient's shoulder with your axilla.
- Localise at the desired area of the spine by varying the angle of your force.

Applicator

- Heel of hand and pisiform, thenar eminence or side of thumb.

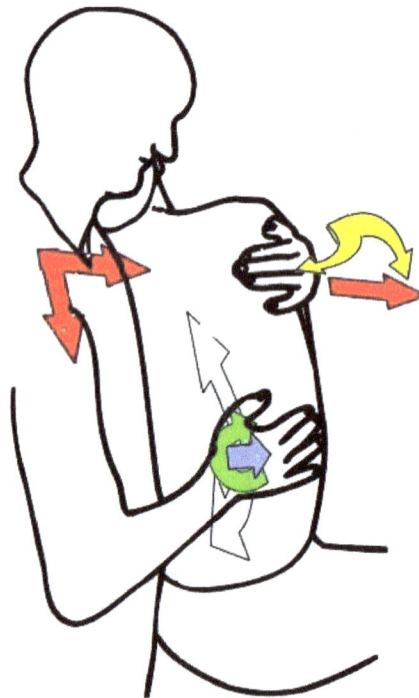

Figure 9.26

Muscle Fibres	⇕	Primary Force	⬇	Secondary Force	↺	Stretch Force	⬇	Contraction Force	⬇

Tissue tension

- Take up the primary tissue tension with your applicator, applying compression and a medial to lateral transverse force on the muscle.
- Take up the secondary tissue tension with your applicator, applying a rotation force (torsion).
- Take up the longitudinal tension by sideshifting and sidebending the patient's spine.
- Rotation away from the applicator can also be utilised effectively to increase longitudinal tension.

Kneading

- Apply a rhythmical cycle of primary, secondary and longitudinal forces.
- When the muscle is at an optimal longitudinal tension increase the primary and secondary forces.
- Your pressure should be just short of discomfort.
- To relax the muscle work with the patients breathing cycle, about 15 breaths per minute.

Active component

- Ask the patient to take a deep breath and hold it in.
- Ask the patient to attempt to straighten their spine from a sidebent position or rotate their spine into your applicator for 3 to 5 seconds using a 10% effort.
- The erector spinae muscles will contract.
- Resist their effort and maintain tissue lockup throughout inhalation.
- Ask the patient to exhale and to relax their muscle contraction.
- As soon as you feel that the patient has relaxed their muscles completely (about 1-3 seconds), take up the tissue slack by increasing the primary, secondary and longitudinal tension.
- Take up the slack after each contraction and during exhalation.
- Repeat 2 or 3 times, or as required.

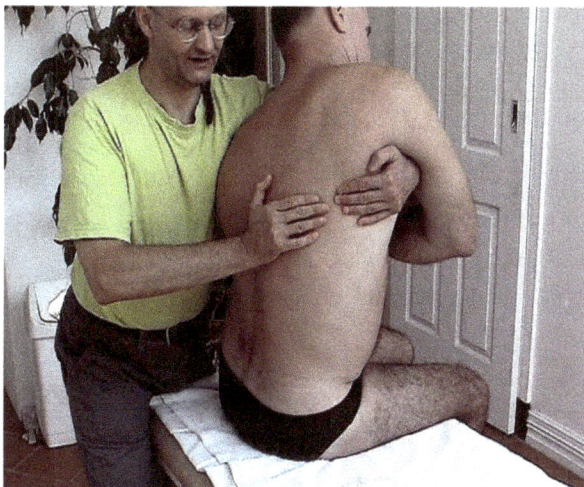

Picture 9.15

Technique 9.16 Kneading of thoracic erector spinae from T3 to T12

Patient

- Seated with legs hanging over the side of the table.
- Ask the patient to be relaxed but sit up straight. Do not allow them to slouch forward.
- The patient's forearms are folded.

Therapist

- Stand at the side of the table, behind and to one side of the patient.
- Rest your forearm on the patient's shoulder.
- Your elbow sits slightly in front of the patient's shoulder to control rotation.
- Lightly grasp the back of the patient's neck.
- Make the shape of your arm, forearm and hand fit as congruently as possible with the patient's shoulder. Keep it snug.
- Place your applicator in the paravertebral gutters just medial to the erector spinae.
- Your fingertips rest on the lateral iliocostalis thoracic muscles.
- To treat the middle and upper thoracic muscle's the emphasis should be on sideshifting the patient by taking them sideways parallel with the floor. The translation of forces goes through the spine and ribs in a horizontal plane.
- When treating the lower thoracic, sidebend the patient more. Do this by pushing down obliquely on the patient's shoulder with your elbow and forearm. Localise at the desired area of the spine by varying the angle of your force.

Applicator

- Side of thumb and all fingertips.
- Alternatively use the heel of the hand, pisiform or thenar eminence.

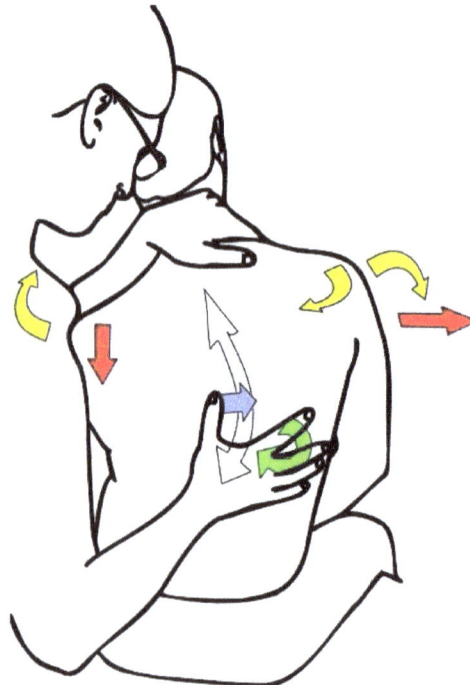

Figure 9.27

Muscle Fibres	⇕	Primary Force	⬇	Secondary Force	↻	Stretch Force	⬇	Contraction Force	⬇

Tissue tension

- Take up the primary tissue tension with your applicator, applying compression and a medial to lateral transverse force on the muscle.
- Take up the secondary tissue tension with your fingertips by applying a rake-like lateral to medial force (for the more lateral iliocostalis) and a rotatory force (for the more medial spinalis and longissimus).
- Take up the longitudinal tension by sideshifting and sidebending the patient's spine.
- Rotation away from the applicator can also be utilised effectively to increase longitudinal tension.
- To keep the patient under optimal control, do not use flexion and extension. Keep the spine in neutral.

Kneading

- Apply a rhythmical cycle of primary, secondary and longitudinal forces.
- When the muscle is at an optimal longitudinal tension, increase the primary and secondary forces.
- Your pressure should be just short of discomfort.
- To relax the muscle, work with the patients breathing cycle, which is about 15 breaths per minute.

Active component

- Ask the patient to take a deep breath and hold it in.
- Ask the patient to attempt to straighten their spine from a sidebent position or to rotate their spine into the applicator for 3 to 5 seconds using a 10% effort.
- The erector spinae muscles will contract.
- Resist their effort and maintain tissue lockup throughout inhalation.
- Ask the patient to exhale and to relax their muscle contraction.
- As soon as you feel that the patient has relaxed their muscles completely (about 1-3 seconds), take up the tissue slack by increasing the primary, secondary and longitudinal tension.
- Take up the slack after each contraction and during exhalation.
- Repeat 2 or 3 times, or as required.

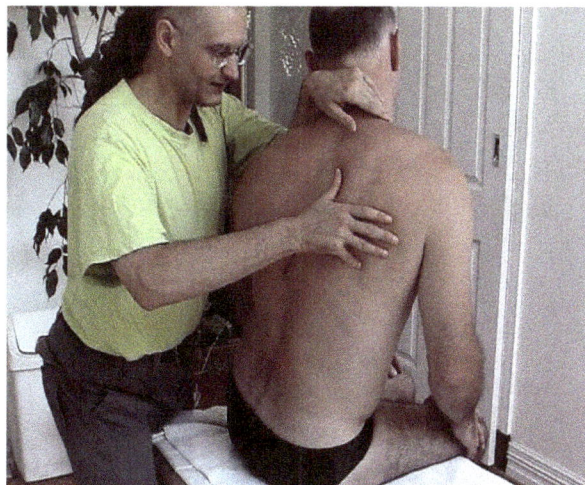

Picture 9.16

Technique 9.17 Kneading of lower thoracic and lumbar from T10 to L5

Patient

- Sidelying near the edge of the table and close to the therapist.
- Their uppermost forearm is flexed 90 degrees and resting at the side of the body. The uppermost arm can be abducted to increase tension on the fascia and some muscles.
- The patient's lowermost arm rests in front of their body. The exact position depends on the patient's body type. It should be positioned so as to prevent trunk rotation but permit sidebending into the table when the appropriate forces are applied.
- If the patient has a scoliosis a pillow may be placed under the apex of the convexity. To treat the shortness the patient should lie with the scoliosis concave up.
- The lowermost leg is flexed 90 degrees at the hip and 90 degrees at the knee.
- The uppermost leg is flexed about 80 degrees and the pull from the abductors helps tilt the pelvis and sidebend the lumbar into the table.

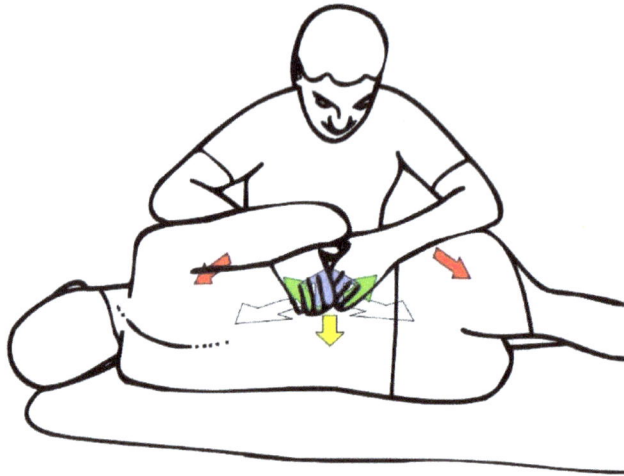

Figure 9.28

Muscle Fibres	⇕	Primary Force	⬇	Secondary Force	↻	Stretch Force	⬇	Contraction Force	⬇

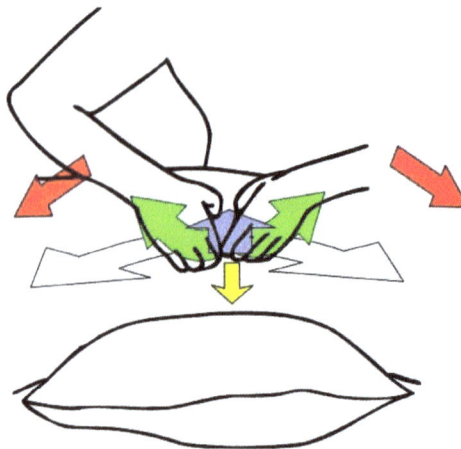

Figure 9.29

Therapist

- Stand by the side of the table facing the patient.
- Lean over the patient's rib cage and shoulder.
- Rest your cephalad forearm on the side of the patient's chest and under their arm and forearm. The patient's arm is draped over your arm.

106

- Rest your caudad forearm on the lateral side of the patient's pelvis, just superior to the greater trochanter. The contact will vary depending on the patient's body type.
- Grasp the uppermost paravertebral muscles with the fingertips of both hands.

Applicator

- All fingertips of one or both hands.

Tissue tension

- Take up the primary tissue tension with compression and a medial to lateral transverse force by pulling up on the paravertebral muscles with your fingertips.
- Take up secondary tissue tension by pushing in an oblique direction with your fingertips.
- Take up the longitudinal tension by starting the technique with the patient's spine sidebent over a pillow placed under the patient's side.
- Take up the longitudinal tension by pushing your forearms lightly on the rib cage and pelvis and then moving your elbows apart in a superior and inferior direction respectively.
- Your forearm pressure on the patient's ribs and pelvis provides stabilisation and leverage.

Kneading

- Apply a rhythmical cycle of primary, secondary and longitudinal forces.
- When the muscle is at an optimal level of longitudinal tension increase the transverse pressure. Alternatively, apply longitudinal and transverse forces simultaneously.
- Pull up on the paravertebral muscles with your fingertips and push your elbows apart.
- Push superiorly on the ribs and push inferiorly on the pelvis with your forearms.
- Your pressure should be just short of discomfort.
- To relax the muscle, work with the patients breathing cycle, about 15 breaths per minute.
- To stimulate, increase your speed to about 40 cycles per minute.

Active component

- Ask the patient to take a deep breath and hold it in.
- Ask the patient to try to straighten their spine by opposing the force of your forearms for 3 to 5 seconds using a 10% effort. The spinal muscles will contract as the patient attempts to move their pelvis superiorly and their shoulder inferiorly.
- Resist their effort and maintain tissue lockup throughout the technique.
- Ask the patient to exhale and to relax their muscle contraction.
- As soon as you feel that the patient has relaxed their spinal muscles completely (about 1-3 seconds), take up the tissue slack by increasing the primary and secondary tension.
- Take up the slack after each contraction and during exhalation.
- Repeat 2 or 3 times, or as required.

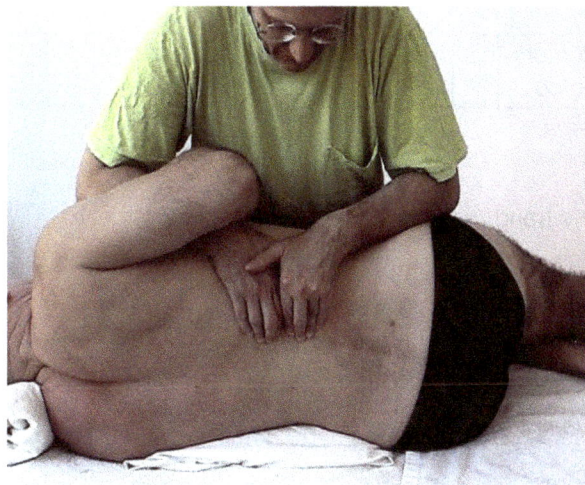

Picture 9.17

Technique 9.18 Kneading of lower thoracic and lumbar from T10 to L5

Patient

- Sidelying with a pillow under the head.
- A pillow may be placed under the side of the lumbar area to help stabilise the spine, or placed at a suitable location at the side of the spine to increase longitudinal tension.
- Their forearms are flexed and their arms rest at the side of the body.
- The patient's lowermost arm should be positioned so as to impede the spine from freely rotating when the applicator pressure is applied. The exact position depends on the patient's body type.
- Both legs are flexed 90 degrees at the hip and about 120 degrees at the knee so the knees protrude off the edge of the table, but the feet rest on the table.

Therapist

- Stand by the side of the table, facing the patient.
- Lean over the patient's lumbar spine.
- Grasp the uppermost paravertebral muscles with the fingertips of both hands.
- Rest the side of your caudad forearm on the iliac crest.
- This forearm acts as a pivot for increasing secondary tension.

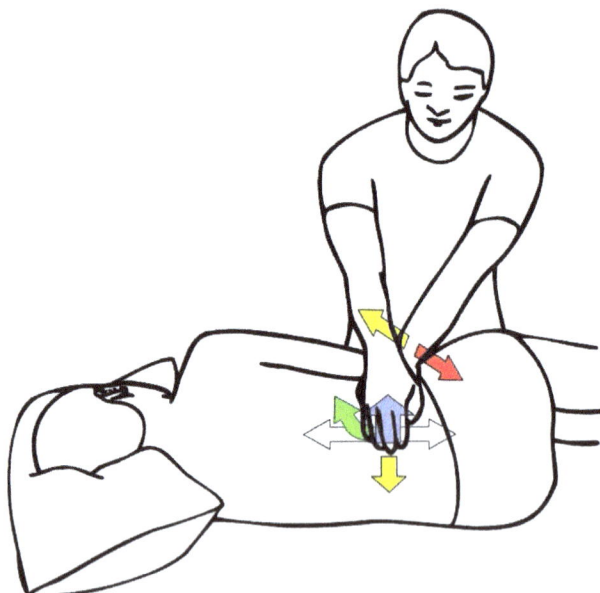

Figure 9.30

Muscle Fibres	⇕	Primary Force	⬇	Secondary Force	↺	Stretch Force	⬇	Contraction Force	⬇

Applicator

- The fingertips of one hand reinforced by the other hand.

Tissue tension

- Take up the primary tissue tension with compression and a transverse force by pulling up on the paravertebral muscles with your fingertips. This is a medial to lateral force.
- Take up the secondary tissue tension by pushing the side of your caudad forearm against the iliac crest, to assist the movement of your fingertips in an obliquely superior and lateral direction.
- Take up the longitudinal tension by pushing inferiorly on the pelvis with both your forearms.

Kneading

- Apply a rhythmical cycle of primary, secondary and longitudinal forces.
- When the muscle is at an optimal level of longitudinal tension increase the transverse pressure.
- As you pull up on the paravertebral muscles with your fingertips push your forearm down on the pelvis.
- Push the pelvis in an inferior direction.
- Your pressure should be just short of discomfort.
- To relax the muscle, work with the patient's breathing cycle, about 15 breaths per minute.
- To stimulate, increase your speed to about 40 cycles per minute.

Active component

- Ask the patient to take a deep breath and hold it in.
- Ask the patient to try to pull up their pelvis (superiorly) for 3 to 5 seconds using a 10% effort. The spinal muscles will contract.
- Resist their effort with the side of your forearm, maintaining tissue lockup throughout the technique.
- Ask the patient to exhale and to relax their muscle contraction.
- As soon as you feel that the patient has relaxed their spinal muscles completely (about 1-3 seconds), take up the tissue slack by increasing the primary and secondary tension.
- Take up the slack after each contraction and during exhalation.
- Repeat 2 or 3 times, or as required.

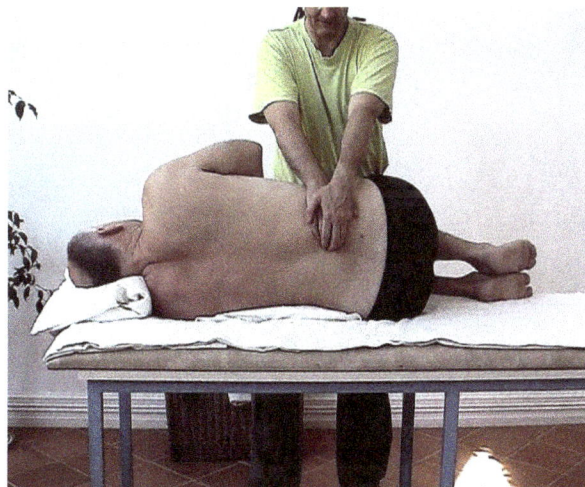

Picture 9.18

10. The intercostal muscles

Anatomy

The muscles arise from the inferior border of ribs 1 to 11. The **external intercostal muscles** are the most superficial and run obliquely, inferiorly and anteriorly, to attach onto the superior border of the adjacent rib below. Their action is to produce inspiration.
The **internal intercostal muscles** are deeper and run obliquely, inferiorly and posteriorly, to attach onto the superior border of the adjacent rib below. Their action is to produce expiration.
Nerve supply: Segmental nerves (anterior division T2 to L1).

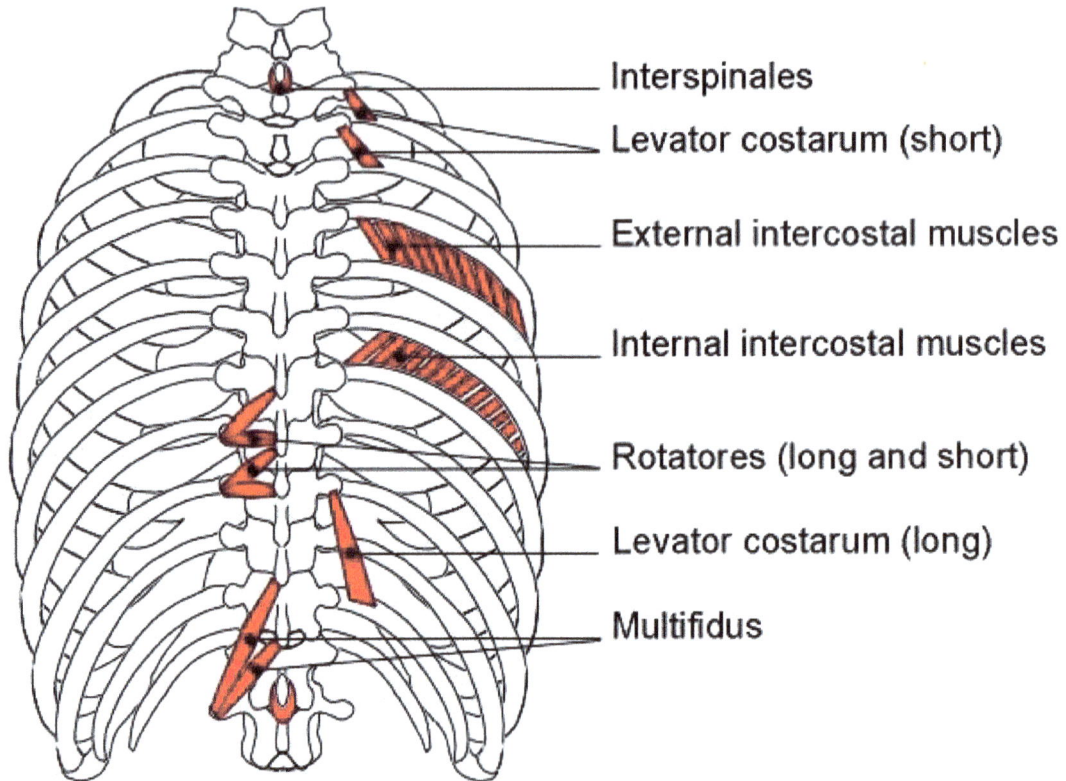

Interspinales
Levator costarum (short)
External intercostal muscles
Internal intercostal muscles
Rotatores (long and short)
Levator costarum (long)
Multifidus

Technique 10.1 Stretch for the intercostal muscles

Patient

- Sidelying and facing the therapist.
- A pillow may be placed under the lateral rib cage.
- The uppermost arm is abducted.
- The lowermost arm is positioned so that the patient is comfortable and well balanced.

Therapist

- Stand by the side of the table, facing the patient.
- Reach over the patient's rib cage with your cephalad hand and grasp the patient's upper group of ribs. Your palm and fingers should mould the contours of the rib cage.
- Place the palm of your caudad hand flat on the lateral aspect of the patient's lower ribs.
- The index finger and thumb of your caudad hand sits in the intercostal space between the two ribs.

110

Applicator

- The index finger and thumb of your caudad hand.
- Contact the muscles with as much of the thumb and side of the index finger as possible.
- Both hands are used to take the ribs apart but only one is the applicator.

Contact

- Start at the most inferior intercostal space and work up the rib cage to about rib 3.
- To influence the mainly pump handle movement of the upper ribs, your applicator should be placed more anteriorly on the rib cage.
- To influence the mainly bucket handle movement of the lower ribs, your applicator should be placed more laterally on the rib cage.

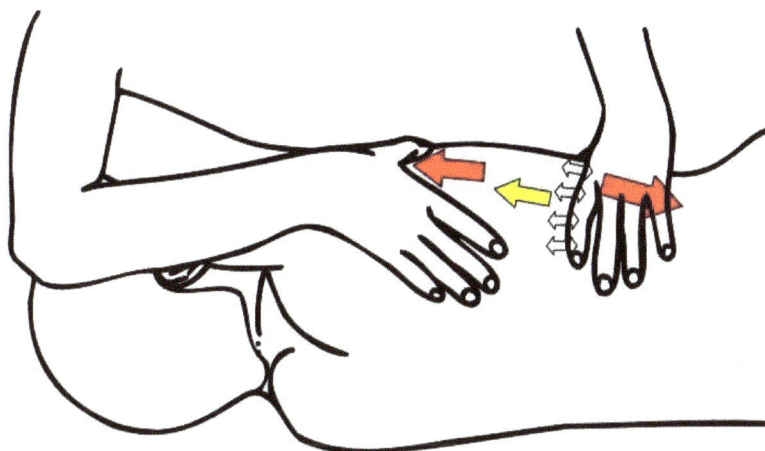

Figure 10.1

Muscle Fibres	⇕	Primary Force	⬇	Secondary Force	↻	Stretch Force	⬇	Contraction Force	⬇

Tissue tension

- The primary tissue tension is compression. Take this up by pushing on the muscle with the full length of the index finger and thumb of your caudad hand.
- The ribs act as levers to stretch the intercostal muscles. Take up the longitudinal tension by pushing the lowermost group of ribs inferiorly and pulling the uppermost group of ribs superiorly or stabilising them.

Inhibition with stretching

- To relax the muscles work with the patient's breathing cycle, about 15 breaths per minute.
- To treat the external intercostals the cephalad hand stabilises the upper rib cage.
- At the end of the patient's cycle of exhalation attempt to increase exhalation even further with a localised inferior force, directed at the target rib by the caudad hand.
- To increase rib excursion of the upper ribs add a posterior force.
- To increase rib excursion of the lower ribs add a medial force.
- Apply a rhythmical cycle of compression with maximum compression at the end of the exhalation cycle.
- The deeper internal intercostals are more difficult to influence with manipulation.
- The caudad hand stabilises the lower rib cage.
- At the end of the patient's cycle of inhalation attempt to increase inhalation even further with a localised superior force directed at the target rib by the cephalad hand.
- Apply a rhythmical cycle of compression with maximum compression at the end of the inhalation cycle.

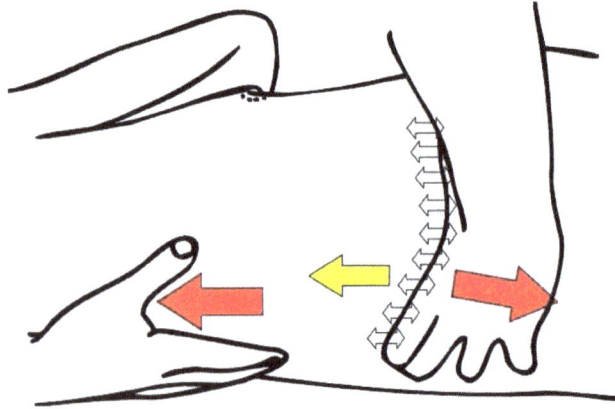

Figure 10.2

Muscle Fibres	↕	Primary Force	⬇	Secondary Force	↺	Stretch Force	⬇	Contraction Force	⬇

Active component

- Ask the patient to take a deep breath in, then a deep breath out.
- Stabilise the patients upper ribs with your cephalad hand.
- Just before the end of exhalation ask the patient to attempt to inhale for 3 to 5 seconds using a 10% effort. The external intercostal will contract.
- Resist their effort to raise their rib cage with pressure from your caudad hand.
- Maintain tissue compression and upper rib stabilisation throughout the technique.
- Ask the patient to cease attempting to inhale against your unyielding resistance.
- Ask the patient to exhale again.
- As soon as you feel that the patient has relaxed their muscle completely, take up the tissue slack by increasing the primary tension (compression) and longitudinal tension.
- The lower rib acts as a lever to increase longitudinal tension on the external intercostals.
- Take up the slack after each contraction and during exhalation.
- Repeat 2 or 3 times, or as required.

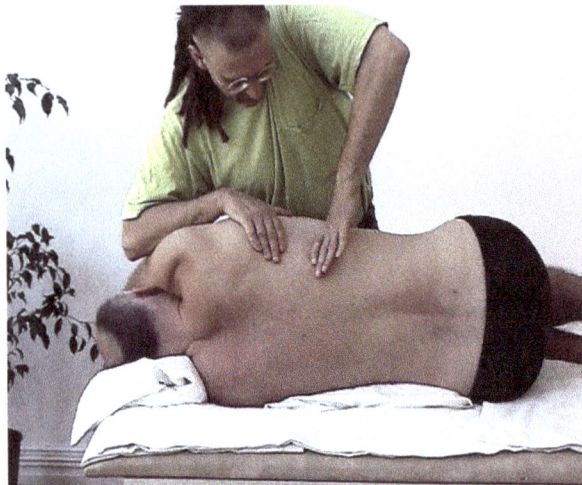

Picture 10.1

11. The abdominal muscles

Anatomy

The abdominal wall consists of a corset of three sheets of muscle and fascia attached to the lateral margin of two long muscles running parasagittally, which attach at the midline. It is important for posture, digestion, defecation, venous return, urination, vomiting, breathing, parturition and fine control of vocal actions such as singing. It works in balance with the erector spinae to support the spine.

Superficial fascia covers most of the abdominal wall. It is made up of two layers, with blood vessels, nerves, lymph nodes and variable levels of fat in between. It passes over the inguinal ligament and below, is continuous with the fascia lata. The deeper of the two layers merges with the linea alba.

Rectus abdominis arises inferiorly by a lateral tendon from the pubic crest and pubic tubercle, and by a medial tendon which merges with the lateral tendon, the interpubic ligament of the symphysis pubis and occasionally with the linea alba. It attaches superiorly on the cartilages of ribs 5, 6 and 7, and occasionally ribs 3 and 4 and the xiphoid process.
Action: It compresses and supports the abdomen and flexes the spine.
Nerve supply: Intercostal nerves 7 to 12

The rectus sheath envelops the rectus abdominis muscle. The fascia is deep and superficial. It attaches at the midline as the linea alba. Laterally the sheath attaches to the oblique muscles. Three tendinous intersections run transversely or zigzag obliquely across the muscle. One occurs at the level of the umbilicus and two occur above it. One or two more may also occur below the umbilicus. They may be incomplete. The tendinous intersections divide the rectus abdominis along it's length into bands with distinct segmental innervation, giving the muscle greater control.

External oblique arises on the lower 8 ribs as muscle. It interdigitates with the fibres of serratus anterior and latissimus dorsi. It runs inferiorly and medially to attach onto the anterior half of the iliac crest, and an aponeurosis. The aponeurosis is a strong tendinous sheet covering the anterior abdomen. It starts where the muscle part of the external oblique ends. This is approximately along a line between the anterior superior iliac spine and the umbilicus. The fibres run inferiorly and medially, extending to the linea alba at the midline, to the pubic symphysis and pubic crest, pubic tubercle and inguinal ligament, inferiorly. The inguinal ligament is a thickening of the aponeurosis, folded internally and with fibres from the rectus sheath forms the floor of the inguinal canal. The external oblique is the most superficial and largest of the group of muscles, which form the lateral abdominal wall. The muscle is palpable, lateral to rectus abdominis. The muscle and aponeurosis are covered in fascia. Digitations of the muscle may be absent or duplicated.

Internal oblique is thinner and deep to the external oblique and so is not directly palpable. It arises on the anterior two-thirds of the iliac crest, the lateral two-thirds of the inguinal ligament and on the thoracolumbar fascia. The fibres arising from the posterior part of the iliac crest run superiorly and laterally to attach onto the lower 4 ribs and are continuous with the internal intercostals. The fibres from the middle of the muscle, arising from the anterior part of the iliac crest diverge, the more posterior fibres running superiorly and medially and the more anterior fibres running horizontally or inferiorly and medially to attach on an aponeurosis. At the lateral border of the rectus abdominis the aponeurosis separates into two layers which wrap around the muscle, reuniting at the linea alba. The aponeurosis of the internal oblique joins with the aponeurosis of the external oblique to form the anterior part of the rectus sheath and joins with the aponeurosis of the transversus abdominis to form the posterior part of the rectus sheath. The fibres arising from the inguinal ligament run inferiorly and medially and form a tendon, which attaches onto the pubic crest. The lower part of the muscle and its aponeurosis may be replaced by fascia. The internal oblique and transversus abdominis may be fused.
Action of the oblique muscles: They compress the abdomen, flex and sidebend the spine and depress the ribs.

Transversus abdominis is the deepest layer and not directly palpable; It arises on the lateral third of the inguinal ligament, the anterior two thirds of the iliac crest, thoracolumbar fascia and cartilages of the lower 6 ribs. It attaches onto aponeurosis and linea alba, pubis and pectineal line. The transversus abdominis may be absent. The lowest part may be replaced by fascia.
Action: Depresses ribs. A constrictor of the abdomen.
Nerve supply: Intercostal nerves 7 to 12 and the Iliohypogastric and Ilioinguinal nerves.

Pyramidalis arises on the pubis and anterior pubic ligament and attaches on the linea alba between the umbilicus and pubis. The muscle may be larger on one side. It may be absent unilaterally or bilaterally, and it may be duplicated.
Action: It tenses the linea alba.
Nerve supply: T12

Clinical indications
The abdominal muscles are rarely short. Some fibres may be relatively short as a result of incorrect exercise which over-emphasises one side of the body, or as a result of a severe rotoscoliosis. Surgery, which results in scarring to the abdominal wall, may cause weakness and shortness.

The abdominal muscles are more commonly hypotonic and therefore weak. The fascia may be over-stretched and become permanently distended by obesity or repeated pregnancy. Laxity of fascia and weakness in the musculature may have consequences on digestive and respiratory systems as well as on postural mechanisms. When the abdominal fascia becomes lax it fails to provide support for the abdominal contents. Digestion is compromised when the connective tissue which supports the abdominal viscera, the mesentery (confirm) becomes over-stretched because the arterial, venous and portal vessel become less efficient in transporting blood. A large area of fat around the abdomen results in changes to the body's centre of gravity, resulting in over activity of the postural muscle, mainly the erector spinae. Respiration is compromised when the diaphragm is affected.

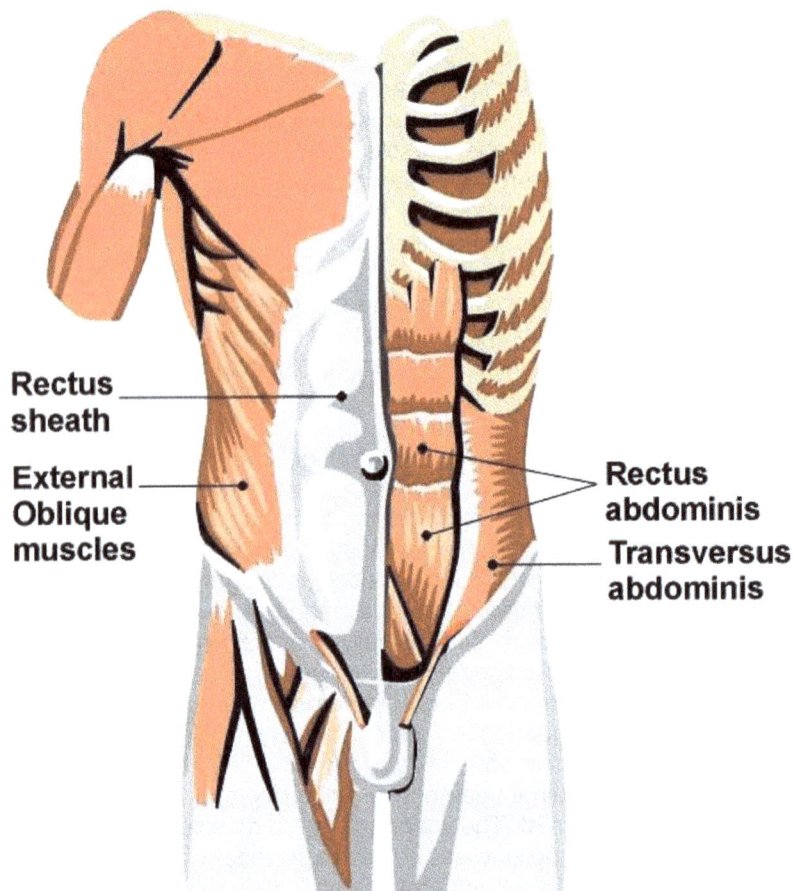

Rectus sheath

External Oblique muscles

Rectus abdominis

Transversus abdominis

Technique 11.1 Friction over abdominal muscles

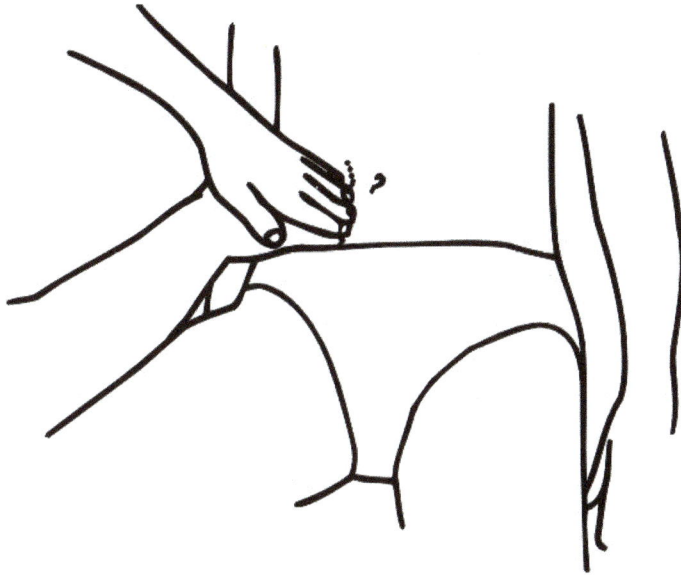

Figure 11.1

- Apply transverse friction to reduce areas of scar tissue
- Use corrective exercises for weakness.

1. Sit ups: unilateral or bilateral.
2. Sustained pelvic tilting.
3. Sidelying leg abduction - unilateral or bilateral.

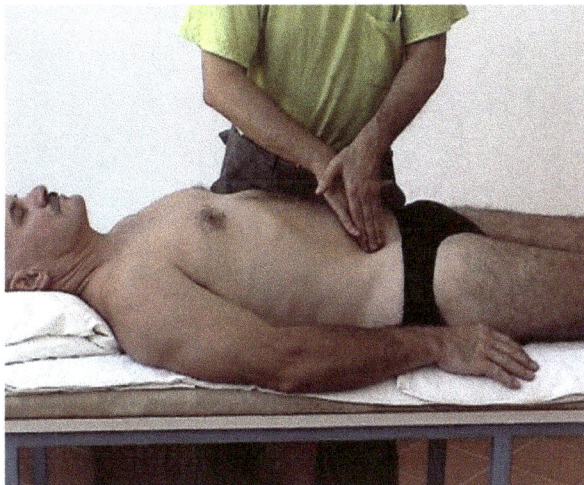

Picture 11.1

12. Supraspinous and interspinous ligaments

Anatomy

The supraspinous and interspinous ligaments are small ligaments running from one vertebra to the next, from the seventh cervical vertebrae to the sacrum. The supraspinous ligaments are stronger, thicker and more superficial than the interspinous ligaments and are more easily palpable.

In the cervical spine the ligamentum nuchae or superior nuchal ligament is the continuation of the supraspinous ligament. It arises on the inion and attaches onto the spinous process of the C7 vertebra (via each cervical spine). It is not distinctly palpable but in flexion is on tension. In the thoracic the sacrospinous and interspinous ligaments are connected to long spinous processes directed inferiorly and posteriorly. They are more exposed in flexion. In the lumbar the sacrospinous and interspinous ligaments are thicker and connected to thick, broad spinous processes that are directed posteriorly and are proportionally larger.

Clinical indications: Motor vehicle accidents cause whiplash injuries to these ligaments in the cervical region and in the lumbar the ligaments they may be strained from the lifting of heavy objects by unprepared or weak muscles.

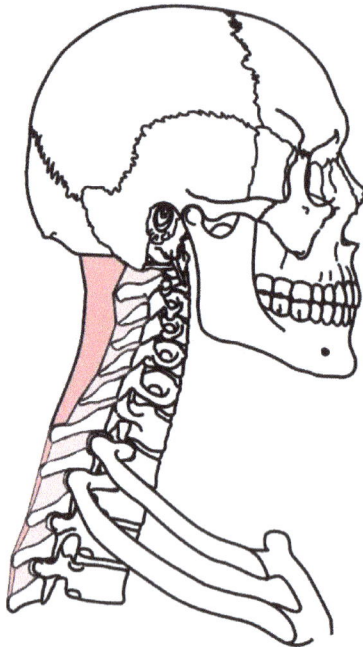

Technique 12.1 Friction over the supraspinous ligament

Patient

- Prone with the head straight in a face hole or rotated away.
- A pillow may be placed under the area you are treating. The ligaments are more accessible with the spine slightly flexed.

Therapist

- Stand at the side of the table, adjacent to the patient's spine.

Applicator

- Tips of thumbs or a T bar.

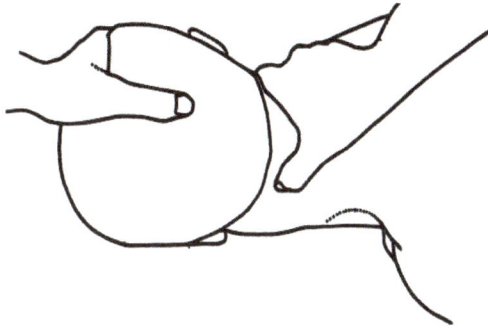

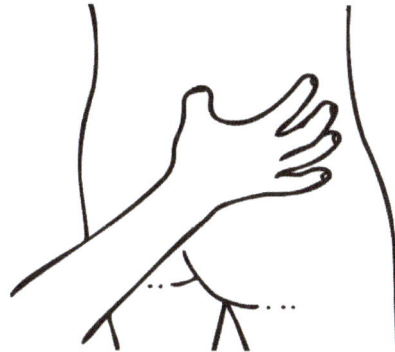

Figure 12.1   Figure 12.2

Transverse Friction

- Place the tips of both thumbs or a small bar between the spinous processes of adjacent vertebrae.
- Apply transverse friction to the supraspinous ligament.
- With your thumb apply a pressure perpendicular to the ligament.
- The cervical and thoracic spinous processes angle about 45 degrees inferiorly so the force should be directed into the intervertebral space 45 degrees superiorly.
- Start light and over 3 to 5 seconds increase to a firm pressure.
- Apply moderately firm pressure over a small area.

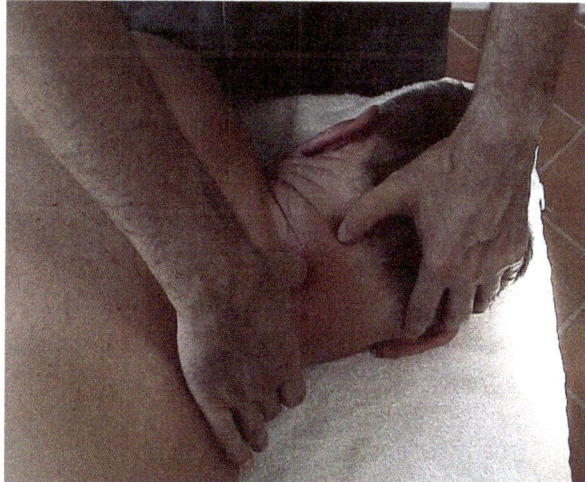

Picture 12.1

13. Trapezius, levator scapulae and rhomboids

Anatomy

Trapezius arises on aponeurosis, firmly anchored at the midline to the occipital bone and skin, the external occipital protuberance, the medial one third of the superior nuchal line of the occiput, the ligamentum nuchae, the spinous processes and supraspinous ligaments of vertebra C7 to T12.

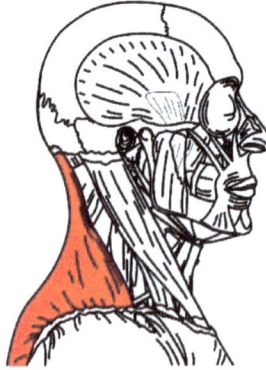

The triangular sheet of trapezius wraps around the shoulder and converges on a U shaped area. The superior fibres attach on the posterior border of the lateral third (sometimes half) of the clavicle; the middle fibres attach on the medial side of the acromion and a superior line along the spine of scapula. The inferior fibres merge into an aponeurosis that attaches onto the medial end of the spine of the scapula. The muscle arises from a broad aponeurosis between C6 and T3. The muscle may merge with the sternocleidomastoid. It may be absent at the occiput and after T8.

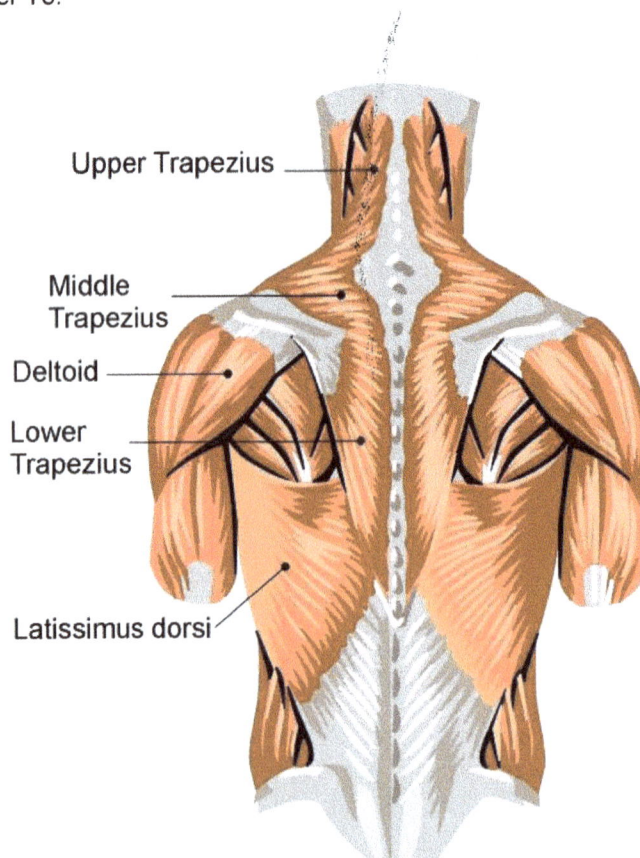

Actions: The muscle supports and stabilises the scapular when the upper limb is active. Working with levator scapulae its upper fibres elevate the scapula, with the rhomboids its middle fibres retract the scapula and with serratus anterior it rotates the scapular to assist with arm elevation. Its upper fibres extend and sidebend the head when the scapula is fixed.
Nerve supply: Accessory nerve (Cranial nerve 11).

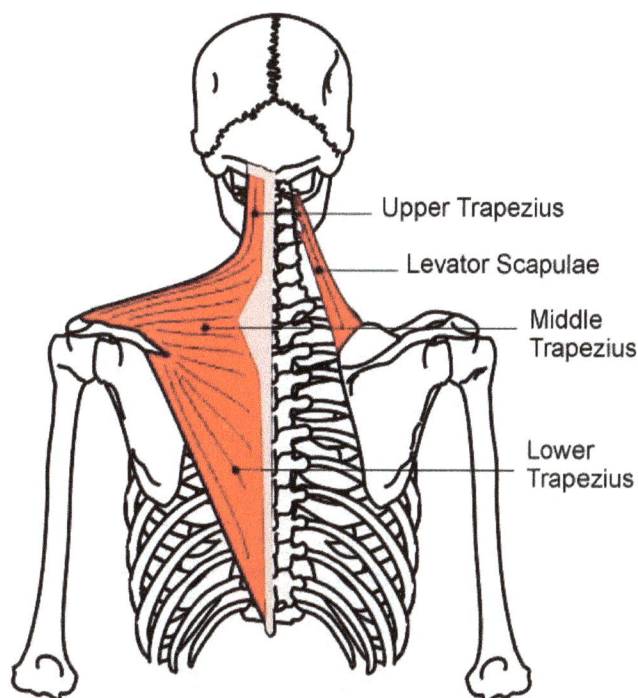

Levator scapulae Tendons arise from the transverse processes of atlas and axis and posterior tubercles of the transverse processes of C3 and C4. The muscle attaches to the medial border of the scapula, between the superior angle and the spine of scapula. Vertebral attachments vary and fibres may attach on the occiput, mastoid process, rib 1 and 2 and merge with adjacent muscles. It lies deep to trapezius.

Actions: The muscle stabilises and moves the scapular when the upper limb is active. It strongly elevates the scapula and is active when carrying a load. With other muscles it draws the scapula medially and rotates the scapula so that the glenoid points down. Levator scapulae extends, rotates, sidebends and helps stabilise the cervical spine.
Nerve supply: C3 and C4 and via the dorsal scapular nerve to C5.

Rhomboids Rhomboid minor arises from the ligamentum nuchae and spinous processes of C7 and T1. Rhomboid major arises from the spinous processes of T2 to T5. Both run inferiorly and laterally to attach onto the medial border of the scapula. Rhomboid minor attaches at the medial end of the spine of the scapula. Rhomboid major muscle fibres may attach on two tendons, inserting on the inferior angle and near the spine of the scapula, or may attach directly on the medial border scapula. Fibres may extend superiorly to the occiput.

Action: Retraction and downward rotation of the scapula.
Nerve supply: Dorsal scapula nerve C4 and **C5**.

Clinical indications: Overuse, headaches, whiplash injuries, torticollis.

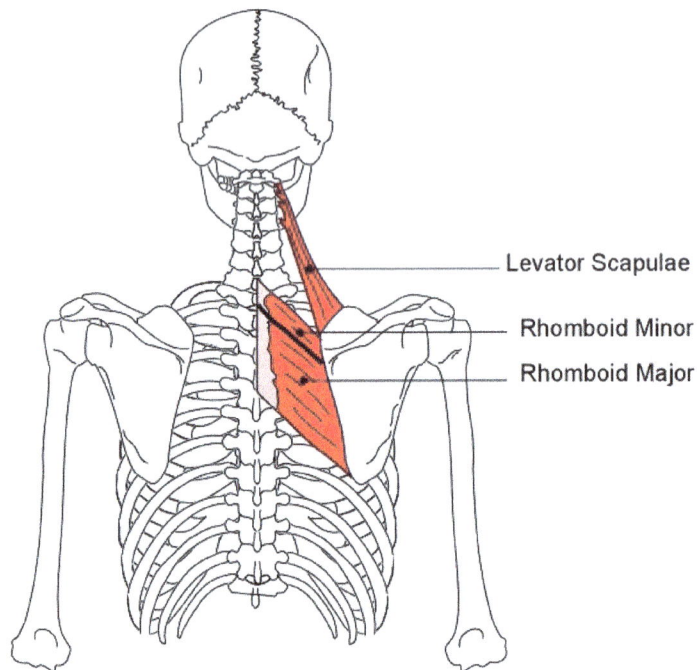

Levator Scapulae

Rhomboid Minor

Rhomboid Major

Technique 13.1 Stretch for trapezius, levator scapulae and the posterior cervical muscles

Patient

- Supine

Therapist

- Stand at the head of the table.
- Support the patient's head in the palm of your hand, and support your hand in the crease between the arm and forearm of your other limb.
- Hold back on the shoulder with your fingers.
- In flexion or neutral the supporting hand can induce variations of sidebending and rotation.

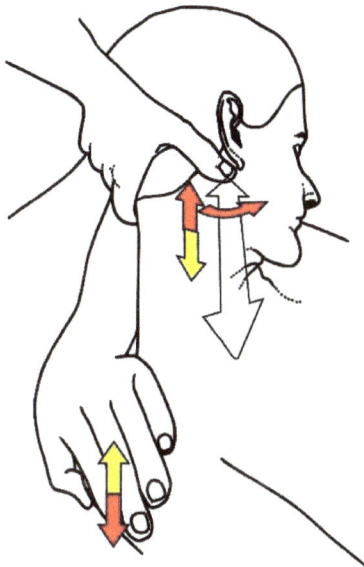

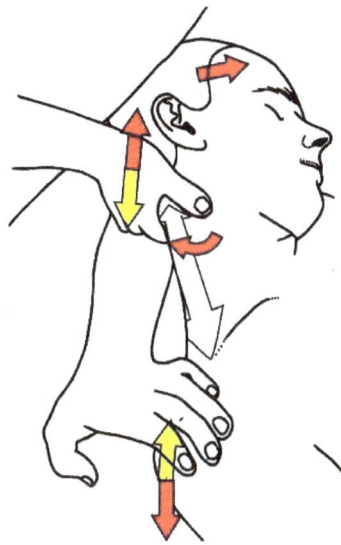

Figure 13.1 Levator scapulae stretch   Figure 13.2 Trapezius stretch

Muscle Fibres	⇕	Primary Force	⬇	Secondary Force	↻	Stretch Force	⬇	Contraction Force	⬇

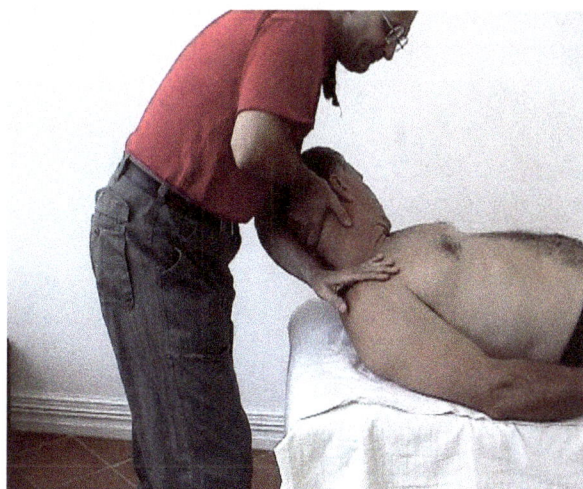

Picture 13.1

Technique 13.2 Strong stretch for trapezius and levator scapulae

Patient

- Supine

Therapist

- Stand at the head of the table.
- Hold back one shoulder with your hand.
- Grasp under the patient's neck with other hand and with the assistance from your chest/abdomen strong variations of flexion, sidebending and rotation can be induced.
- Care should be taken not to place stress on the sub-occipital muscles. A hand wrap around the sub-occipital area helps supports the head in a neutral position.

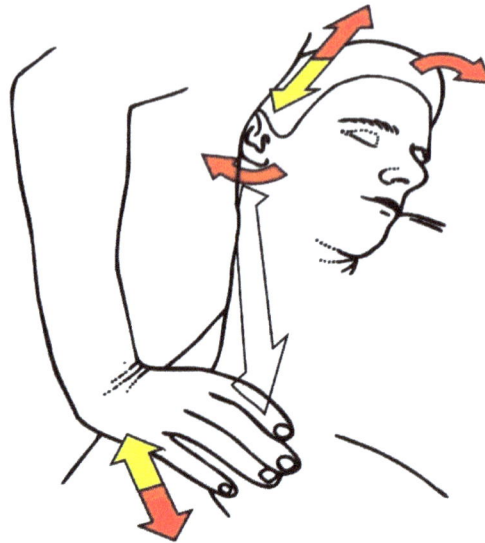

Figure 13.3 Trapezius stretch

Muscle Fibres	⇕	Primary Force	⬇	Secondary Force	↺	Stretch Force	⬇	Contraction Force	⬇

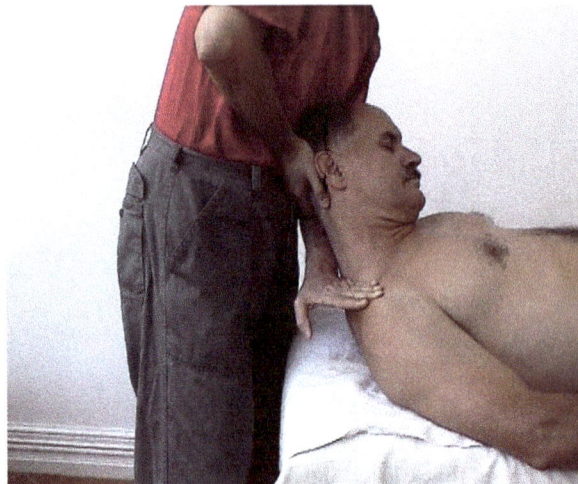

Picture 13.2

Technique 13.3 Stretch for trapezius, levator scapulae and the posterior cervical muscles

Patient

- Supine

Therapist

- Stand at the head of the table.
- Your arms are crossed under the patient's head and your fingers hold back on the patient's shoulders.
- Produce flexion or combined flexion with sidebending or flexion with rotation.

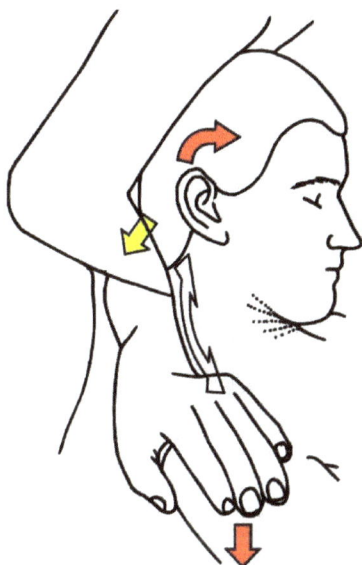

Figure 13.4 Posterior cervical stretch   Figure 13.5 Levator scapulae stretch

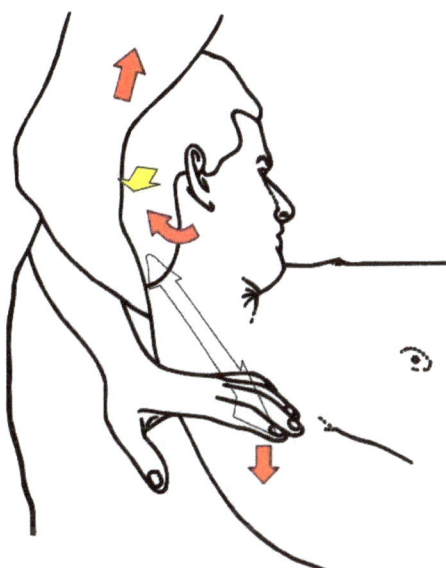

Muscle Fibres	⇕	Primary Force	⬇	Secondary Force	↻	Stretch Force	⬇	Contraction Force	⬇

- These levers may be used as a stretch, articulation, isometric or isokinetic procedure and as a cross fibre kneading or inhibition technique.
- Take care not to pull the patient's hair.

Active component

- Ask the patient to take a deep breath and hold it in.
- Ask the patient to extend or sidebend their head for 3 to 5 seconds using a 10% effort.
- Alternatively, ask the patient to shrug their shoulder.
- Resist the patient's effort and maintain tissue lockup throughout the technique.
- Ask the patient to exhale and to relax their muscle contraction.
- As soon as you feel that the patient has relaxed their muscles completely (about 1-3 seconds), take up the tissue slack by increasing the primary and secondary tension.
- Take up the slack after each contraction and during exhalation.
- Repeat 2 or 3 times, or as required.

Technique 13.4 Kneading and stretch for upper trapezius and cervical fascia

Patient

- Prone with head rotated towards the side you are standing.
- The shoulders are depressed.

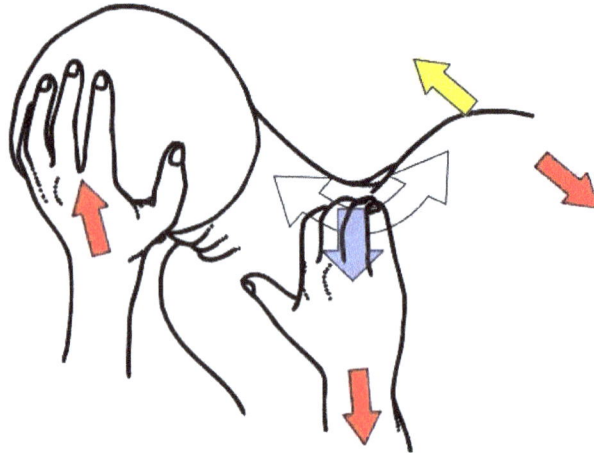

Figure 13.6

Muscle Fibres	⇕	Primary Force	⬇	Secondary Force	↻	Stretch Force	⬇	Contraction Force	⬇

Therapist

- Stand at the side of the table adjacent to the patient's shoulder.
- Place the palm of your cephalad hand over the crown and side of the patient's head.
- Reach into the supraclavicular fossa on the opposite side of the spine and grasp the anterior shoulder myofascia with your caudad hand.

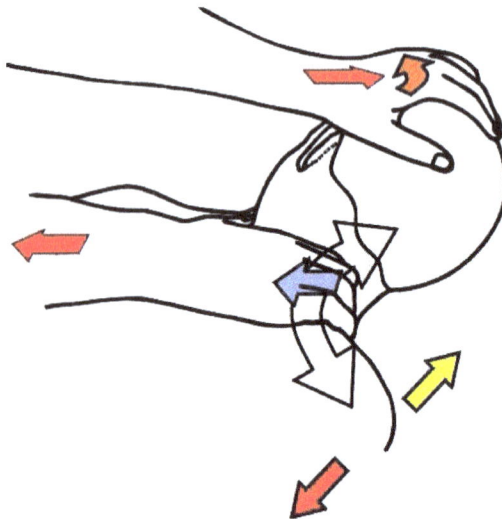

Figure 13.7

Muscle Fibres	⇕	Primary Force	⬇	Secondary Force	↻	Stretch Force	⬇	Contraction Force	⬇

124

Stretch

- Stabilise the patient's head with your cephalad hand.
- With your caudad hand slowly pull on the fascia and drag your fingertips across the skin.
- Cover the fascia overlying the upper trapezius and cervical area.
- Depending on the height of the table, this technique may be done more efficiently by keeping both your elbows extended, leaning back and using your body weight.

Active component

- Ask the patient to take a deep breath and hold it in.
- Ask the patient to shrug their shoulder or push (extend) their head back up and off the table for 3 to 5 seconds using a 10% effort.
- Resist the patient's effort and maintain tissue lockup throughout the technique.
- Ask the patient to exhale and to relax their muscle contraction.
- As soon as you feel that the patient has relaxed their muscles completely (about 1-3 seconds), take up the tissue slack by increasing the primary and secondary tension.
- Take up the slack after each contraction and during exhalation.
- Repeat 2 or 3 times, or as required.

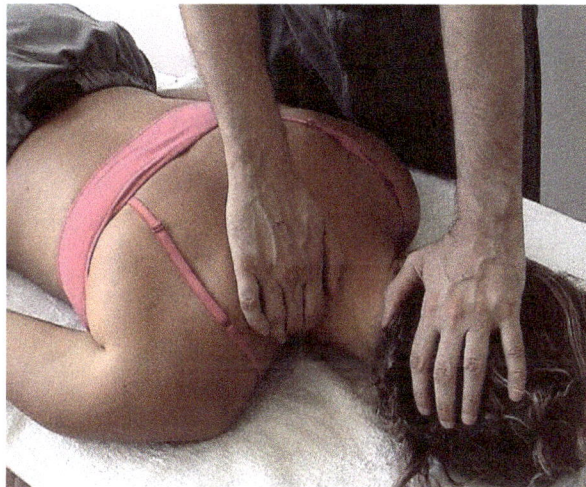

Picture 13.3

Technique 13.5 Inhibition for upper trapezius and stretch for cervical fascia

Patient

- Supine with the head straight, or for unilateral treatment of the trapezius, sidebend the head.
- A rolled up towel may be placed under the patient's thoracic spine, or for unilateral treatment of the trapezius, the towel may be placed under one of the patient's scapula.

Therapist

- Stand at the head of the table.
- Place the heal of your left hand on the patient's left acromion process and the heal of your right hand on the patient's right acromion process.

Applicator

- The pad or tip of one or both thumbs.

Tissue tension

- Take up the tissue tension by gradually increasing your thumb pressure on the muscle.
- Your pressure is directed perpendicular to the muscle.
- Make sure the force goes through your thumbs and not your fingers.

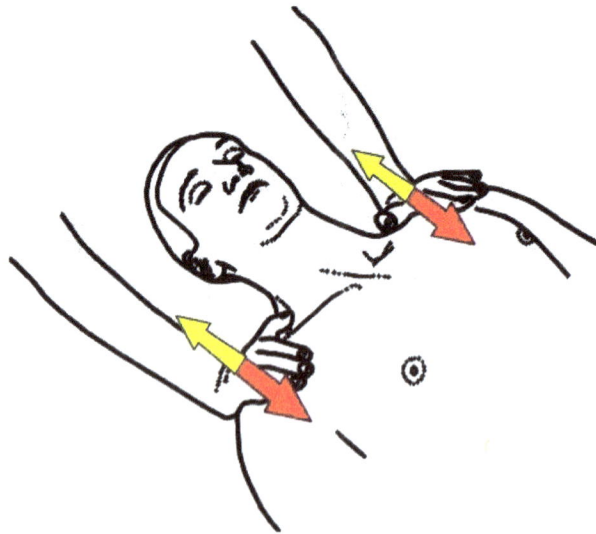

Figure 13.8

Muscle Fibres	⇕	Primary Force	⬇	Secondary Force	↻	Stretch Force	⬇	Contraction Force	⬇

Inhibition

- Apply pressure (compression) on the area of muscle covered by your thumb.
- Use one thumb for unilateral inhibition or both thumbs for bilateral inhibition.
- Your pressure should be just short of discomfort.
- To relax the muscle work with the patients breathing cycle, about 15 breaths per minute.
- Maintain some compression throughout the technique, but increase it during exhalation.

Stretch

- Press on both shoulders simultaneously with both your hands for a bilateral stretch.
- Keep both your elbows extended and use you body weight.
- Inferior pressure stretches the upper trapezius and fascia.
- Sidebend the patient's head away from the side you are treating if you want to apply a unilateral stretch.

Active component

- Ask the patient to take a deep breath and hold it in.
- Ask the patient to shrug their shoulders or push (extend) their head back into the table, or push their head sideways for 3 to 5 seconds using a 10% effort.
- Resist the patient's effort and maintain tissue lockup throughout the technique.
- Ask the patient to exhale and to relax their muscle contraction.
- As soon as you feel that the patient has relaxed their muscles completely (about 1-3 seconds), take up the tissue slack by increasing the primary tension (compression) and longitudinal tension by further depressing the scapula or sidebending the head.
- Take up the slack after each contraction and during exhalation.
- Repeat 2 or 3 times, or as required.

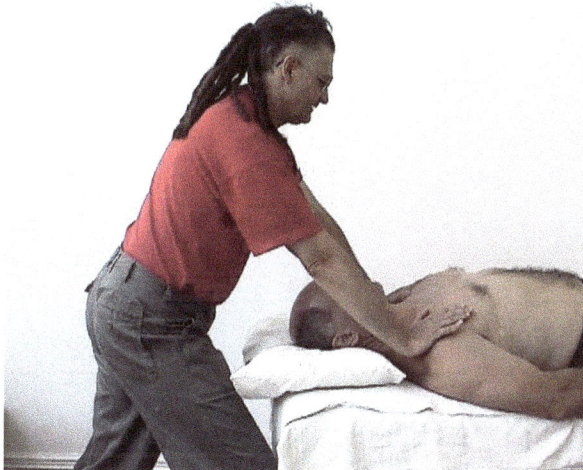

Picture 13.4

Technique 13.6 Kneading of trapezius, levator scapulae and rhomboids

Patient

- Prone with their head rotated away from the side you are standing.

Therapist

- Stand at the side of the table adjacent to the patient's shoulder.
- Grasp the trapezius on the side of the spine you are standing. Grasp it between the fingertips and thumb of your cephalad hand.
- You may use the fingers of your caudad hand to reinforce the thumb of your cephalad hand.

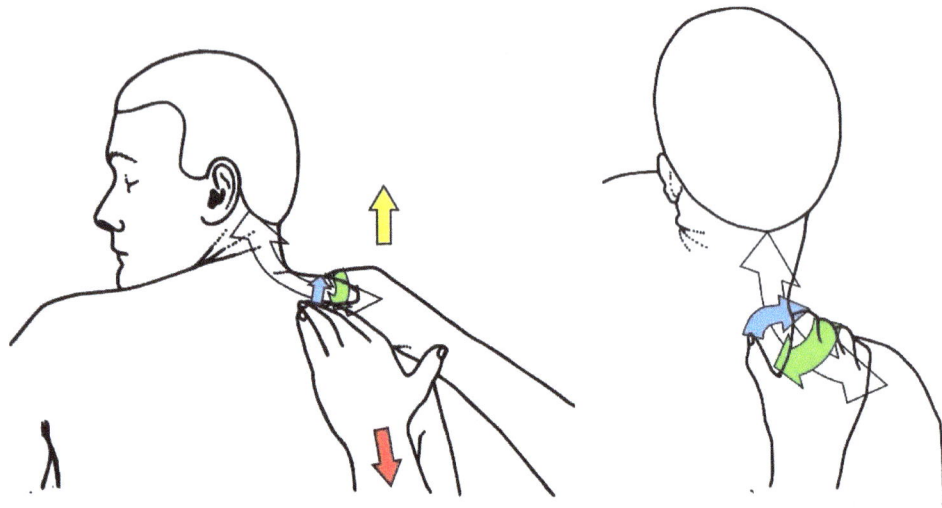

Figure 13.9   Figure 13.9b

Muscle Fibres	⇕	Primary Force	⬇	Secondary Force	↻	Stretch Force	⬇	Contraction Force	⬇

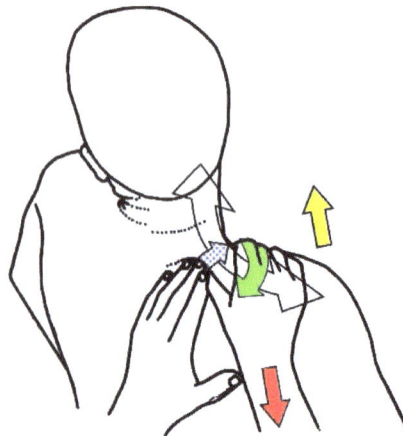

Figure 13.10

Applicator

- The fingertips and thumb of your cephalad hand.
- Use the pad or the lateral side of your thumb on the trapezius. The tip of your thumb is useful for working on the very superior fibres of trapezius and to reach the rhomboids or levator scapula muscles which lie deeper.
- The fingers of your caudad hand may be used to reinforce the thumb of your cephalad hand.

Tissue tension

- Take up the primary tissue tension. This is a transverse force done by flexing your thumb.
- Your force is perpendicular to the muscle and in an anterior and superior direction.
- Secondary tension is taken up by pulling back on the muscle with your fingertips.
- Longitudinal tension is taken up by starting the technique with the shoulder depressed.
- Further longitudinal tension is taken up by flexing and sidebending the patient's head, away from the shoulder being treated.

Kneading

- Maintain longitudinal tension by gently pushing down on the shoulder with the hypothenar eminence of your cephalad hand.
- Apply cross fibre kneading to the muscle with your applicator.
- Pull posteriorly on the muscle with the fingertips of your cephalad hand, and push anteriorly and superiorly with the thumb of your cephalad hand.
- The push may be assisted with the fingers of your caudad hand.
- Combine the fingertips and thumb action to apply a rhythmical cycle of primary and secondary forces.
- Your fingertips remain hooked over the anterior of the trapezius.
- Work across the trapezius fibres from the occiput to the acromion process, then down to the middle thoracic.
- The grip between your fingers and thumb becomes narrower as you go superiorly.
- Depending on the size of the patient and the size of your hand, cover as much of the middle trapezius as you can reach.
- Press more firmly and through the trapezius with your thumb to treat the levator scapula and rhomboids.
- Your pressure should be just short of discomfort.
- To relax the muscle, work with the patients breathing cycle, about 15 breaths per minute.
- To stimulate, increase your speed to about 40 cycles per minute.

Active component

- Ask the patient to take a deep breath and hold it in.
- Ask the patient to lift their head back and up off the table (extend or sidebend their head) for 3 to 5 seconds using a 10% effort.
- Alternatively, ask the patient to shrug their shoulder.
- Resist the patient's effort and maintain tissue lockup throughout the technique.
- Ask the patient to exhale and to relax their muscle contraction.
- As soon as you feel that the patient has relaxed their muscles completely (about 1-3 seconds), take up the tissue slack by increasing the primary and secondary tension.
- Take up the slack after each contraction and during exhalation.
- Repeat 2 or 3 times, or as required.

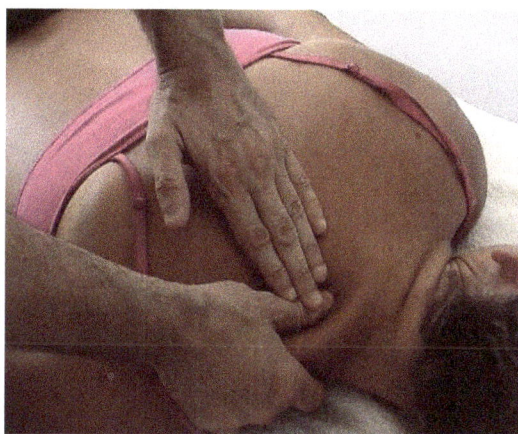

Picture 13.5

Technique 13.7 Bilateral or unilateral kneading of trapezius, levator scapulae and the rhomboids and fascial stretch

Patient

- Seated in a chair or low table.
- Ask the patient to be relaxed but sit up straight. Do not allow them to slouch.
- This technique utilises gravity and may be used if the patient is uncomfortable while prone.

Therapist

- Stand behind the patient.
- With both hands grasp the upper trapezius bilaterally.

Applicator

- The fingertips and thumb of your both hand.
- The pad or lateral side of the thumb is used on the trapezius.
- The tip of the thumb is used on the very superior fibres of trapezius and to reach the deeper rhomboids or levator scapula muscles.

Tissue tension

- Take up the primary tissue tension. This is a transverse force done by flexing both your thumbs.
- Your force is perpendicular to the muscle and in an anterior and superior direction.
- Secondary tension is taken up by pulling back on the muscle with your fingertips.
- Longitudinal tension is taken up by starting the technique with the shoulder depressed.
- Further longitudinal tension may be taken up by flexing the patient's head.

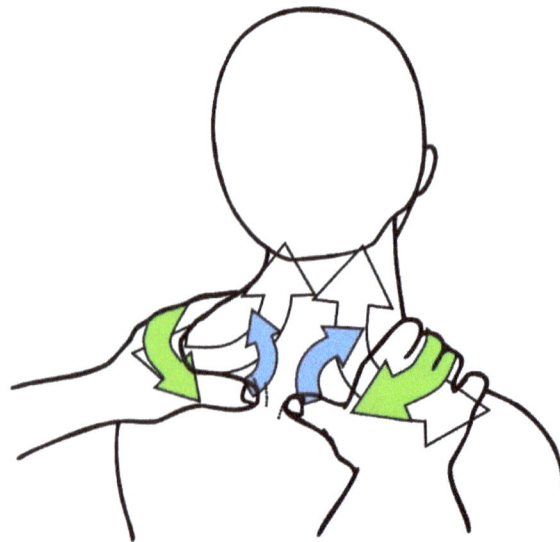

Figure 13.11

Muscle Fibres	⇕	Primary Force	⬇	Secondary Force	↻	Stretch Force	⬇	Contraction Force	⬇

Kneading

- Maintain longitudinal tension by gently pushing down on the shoulder with the hypothenar eminence of your hands.
- Pull posteriorly on the muscle with your fingertips while pushing anteriorly and superiorly with your thumbs.
- Combine the fingertips and thumb action to apply a rhythmical cycle of primary and secondary forces.
- Your fingertips remain hooked over the anterior of the trapezius.
- Work across the trapezius fibres from the occiput to the acromion process, then down to the middle thoracic.
- The grip between your fingers and thumbs becomes narrower as you go superiorly.
- Depending on the size of the patient and the size of your hand, cover as much of the middle trapezius as you can reach.
- Press through trapezius with your thumb to treat levator scapula and rhomboids.
- Your pressure should be just short of discomfort.
- To relax the muscle, work with the patients breathing cycle, about 15 breaths per minute.
- To stimulate, increase your speed to about 40 cycles per minute.

Active component

- Ask the patient to take a deep breath in and hold it.
- Ask the patient to shrug their shoulder for 3 to 5 seconds using a 10% effort.
- Resist the patient's effort and maintain tissue lockup throughout the technique.
- Ask the patient to exhale and to relax their muscle contraction.
- As soon as you feel that the patient has relaxed their muscles completely (about 1-3 seconds), take up the tissue slack by increasing the primary and secondary tension.
- Maintain longitudinal tension by gently pushing down on the shoulders with your hands.
- Take up the slack after each contraction and during exhalation.
- Repeat 2 or 3 times, or as required.

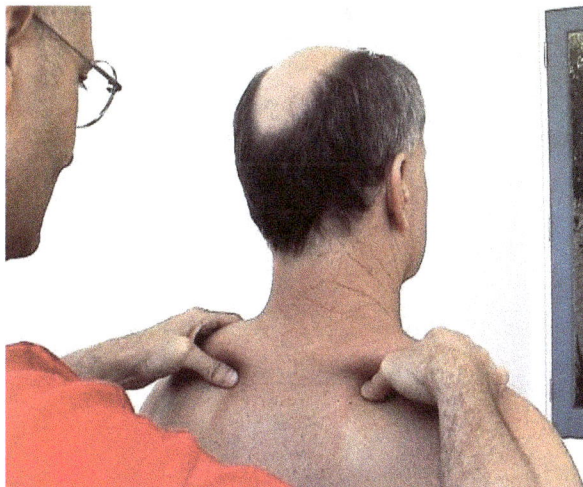

Picture 13.6

Technique 13.8 Unilateral kneading for trapezius, levator scapulae or rhomboids and fascial stretch

Patient

- Seated in a chair or low table.
- Ask the patient to be relaxed but sit up straight. Do not allow them to slouch.
- This technique utilises gravity and may be used if the patient is uncomfortable while prone.

Therapist

- Stand behind the patient.
- Place the palm of one hand on the crown of the patient's head and spread the fingers widely so as to be able to control head movement.
- Place the fingertips of the other hand in the supraclavicular fossa, just anterior to the trapezius. Place the thumb on the muscle to be treated.

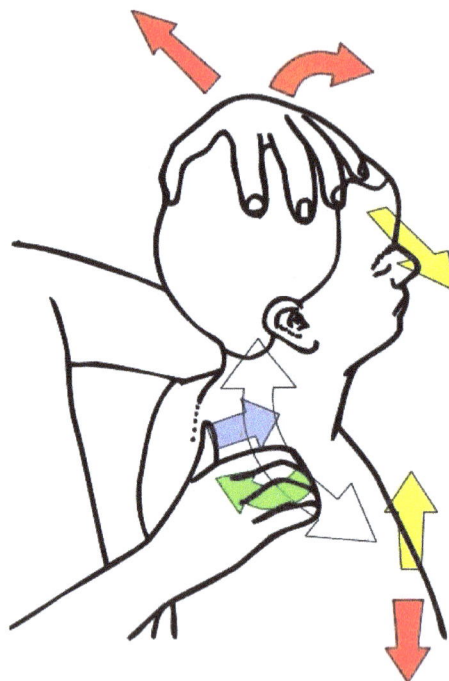

Figure 13.12

Muscle Fibres	⇕	Primary Force	⬇	Secondary Force	↻	Stretch Force	⬇	Contraction Force	⬇

Applicator

- The fingertips and thumb of one hand.
- The pad or lateral side of the thumb is used on the trapezius and the tip of the thumb is used to reach the deeper rhomboids or levator scapula muscles.

Tissue tension

- Take up the primary tissue tension. This is a transverse force done by flexing your thumb.
- Your force is perpendicular to the muscle, in an anterior and superior direction.
- Secondary tension is taken up by pulling back on the muscle with your fingertips.
- Longitudinal tension is taken up by starting the technique with the shoulder depressed.
- Further longitudinal tension is taken up by flexing and sidebending the patient's head, away from the shoulder being treated (to the left in the diagram).

Kneading

- Apply posterior to anterior cross fibre kneading to trapezius with the side or pad of your thumbs, or to the deeper levator scapulae and rhomboids with the tip of your thumb.
- Apply anterior to posterior stretching of the fascia by pulling back with your fingertips.
- Combine the fingertips and thumb action to apply a rhythmical cycle of primary and secondary forces.
- Maintain some longitudinal tension by gently pushing down on the shoulder with the hypothenar eminence of your hand.
- Circumduct the patient's head and at the point of optimal longitudinal tension increase the primary and secondary forces.
- Cover the entire muscle, working as far inferiorly as your hand can reach.
- Your pressure should be just short of discomfort.
- To relax the muscle, work with the patients breathing cycle, about 15 breaths per minute.
- To stimulate, increase your speed to about 40 cycles per minute.

Active component

- Ask the patient to take a deep breath and hold it in.
- Ask the patient to extend or sidebend their head for 3 to 5 seconds using a 10% effort.
- Alternatively, ask the patient to shrug their shoulder.
- Resist the patient's effort and maintain tissue lockup throughout the technique.
- Ask the patient to exhale and to relax their muscle contraction.
- As soon as you feel that the patient has relaxed their muscles completely (about 1-3 seconds), take up the tissue slack by increasing the primary and secondary tension.
- Take up the slack after each contraction and during exhalation.
- Repeat 2 or 3 times, or as required.

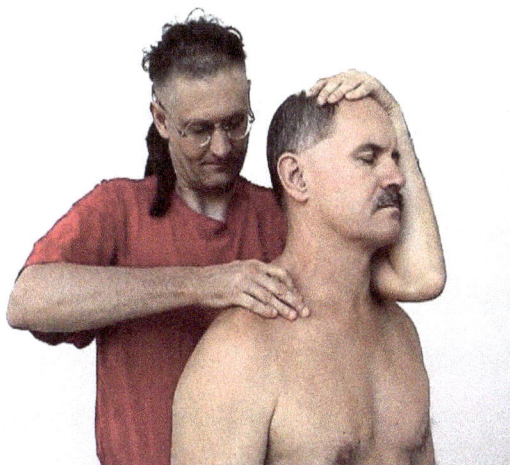

Picture 13.7

Technique 13.9 Kneading and articulation of trapezius, levator scapulae and rhomboids

Patient

- Supine with their head straight.
- A thin pillow or folded towel may be placed under their head to prevent extension.

Therapist

- Stand at the side of the table, adjacent to the patient's rib cage and facing the patient's head.
- Grasp and stabilise the patients forehead with your cephalad hand.
- The fingertips of your caudad hand hook around the muscle on the opposite side.

Applicator

- The fingertips of your caudad hand.

Tissue tension

- Take up the primary tissue tension with compression and using a transverse force.
- Your fingertips remain hooked over the posterior aspect of the muscle.
- For greatest efficiency your caudad forearm should remain extended. However the height of the table may require that you flex it slightly.
- Lean back and using your shoulder and body weight, pull the muscle towards you.
- Pull your fingertips into, and then across, the fibres of the muscle.
- To treat levator scapula and rhomboids you must work through trapezius and so you will need to press more firmly.
- Longitudinal tension is taken up by starting the technique with the shoulder depressed.

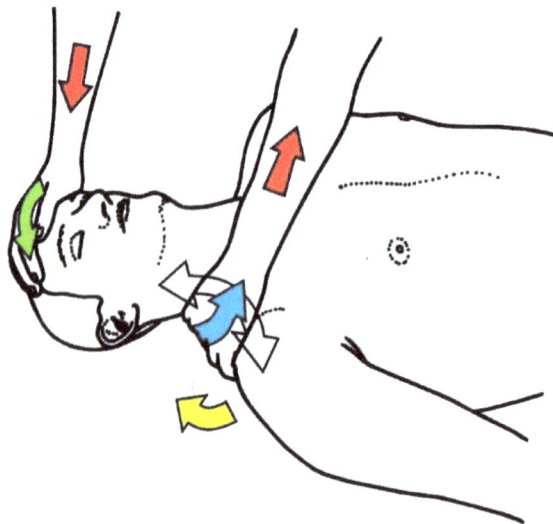

Figure 13.13

Muscle Fibres	⇕	Primary Force		Secondary Force	↻	Stretch Force		Contraction Force	

Kneading

- Maintain longitudinal tension by pushing inferiorly on the patient's shoulder with your caudad hand.
- Apply cross fibre kneading to the muscle by pulling on the muscle with your fingertips.
- Your force is perpendicular to the muscle, generally in an anterior direction.

134

- For the most superior fibres of the upper trapezius work in a lateral direction. For levator scapulae, rhomboids and the most inferior fibres of the upper trapezius work in a superior and lateral direction. For middle trapezius work in a superior direction.
- Work across the fibres from the occiput to the acromion process and down to the middle thoracic.
- Depending on the size of the patient and the size of your hand cover as much of the middle trapezius as you can reach.
- The cephalad hand may be used to hold the patient's head in a fixed position.
- Alternatively, the patient's head may be used as a lever to increase secondary tension.
- Push against the side of the patient's head and roll their head away from you.
- With your caudad hand hold back on the muscle and at the point of optimum tension increase the primary tension by pulling the muscles towards you.
- Use a synchronised push-pull action with both hands.
- Your pressure should be just short of discomfort.
- To relax the muscle, work with the patients breathing cycle, about 15 breaths per minute.
- To stimulate, increase your speed to about 40 cycles per minute.

Active component

- Ask the patient to take a deep breath in and hold it.
- Ask the patient to shrug their shoulder for 3 to 5 seconds using a 10% effort.
- Resist the patient's effort and maintain tissue lockup throughout the technique.
- Ask the patient to exhale and to relax their muscle contraction.
- As soon as you feel that the patient has relaxed their muscles completely (about 1-3 seconds), take up the tissue slack by increasing the primary and secondary tension.
- Take up the slack after each contraction and during exhalation.
- Repeat 2 or 3 times, or as required.

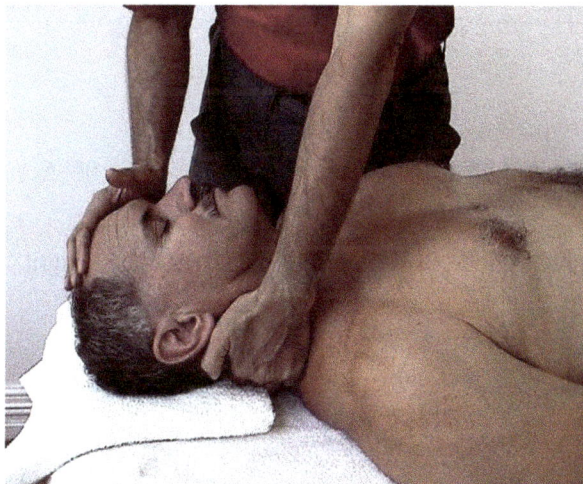

Picture 13.8

Technique 13.10 Bilateral kneading of trapezius, levator scapulae and rhomboids and fascia stretch

Patient

- Seated on a chair or low table with forearms folded.
- Their forehead rests on their forearms.

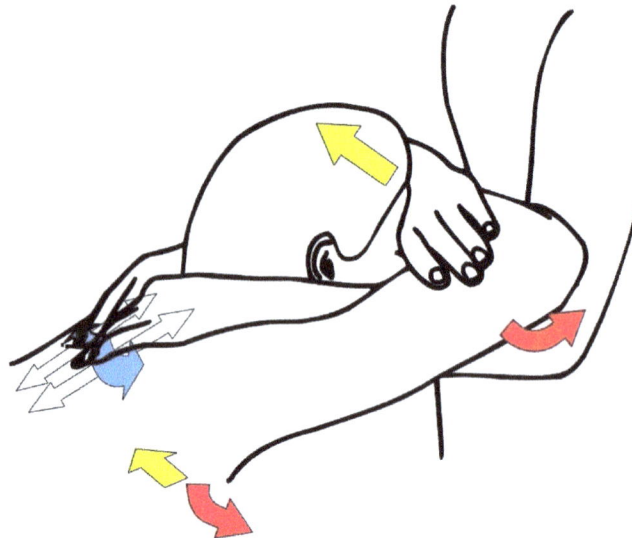

Figure 13.14

Muscle Fibres	⇕	Primary Force	⬇	Secondary Force	↻	Stretch Force	⬇	Contraction Force	⬇

Therapist

- Stand by the side of the table, facing the patient.
- Feed your hands between the patient's folded arms and their neck.
- Place your fingertips on a muscle on either side of the spine.
- The patient places their folded forearms on your forearms
- The patient leans forward and you support the patient's body weight.

Applicator

- Fingertips of both hands.

Tissue tension

- Take up the primary tissue tension with compression and a transverse force on the muscle.
- Your fingertips move superiorly and laterally across the fibres of trapezius and the deeper levator scapulae and rhomboids.
- Take up secondary tissue tension with extension of the patient's shoulders and spine.
- With sideshifting (sidebending) and rotation you can place emphasis on one side of the spine.

Kneading

- Apply a rhythmical cycle of primary and secondary forces.
- Your pressure should be just short of discomfort.
- To relax the muscle, work with the patient's breathing cycle, about 15 breaths per minute.

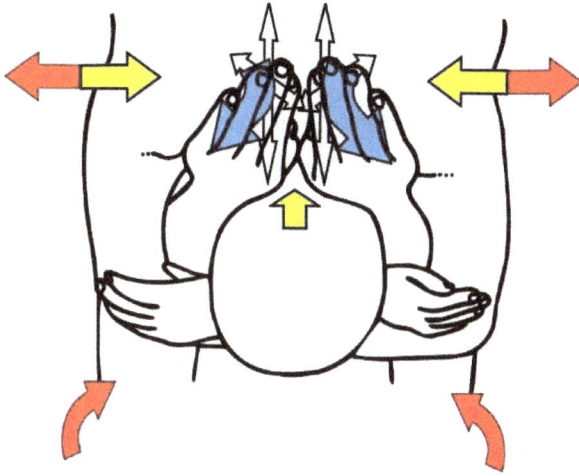 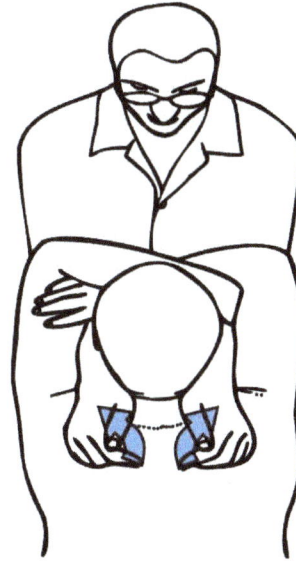

Figure 13.15   Figure 13.16

Muscle Fibres	↕	Primary Force	⬇	Secondary Force	↻	Stretch Force	⬇	Contraction Force	⬇

Active component

- Ask the patient to take a deep breath and hold it in.
- Ask the patient to attempt to squeeze their shoulder blades together for 3 to 5 seconds using a 10% effort.
- The muscles will contract.
- Resist their effort and maintain tissue lockup throughout inhalation.
- Ask the patient to exhale and to relax their muscle contraction.
- As soon as you feel that the patient has relaxed their muscles completely (about 1-3 seconds), take up the tissue slack by increasing the primary and secondary tension.
- Take up the slack after each contraction and during exhalation.
- Repeat 2 or 3 times, or as required.

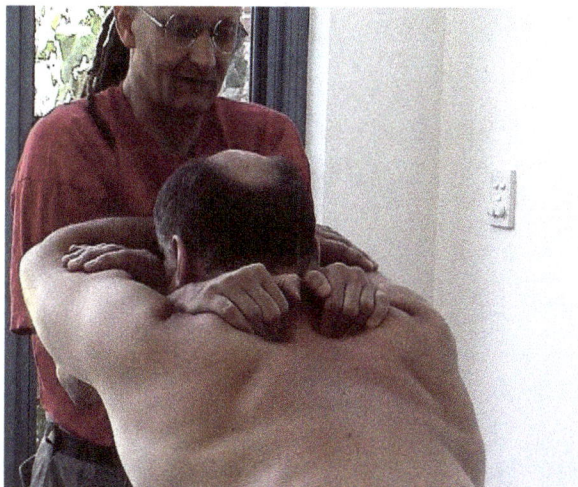

Picture 13.9

Technique 13.11 Kneading of trapezius, rhomboid and levator scapulae, and fascia stretch, using the scapula as a lever

Patient

- Supine with the head resting on a pillow or folded towel.
- The head, cervical and upper thoracic spine is sidebent away from the side you are standing.
- A rolled up towel may be placed under the patient's scapula.

Therapist

- Stand at the side of the table, adjacent to the patient's rib cage.
- Reach over the patient's shoulder and grasp the superior and medial scapular on the side you are standing, with the thumb and index finger of your caudad hand.
- Your other fingertips make contact with the muscle to be treated.
- Grasp the patient's wrist with your cephalad hand.
- Lift the patient's hand until the forearm is extended at the elbow and the arm points almost vertically towards the ceiling.

Applicator

The flexed middle, ring and little finger of your caudad hand.

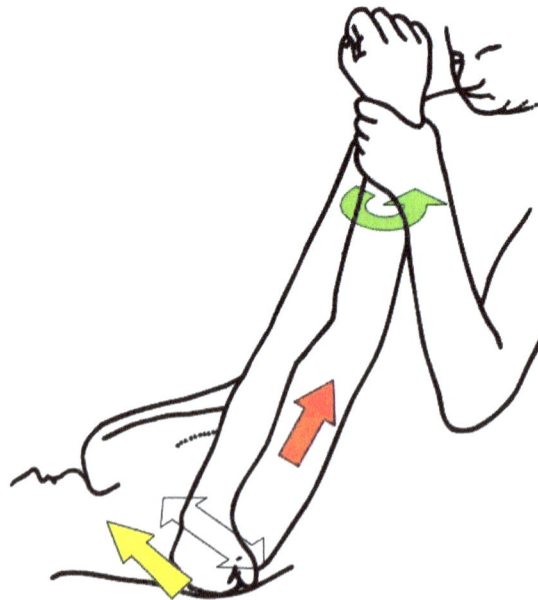

Figure 13.17

Muscle Fibres	⇕	Primary Force	⬇	Secondary Force	↻	Stretch Force	⬇	Contraction Force	⬇

Tissue tension

- Take up the primary tissue tension with compression by gradually increasing your fingertip pressure on the muscle.
- Hook your fingertips around the muscle and apply a transverse force.
- Your pressure is directed perpendicular to the muscle fibres, which for trapezius, rhomboid and levator scapulae is superior and lateral.
- Make sure your force goes through the muscle and not the scapula.
- Longitudinal tension is taken up by appropriate positioning of the scapula.

Kneading

- Apply a primary force of compression and a transverse force on the muscle with the middle, ring and little fingertips of your caudad hand.
- Longitudinal tension is produced by increasing scapula protraction, depression and downward rotation.
- Move the scapula inferiorly (depression) and laterally (protraction) with the index finger and thumb of your caudad hand.
- Pull the patient's arm up towards the ceiling with your cephalad hand to take the scapula laterally into protraction. To take the scapula into downward rotation, externally rotate the arm with your cephalad hand.
- Circumduct the patient's shoulder and at the point of optimal longitudinal tension increase the primary forces on the muscle.
- Cover the entire muscle, working as far inferiorly as your hand can reach.
- Your pressure should be just short of discomfort.
- To relax the muscle, work with the patients breathing cycle, about 15 breaths per minute.
- To stimulate, increase your speed to about 40 cycles per minute.

Active component

- Ask the patient to take a deep breath and hold it in.
- Ask the patient to shrug their shoulders or pull back their shoulders back towards the table for 3 to 5 seconds using a 10% effort.
- Resist the patient's effort and maintain tissue lockup throughout the technique.
- Ask the patient to exhale and to relax their muscle contraction.
- As soon as you feel that the patient has relaxed their muscles completely (about 1-3 seconds), take up the tissue slack by increasing the primary and longitudinal tensions.
- Take up the slack after each contraction and during exhalation.
- Repeat 2 or 3 times, or as required.

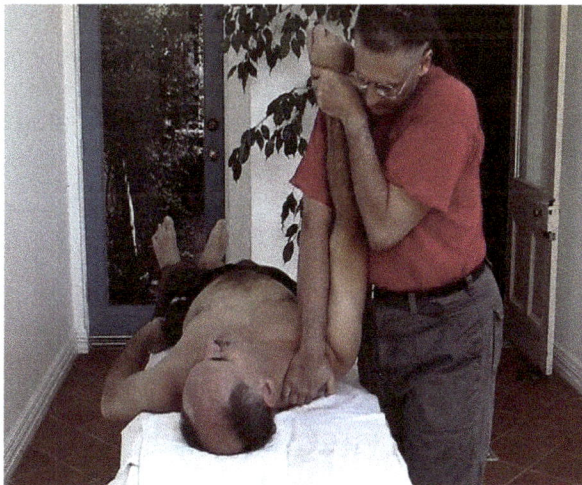

Picture 13.10

139

14. Subscapularis, rhomboid, levator scapulae and upper, middle and lower trapezius

Anatomy

Subscapularis arises from the medial two-thirds of the subscapular fossa and its tendon attaches on the lesser tubercle of humerus. Its fibres are deep and run laterally as part of the posterior axilla. It is not palpable. In flexible individuals however, some of its medial fibres may be accessible.

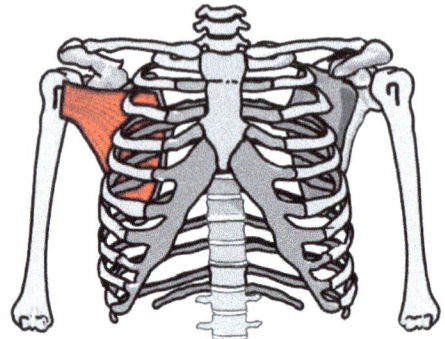

Action: Internal rotation and horizontal flexion of the humerus.
Clinical indications: Postural and tendon strain.
Nerve supply: Subscapular nerve C5 and 6.

Technique 14.1 Kneading of the interscapular and subscapular muscles using the scapula as a lever

Patient

- Prone with their head facing away from the side you are standing.
- Their arm is resting at their side.
- If the patient has normal mobility, then you will be able to flex their forearm and place their hand behind their back.

Therapist

- Stand at the side of the table level with the patient's rib cage.
- Firmly grasp the end of the shoulder over the deltoid area with your cephalad hand.
- Lift the shoulder off the table and push it medially to produce winging.
- The fingertips of your caudad hand can now access the medial area between the scapula and the rib cage.

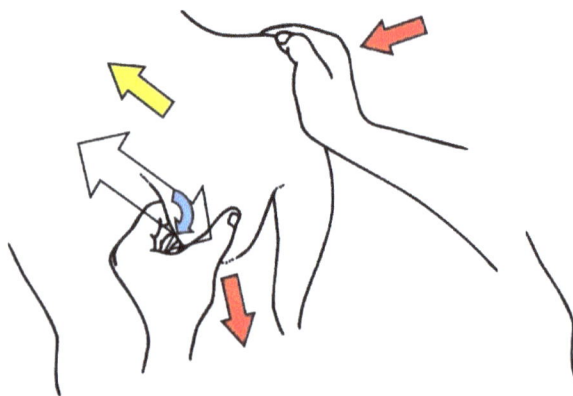

Figure 14.1

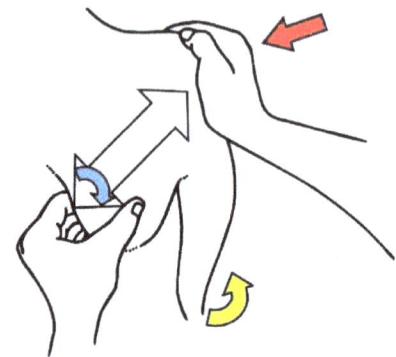

Figure 14.2

Muscle Fibres	⇕	Primary Force	⬇	Secondary Force	↻	Stretch Force	⬇	Contraction Force	⬇

You may be able to place your knee or a pillow under the patient's shoulder to maintain the winging of the scapula. This will save you having to exert effort in holding the winging, freeing your hands for better positioning of the scapula or for directly working on the muscle (see Fig 14.5).

Applicator

- The fingertips or thumb of your caudad hand.

Tissue tension

- Take up the primary tissue tension with compression by increasing your fingertip pressure and add a transverse force to the muscle by flexing your fingertips.
- Work perpendicular to the muscle. This will be in an inferior, medial or lateral direction, depending on which variation of the technique you are doing in this section.
- Longitudinal tension is taken up on the interscapular muscles by protracting and depressing the scapula
- Longitudinal tension is taken up on subscapularis by starting the technique with the arm externally rotated at the shoulder.
- Keep the muscle exposed by maintaining some winging of the scapula during the technique by holding the shoulder or supporting it with your knee or a pillow.

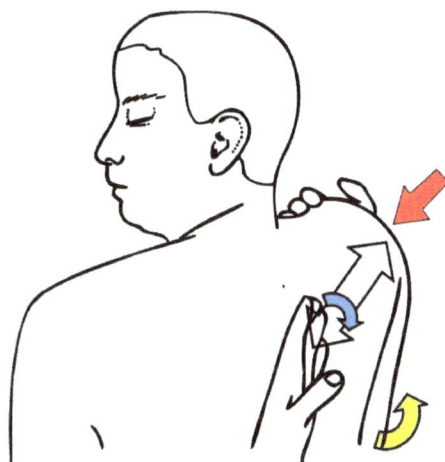

Figure 14.3

Muscle Fibres	⇕	Primary Force	⬇	Secondary Force	↻	Stretch Force	⬇	Contraction Force	⬇

Kneading

- With the fingertips or thumb of your caudad hand apply a rhythmical cycle of primary, secondary and longitudinal forces.
- Sometimes the objective of exposing the muscle for better direct manipulation by the applicator will conflict with the objective of increasing longitudinal tension.
- Work across the fibres of the interscapular and subscapular muscles.
- With your thumb or fingertips knead the muscle under the scapula.
- Here are three options for applying cross fibre kneading to the muscle.

1. Articulate the shoulder in a circular motion while maintaining fixed fingertip or thumb pressure on the muscle.
2. Articulate the shoulder in a circular motion and when the muscle is at an optimal longitudinal tension, increase the primary forces.
3. Maintain the shoulder in a fixed winged position and apply a rhythmical cycle of primary forces.

- Press more firmly through trapezius with your thumb to treat levator scapula, rhomboid and subscapularis.
- Your pressure should be just short of discomfort.
- To relax the muscle, work with the patient's breathing cycle, about 15 breaths per minute.
- To stimulate, increase your speed to about 40 cycles per minute.

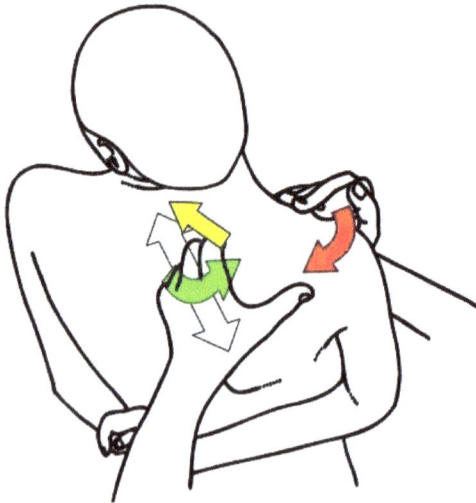
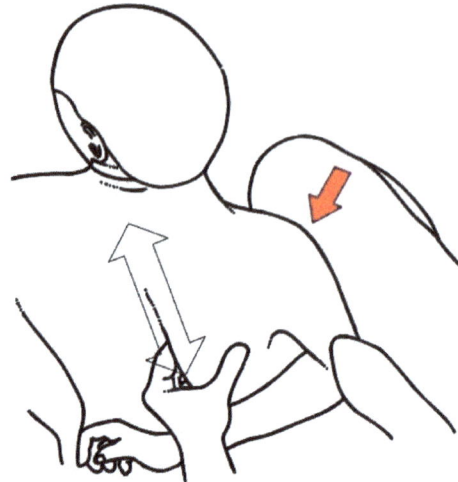

Figure 14.4   Figure 14.5

Muscle Fibres	⇕	Primary Force	⬇	Secondary Force	↺	Stretch Force	⬇	Contraction Force	⬇

Active component

- Ask the patient to take a deep breath and hold it in.
- To activate subscapularis ask the patient to rotate their arm into the table (internal rotation). To activate the interscapular muscles ask the patient to either lift their head back and up off the table, to shrug their shoulder or to squeeze their shoulder in towards their spine for 3 to 5 seconds using a 10% effort.
- Resist the patient's effort and maintain tissue lockup throughout the technique.
- Ask the patient to exhale and to relax their muscle contraction.
- As soon as you feel that the patient has relaxed their muscles completely (about 1-3 seconds), take up the tissue slack by increasing the primary, secondary and longitudinal tension.
- Take up the slack after each contraction and during exhalation.
- Repeat 2 or 3 times, or as required.

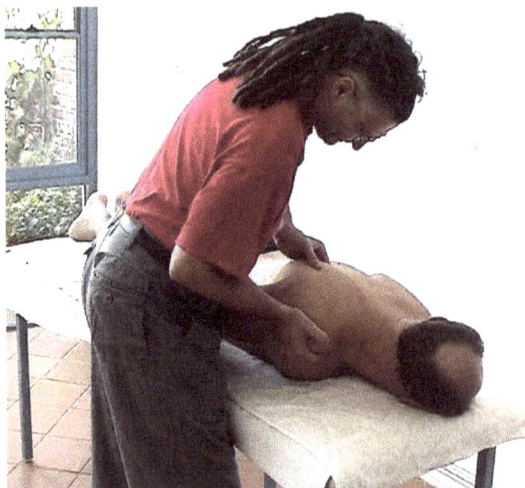

Picture 14.1

Technique 14.2 Stretch and kneading using and the scapula as a lever

Patient

- Sidelying near to the edge of the table nearest the therapist.
- The trunk should remain perpendicular to the table.
- The forearm that the patient is lying on is flexed at the elbow and rests against the front of the chest.
- The uppermost forearm is flexed and rests against the side of their chest.

Therapist

- Stand at the side of the table, in front of the patient.
- Reach under the arm and flexed forearm with your caudad hand and reach over the shoulder with your cephalad hand.
- To wing the scapula and expose the subscapularis muscle, press downward on the head of the humerus with your sternum.
- Grasp under the medial border of the scapula.
- Position the scapula so that the appropriate muscle is on stretch or exposed.
- While one hand controls the scapula the fingers of the other hand can now work across the muscle fibres.

Applicator

- The fingertips of either or both hands.

Tissue tension

- Take up the primary tissue tension with compression by gradually increasing your fingertip pressure on the muscle.
- Hook your fingertips around the muscle and apply a transverse force.
- Your pressure is directed perpendicular to the muscle fibres, which for upper trapezius, rhomboid and levator scapulae is superior and lateral. The pressure for middle trapezius and subscapularis is superior and for the lower trapezius is inferior and lateral.
- Longitudinal tension is taken up by appropriate positioning of the scapula.

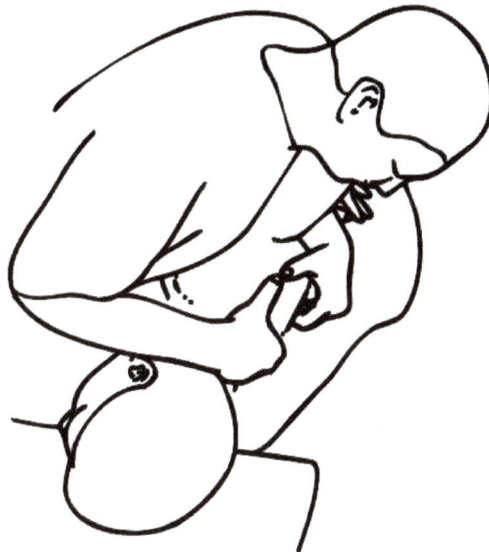

Figure 14.6

Muscle Fibres	⇕	Primary Force	⬇	Secondary Force	↺	Stretch Force	⬇	Contraction Force	⬇

143

- Longitudinal tension is produced in:

1. Rhomboids, levator scapulae and upper trapezius by increasing scapula protraction, depression and downward rotation; middle trapezius by increasing scapula protraction.
2. Lower trapezius by increasing scapula protraction, elevation and downward rotation.
3. Subscapularis by increasing shoulder external rotation.

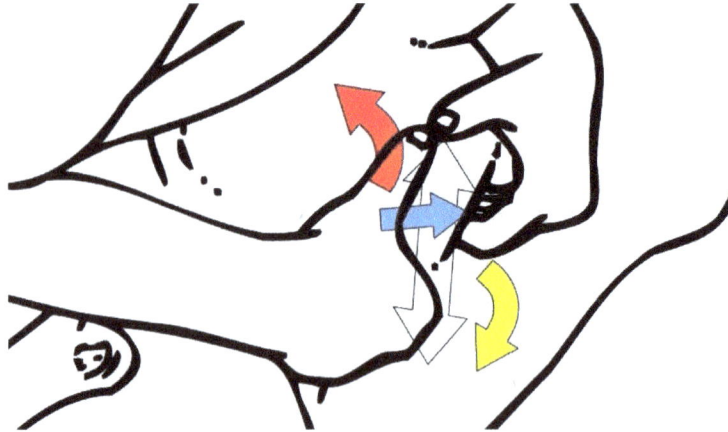

Figure 14.7

Muscle Fibres		Primary Force		Secondary Force		Stretch Force		Contraction Force	

Kneading

- Apply a primary force of compression and a transverse force on the muscle with the fingertips of your hand.
- The scapula held in one or both hands and wedged between your hands and the body of your sternum.
- Circumduct the patient's shoulder and at the point of optimal longitudinal tension increase the primary forces on the muscle.

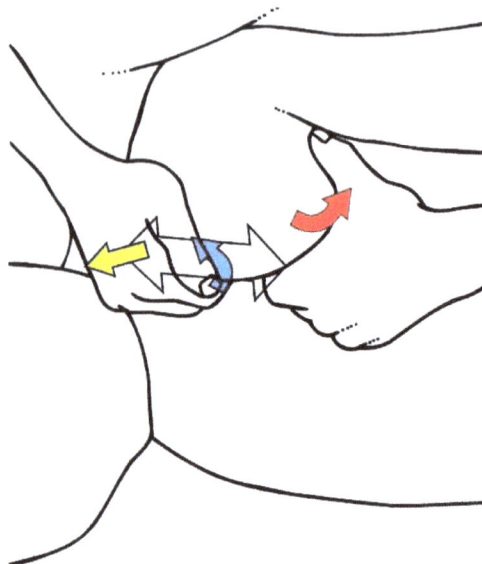

Figure 14.8

Muscle Fibres		Primary Force		Secondary Force		Stretch Force		Contraction Force	

- Apply kneading to rhomboids, levator scapulae, subscapularis or trapezius.
- Cover the entire muscle.
- Your pressure should be just short of discomfort.
- To relax the muscle, work with the patient's breathing cycle, about 15 breaths per minute.
- To stimulate, increase your speed to about 40 cycles per minute.

Active component

- Ask the patient to take a deep breath in and hold it.
- To activate subscapularis ask the patient to internally rotate their arm by pushing their hand against the abdomen.
- To activate the interscapular muscles ask the patient to lift their head up off the table, shrug their shoulder, squeeze their shoulder in towards their spine or pull their shoulder down towards their feet for 3 to 5 seconds using a 10% effort.
- Resist the patient's effort and maintain tissue lockup throughout the technique.
- Ask the patient to exhale and to relax their muscle contraction.
- As soon as you feel that the patient has relaxed their muscles completely (about 1-3 seconds) take up the tissue slack by increasing the primary and longitudinal tensions.
- Take up the slack after each contraction and during exhalation.
- Repeat 2 or 3 times or as required.

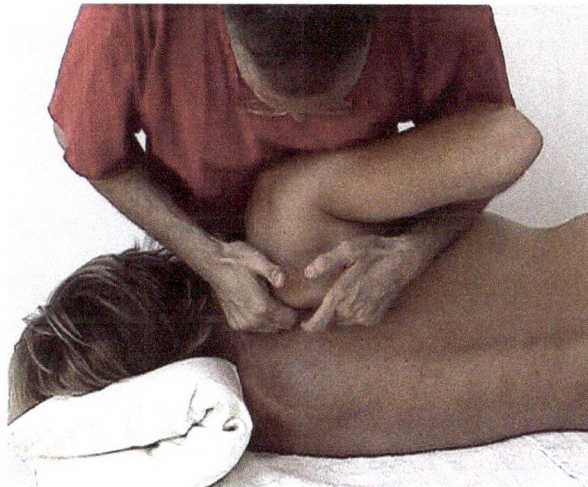

Picture 14.2

Technique 14.3 Kneading using the humerus and scapula as a lever

Patient
- Sidelying near to the edge of the table closest to the therapist and facing the therapist.
- The trunk should remain perpendicular to the table.
- The forearm of the arm that the patient is lying on is flexed at the elbow and rests against the front of their chest.

Therapist

- Stand at the side of the table, in front of the patient and adjacent to their rib cage.
- The patient's uppermost arm is partially abducted and draped over your cephalad arm.
- Further abduct and extend the patient's arm with your cephalad shoulder.
- Position and control the patient's scapula with one or both hands.

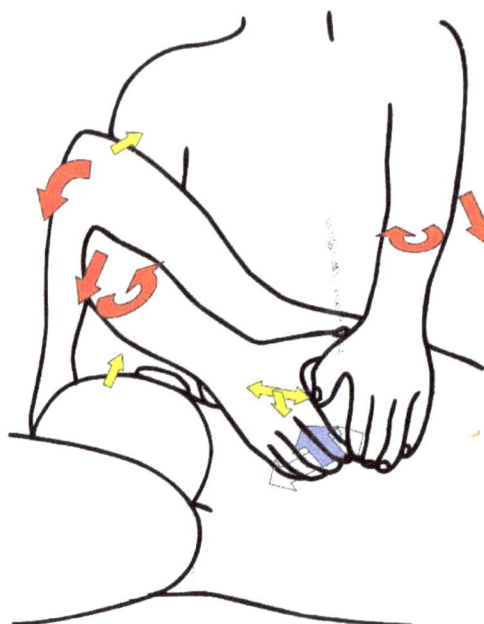

Figure 14.9

Muscle Fibres	⇕	Primary Force	⬇	Secondary Force	↻	Stretch Force	⬇	Contraction Force	⬇

Applicator

- All fingertips of one or both hands.

Tissue tension

- Take up the primary tissue tension with compression and add a transverse force by pulling on muscles with your fingertips.
- Take up the secondary tissue tension by increasing abduction and extension of the patient's arm with your cephalad shoulder.
- To increase longitudinal tension a pillow can be placed under the patient's rib cage to sidebend their thoracic and cervical spine towards the table.

Kneading

- Apply a rhythmical cycle of primary and secondary forces.
- When the muscle is at an optimal level of secondary tension add compression and increase the transverse pressure.
- Your pressure should be just short of discomfort.
- To relax the muscle, work with the patient's breathing cycle, about 15 breaths per minute.
- To stimulate, increase your speed to about 40 cycles per minute.

Active component

- Ask the patient to take a deep breath and hold it in.
- Ask the patient to try to lift their head up off the table, shrug their shoulder, squeeze their shoulder in towards their spine, bring their arm down to their side or pull their shoulder down towards their feet for 3 to 5 seconds using a 10% effort. The interscapular muscles will contract.
- Resist their effort and maintain tissue lockup throughout the technique.
- Ask the patient to exhale and to relax their muscle contraction.
- As soon as you feel that the patient has relaxed their spinal muscles completely (about 1-3 seconds), take up the tissue slack by increasing the primary and secondary tension.
- Take up the slack after each contraction and during exhalation.
- Repeat 2 or 3 times, or as required.

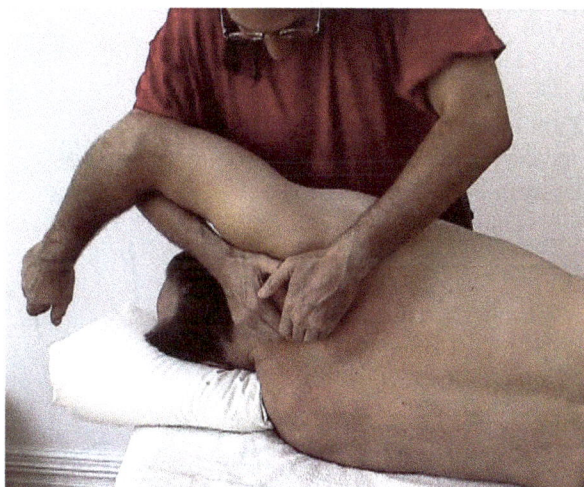

Picture 14.3

15. Supraspinatus

Anatomy

The **Supraspinatus** arises from the medial two thirds of the supraspinatus fossa, passes under the acromion and it's tendon attaches on the top of the greater tubercle of humerus. It is palpable deep to trapezius. The tendon merges with the capsule of the shoulder joint and is the most frequently strained of the rotator cuff muscles.

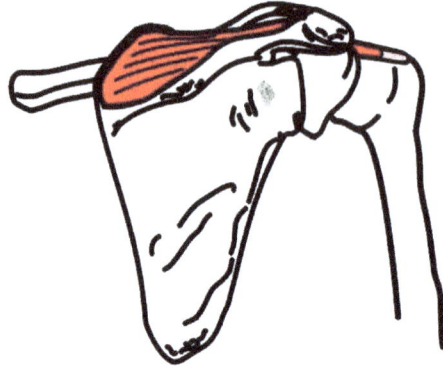

Action: Starter of abduction and stabiliser.
Clinical indications: Partial or complete rupture of the tendon, subacromial bursitis.
Nerve supply: Suprascapular nerve C4, **5** & 6

Technique 15.1 Inhibition for supraspinatus

Patient

- Prone with their head rotated away from you.

Therapist

- Stand by the side of the table, near to the head end.
- Grasp the patient's forearm and flex their elbow to ninety degrees.
- Place the patient's forearm behind their back.

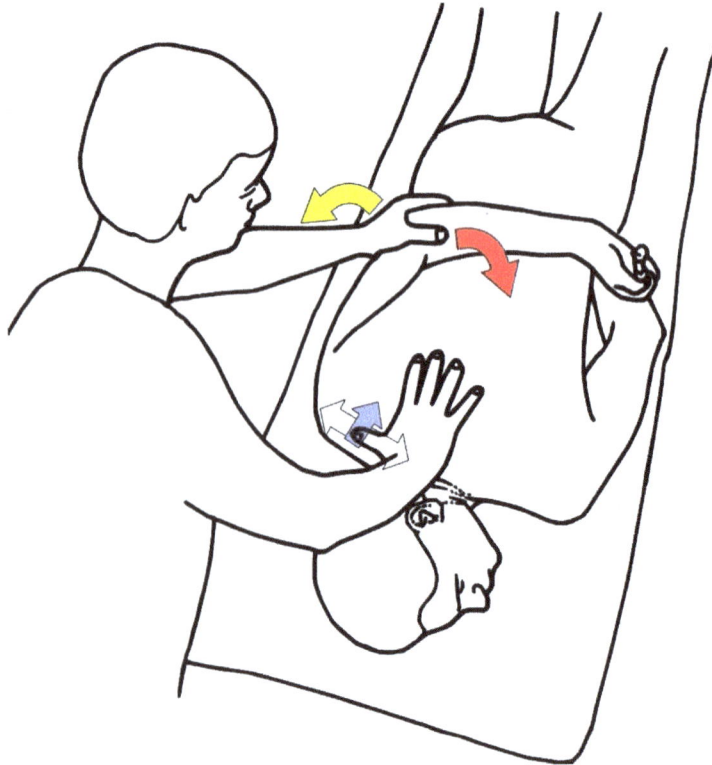

Figure 15.1

Muscle Fibres	⇕	Primary Force	⬇	Secondary Force	↻	Stretch Force	⬇	Contraction Force	⬇

148

- Grasp the patient's elbow with your caudad hand.
- The applicator of your cephalad hand makes contact on the muscle to be treated.

Applicator

- Pad of thumb.

Tissue tension

- Take up the primary tissue tension with your applicator applying compression on the muscle.
- Take up the longitudinal tension with adduction of the shoulder, applied by the caudad hand on the patient's elbow.

Inhibition

- Apply compression on the area of muscle covered by your thumb.
- Your pressure should be just short of discomfort.
- To relax the muscle work with the patients breathing cycle, about 15 breaths per minute.
- Maintain some compression throughout the technique, but increase it during exhalation.

Active component

- Ask the patient to take a deep breath and hold it in.
- Ask the patient to attempt to push their elbow sideways (abduct their arm) for 3 to 5 seconds using a 10% effort. The supraspinatus muscles will contract.
- Resist their effort and maintain tissue compression throughout inhalation.
- Ask the patient to exhale and to relax their muscle contraction.
- As soon as you feel that the patient has relaxed their muscle completely (about 1-3 seconds), take up the tissue slack by increasing compression and positioning the arm in further adduction. You may need to lift the elbow slightly if the forearm sticks to the patients skin.
- Take up the slack after each contraction and during exhalation.
- Repeat 2 or 3 times, or as required.

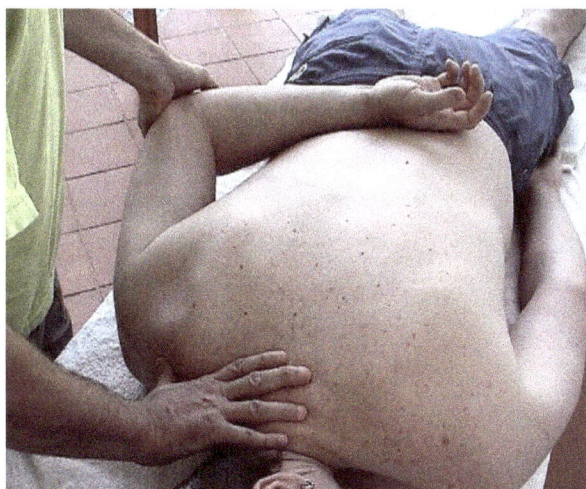

Picture 15.1

16. Infraspinatus

Anatomy

Infraspinatus arises from the medial two thirds of the infraspinatus fossa and the tendon attaches to the middle of the greater tubercle of the humerus. The muscle is palpable but the medial fibres are deep to trapezius and the lateral fibres are covered by posterior deltoid. Sometimes it is merged with teres minor. The tendon merges with the capsule of the shoulder joint but sometime it is separated from the capsule by a bursa.
Actions: External rotation and horizontal extension of the shoulder. A stabiliser of the shoulder joint.
Clinical indications: Overuse, bursitis and tendon strain.
Nerve supply: Suprascapular nerve C**5** & 6.

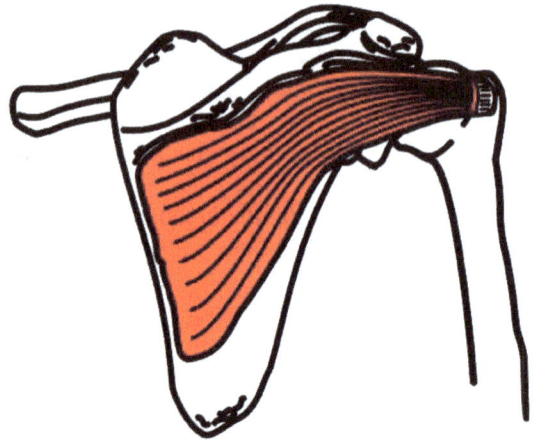

Technique 16.1 Kneading of infraspinatus

Patient

- Prone with their head rotated away from the side you are standing.

Therapist

- Stand at the head of the table, near to the muscle on the side you are treating.
- Grasp the patient's wrist with your caudad hand. Abduct the patient's shoulder ninety degrees and flex their elbow ninety degrees.
- The applicator of your cephalad hand makes contact on the muscle to be treated.

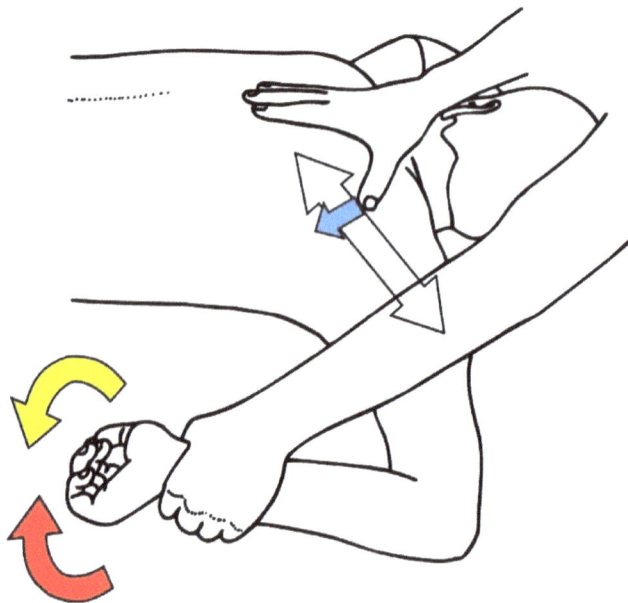

Figure 16.1

Muscle Fibres	⇕	Primary Force	⬇	Secondary Force	↻	Stretch Force	⬇	Contraction Force	⬇

150

Applicator

- The lateral side of your thumb or your pisiform bone.

Tissue tension

- Take up the primary tissue tension with your applicator, applying compression and a transverse pressure on the muscle.
- Take up the longitudinal tension with internal rotation of the shoulder, applied by the caudad hand.

Kneading

- Apply a rhythmical cycle of primary and longitudinal forces.
- When the muscle is at an optimal longitudinal tension increase the primary forces.
- Your pressure should be just short of discomfort.
- To relax the muscle, work with the patient's breathing cycle, about 15 breaths per minute.
- To stimulate, increase your speed to about 40 cycles per minute.

Active component

- Ask the patient to take a deep breath and hold it in.
- Ask the patient to attempt to push their wrist down towards the floor for 3 to 5 seconds using a 10% effort. The infraspinatus will contract.
- Resist their effort and maintain tissue lockup throughout inhalation. You may need to place your forearm against their forearm to prevent their elbow from lifting up (horizontal extension at the shoulder).
- Ask the patient to exhale and to relax their muscle contraction.
- As soon as you feel that the patient has relaxed their infraspinatus muscle completely (about 1-3 seconds), take up the tissue slack by increasing the primary and longitudinal tension.
- Take up the slack after each contraction and during exhalation.
- Repeat 2 or 3 times, or as required.

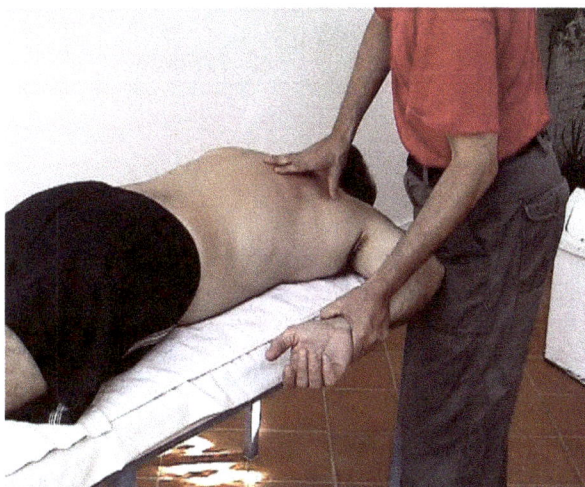

Picture 16.1

Technique 16.2 Stretch for infraspinatus and teres minor

Patient

- Sidelying with the patient's uppermost hand behind their back.

Therapist

- Stand at the side of the table facing the patient.
- Reach over the patient and grasp their elbow with your caudad hand.
- Grasp the patient's shoulder with your cephalad hand.

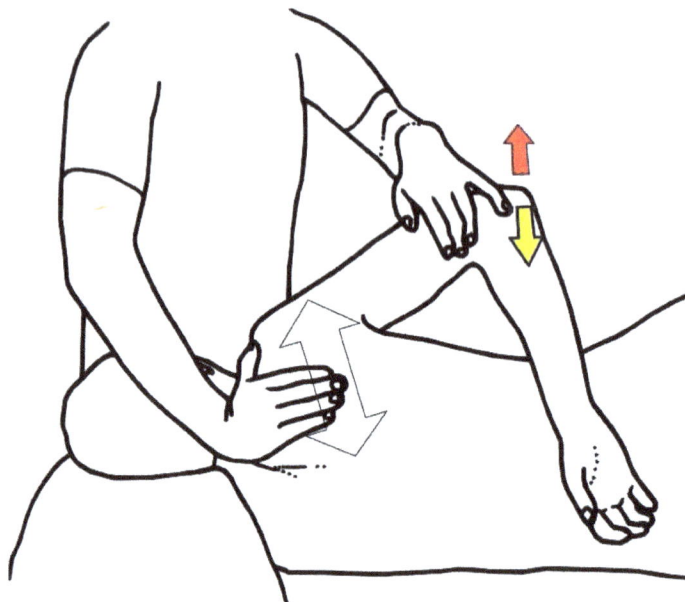

Figure 16.2

Muscle Fibres	↕	Primary Force	⬇	Secondary Force	↻	Stretch Force	⬇	Contraction Force	⬇

Tissue tension

- Hold the patient's scapula firmly against their rib cage.
- Pull the patient's elbow forwards towards you.
- Take up the longitudinal tension with shoulder internal rotation.
- Apply a slow rhythmical cycle of longitudinal force.
- A stronger stretch can be obtained by slightly abducting the patient's arm.

Active component

- Ask the patient to take a deep breath and hold it in.
- Ask them to attempt to push their elbow backwards for 3 to 5 seconds using a 10% effort.
- The infraspinatus and teres minor will contract.
- Resist their effort and maintain tissue lockup throughout inhalation.
- Ask the patient to exhale and to relax their muscle contraction.
- As soon as you feel that the patient has relaxed their muscles completely (about 1-3 seconds), take up the tissue slack by increasing the longitudinal tension.
- Take up the slack after each contraction and during exhalation.
- Repeat 2 or 3 times, or as required.

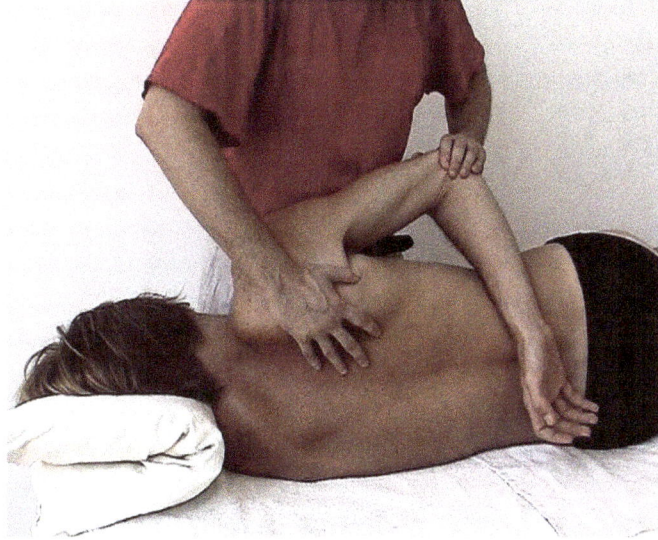

Picture 16.2

17. Teres minor

Anatomy

Teres minor arises as a muscle from the upper two thirds of a strip along the posterior and lateral border of the scapula and the tendon attaches to the lower part of the greater tubercle of the humerus. It is palpable but its medial fibres are deep to the upper borders of latissimus dorsi and laterally it is covered by posterior deltoid. The tendon merges with the capsule of the shoulder joint.

Action: External rotation and horizontal extension of the humerus.
Nerve supply: Axillary nerve C**5** and 6.

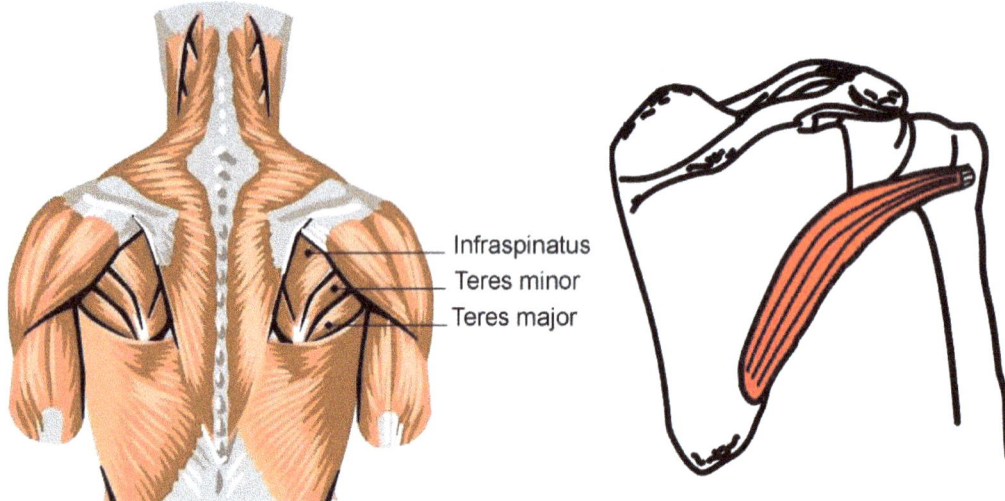

Infraspinatus
Teres minor
Teres major

Technique 17.1 Kneading of teres minor

Patient

- Prone with their head rotated away from the side you are standing.

Therapist

- Stand at the side of the table, at the level of the patient's shoulder.
- Grasp the patient's arm with your cephalad hand.
- Abduct the patient's shoulder 90 degrees.
- The applicator of your caudad hand makes contact on the muscle to be treated.

Applicator

- The tip or pad of the thumb of your caudad hand.

Tissue tension

- With the applicator of your caudad hand take up the primary tissue tension by applying compression and a transverse force on the muscle.
- With your cephalad hand take up the longitudinal tension with internal rotation and further abduction of the shoulder.

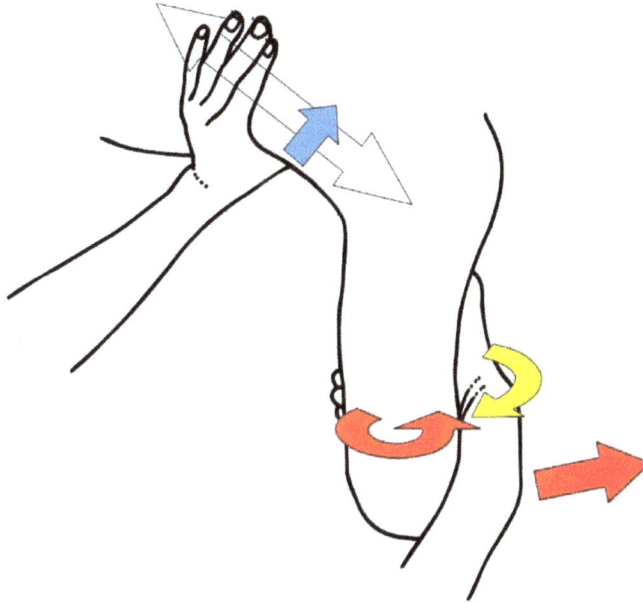

Figure 17.1

Muscle Fibres	↕	Primary Force	⬇	Secondary Force	↺	Stretch Force	⬇	Contraction Force	⬇

Kneading

- Apply a rhythmical cycle of primary and longitudinal forces.
- When the muscle is at an optimal longitudinal tension increase the primary forces.
- Your pressure should be just short of discomfort.
- To relax the muscle, work with the patient's breathing cycle, about 15 breaths per minute.
- To stimulate, increase your speed to about 40 cycles per minute.

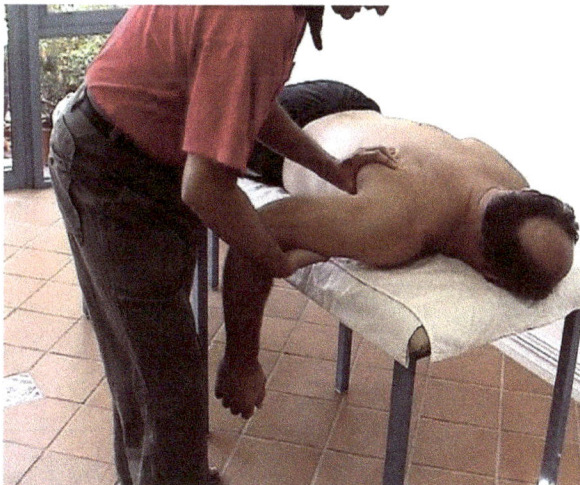

Picture 17.1

Technique 17.2 Kneading of teres minor

Patient

- Prone with their head rotated away from the side you are standing.

Therapist

- Stand at the side of the table, at the level of the patient's lower rib cage.
- Grasp the patient's wrist with your cephalad hand. Abduct the patient's shoulder 90 degrees and flex their elbow 90 degrees.
- The applicator of your caudad hand makes contact on the muscle to be treated.
- Grasp the muscle through latissimus dorsi.

Applicator

- The thumb and fingertips of your caudad hand.

Tissue tension

- Take up the primary tissue tension with your thumb applying compression and transverse pressure on the muscle.
- Take up the secondary tension with your fingers applying rotation (torsion) pressure on the muscle.
- With your cephalad hand take up the longitudinal tension with internal rotation and further abduction of the shoulder.

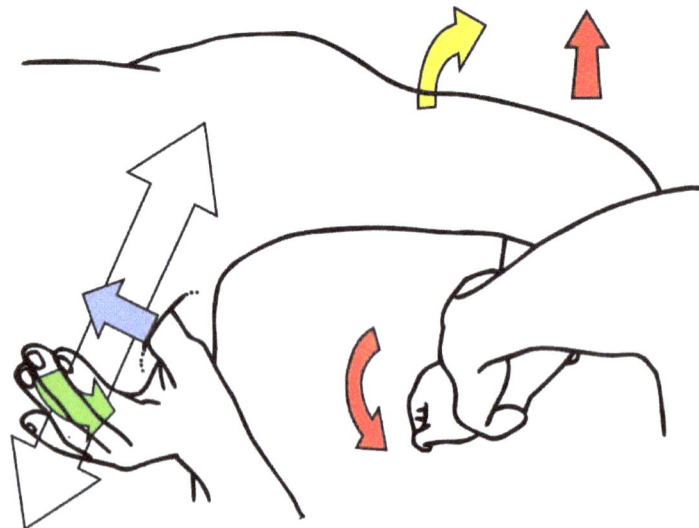

Figure 17.2

Muscle Fibres		Primary Force		Secondary Force		Stretch Force		Contraction Force	

Kneading

- Apply a rhythmical cycle of primary, secondary and longitudinal forces.
- When the muscle is at an optimal longitudinal tension increase the primary and secondary forces.
- Your pressure should be just short of discomfort.
- To relax the muscle, work with the patients breathing cycle, about 15 breaths per minute.
- To stimulate, increase your speed to about 40 cycles per minute.

Active component

- Ask the patient to take a deep breath and hold it in.
- Ask the patient to attempt to push their wrist down towards the floor and up towards their head or rotate their arm outwards (external rotation) for 3 to 5 seconds using a 10% effort. Teres minor will contract.
- Resist their effort and maintain tissue lockup throughout inhalation.
- Ask the patient to exhale and to relax their muscle contraction.
- As soon as you feel that the patient has relaxed the muscle completely (about 1-3 seconds), take up the tissue slack by increasing the primary, secondary and longitudinal tension.
- Take up the slack after each contraction and during exhalation.
- Repeat 2 or 3 times, or as required.

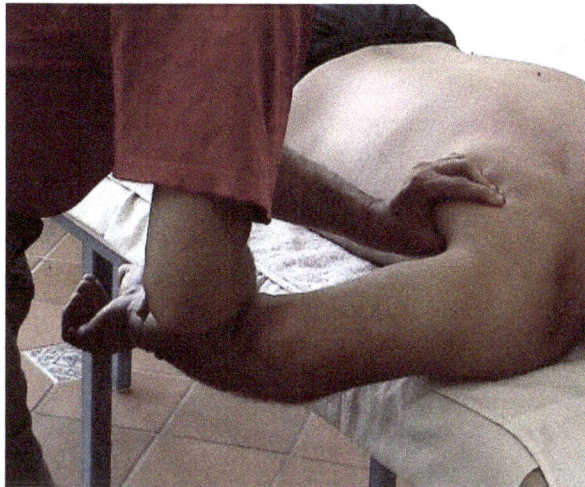

Picture 17.2

18. Pectoralis major

Anatomy

Pectoralis major is a thick triangular muscle which defines the anterior axillary fold. It can be emphasised by pressing the hands on the hips. Its upper part, the clavicular fibres, arises from the medial half of the clavicle. Its lower part, the sternocostal fibres, arises from the anterior surface of the sternum and costal cartilages of ribs 2 to 6. It merges with the aponeurosis of the external oblique muscle. The two heads unite on a narrow flat tendon about 5 cm wide, which passes deep to the deltoid to insert on the lateral crest of the bicipital groove/intertubercular sulcus of the humerus. Fibres from the tendon form a cover over the bicipital groove and some merge with the capsular ligaments.

Superficial to pectoralis major are deep and superficial layers of fascia, platysma, supraclavicular nerves and mammary glands. Deep to pectoralis major is the sternum, ribs, costal cartilages, clavipectoral fascia, subclavius, serratus anterior, intercostal and pectoralis minor muscle.

Action: Clavicular fibres: Flexion, medial rotation, and horizontal flexion of the humerus. Sternocostal fibres: Extension, adduction, medial rotation and horizontal flexion of the humerus. Forced inhalation.
Clinical indications: Shortness resulting in postural dysfunctions and muscle or tendon strain.
Nerve supply: Medial and lateral pectoral nerves. C5 and **6** supply the clavicular fibres. C**7**, **8** and T1 supply the sternocostal fibres.

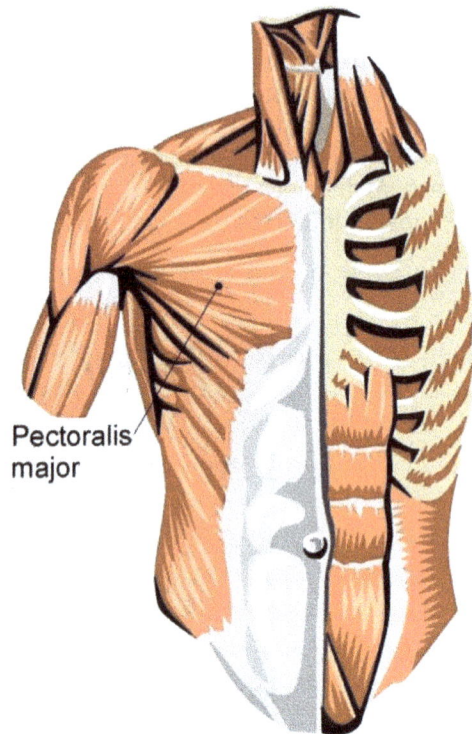

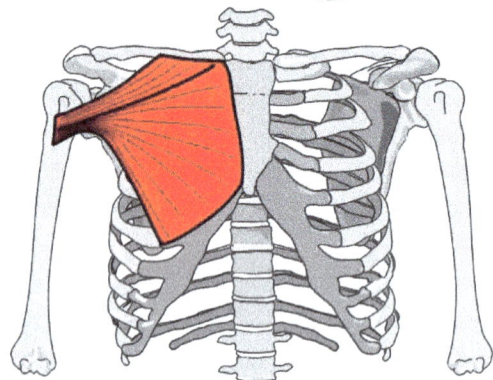

Pectoralis major

Technique 18.1 Stretch for pectoralis major and minor and fascia

Patient

- Seated with legs straight along the length of the table.
- The fingers of both hands are interlaced behind the head.

Therapist

- Stand at the head of the table.
- Flex your hip and knee and place your thigh and leg on the table so that your knee points down the middle of the table.
- You should be standing on one leg.
- Ask the patient to slowly curl back down to the table until they rest over your thigh.
- Reach over the front of the patient's arms and forearms.
- Grasp the patient's scapulae, one in either hand.

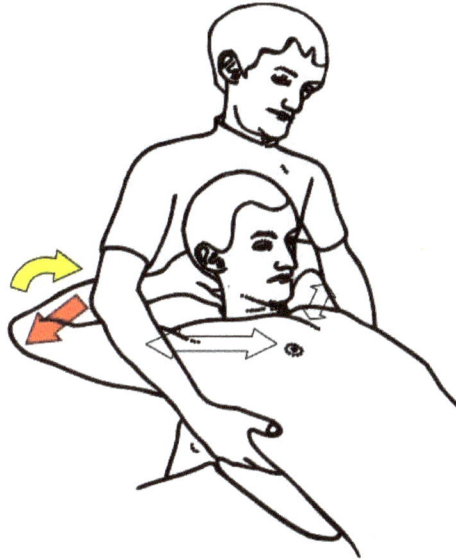

Figure 18.1

Muscle Fibres	↕	Primary Force	⬇	Secondary Force	↻	Stretch Force	⬇	Contraction Force	⬇

Tissue tension

- Take up the longitudinal tension with shoulder abduction and traction.
- Hold back on the patient's shoulders with your forearms.
- Use sideshifting (sidebending) to emphasise one side.
- Apply a slow rhythmical cycle of longitudinal forces.

Active component

- Ask the patient to take a deep breath and hold it in.
- Ask the patient to attempt to push both their elbows forwards and downwards towards their feet for 3 to 5 seconds using a 10% effort.
- The pectoralis major and minor will contract.
- Resist their effort and maintain tissue lockup throughout inhalation.
- Ask the patient to exhale and to relax their muscle contraction.
- As soon as you feel that the patient has relaxed their muscles completely (about 1-3 seconds), take up the tissue slack by increasing the longitudinal tension.
- Take up the slack after each contraction and during exhalation.
- Repeat 2 or 3 times, or as required.

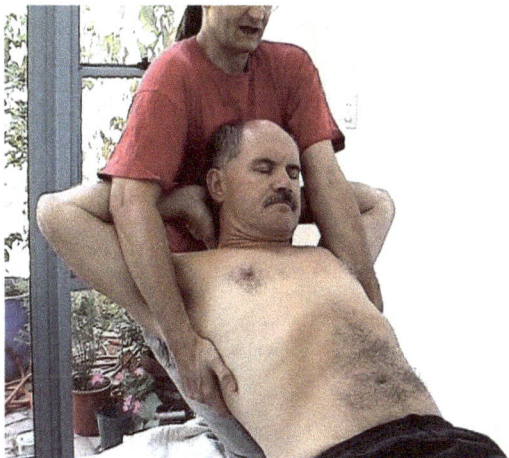

Picture 18.1

Technique 18.2 Stretch for upper pectoralis major and cervical pectoral fascia

Patient

- Supine with the head straight.
- A rolled up towel or your thigh flexed at the knee may be placed under the patient's thoracic spine.
- For unilateral treatment of pectoralis major a towel may be placed under one of the patient's scapula, or the patient positioned so that one shoulder hangs over the edge of the table.

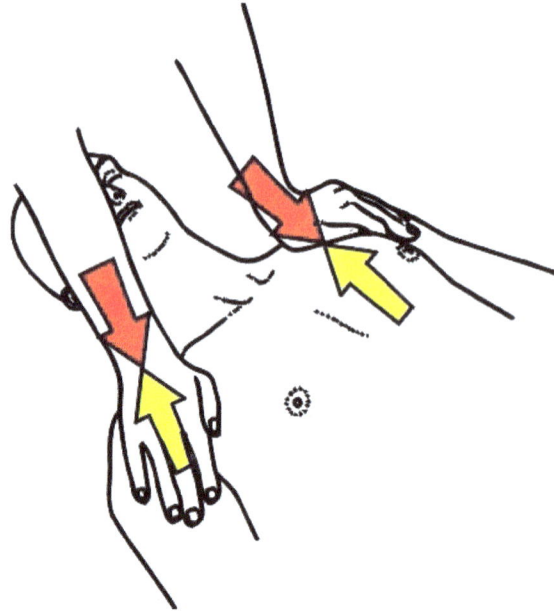

Figure 18.2

Muscle Fibres	⇕	Primary Force	⬇	Secondary Force	↻	Stretch Force	⬇	Contraction Force	⬇

Therapist

- Stand at the head of the table.
- Place the heal of your left hand just in front of the patient's left acromion process and the heal of your right hand just in front of the patient's right acromion process.

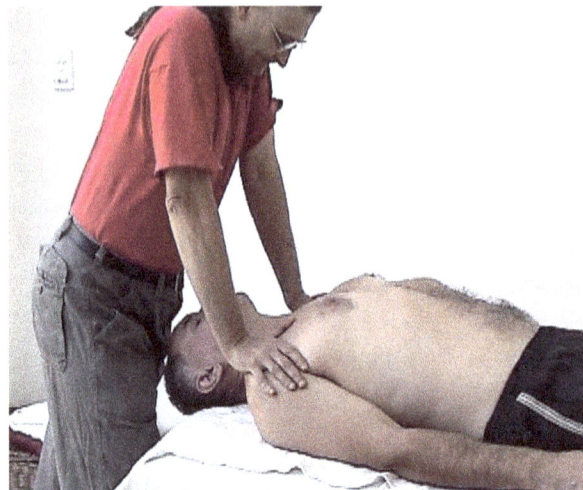

Picture 18.2

160

Stretch

- Press with your hands on both shoulders simultaneously for a bilateral stretch, or emphasis one side for a unilateral stretch.
- Keep both your elbows extended and use your body weight.
- Inferior and posterior pressure stretches the clavicular part of pectoralis major.
- Posterior pressure stretches the sternal-costal part of pectoralis major and fascia.

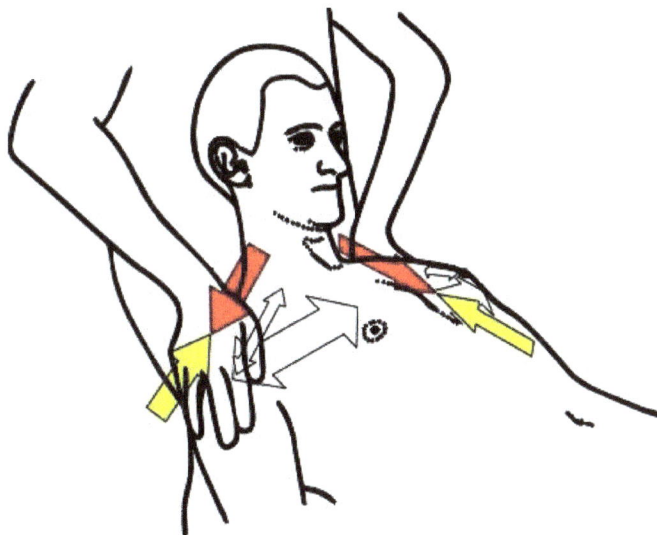

Figure 18.3

Muscle Fibres	⇕	Primary Force	⬇	Secondary Force	↻	Stretch Force	⬇	Contraction Force	⬇

Active component

- Ask the patient to take a deep breath and hold it in.
- Ask the patient to attempt to lift their shoulders up and off the table for 3 to 5 seconds using a 10% effort.
- Resist the patient's effort and maintain tissue lockup throughout the technique.
- Ask the patient to exhale and to relax their muscle contraction.
- As soon as you feel that the patient has relaxed their muscles completely (about 1-3 seconds), take up the tissue slack by increasing the primary tension (compression) and longitudinal tension by further depressing the scapula or sidebending the head.
- Take up the slack after each contraction and during exhalation.
- Repeat 2 or 3 times, or as required

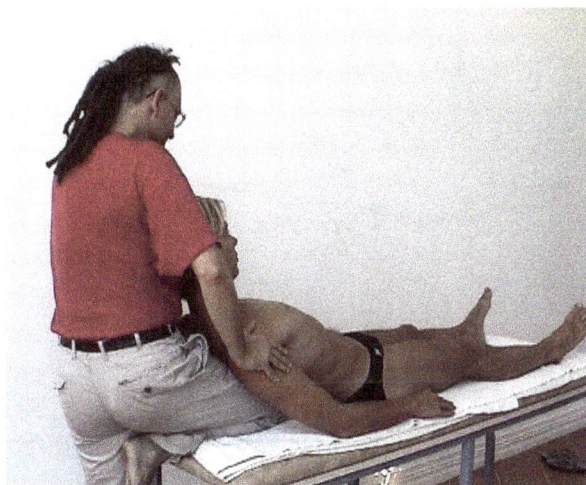

Picture 18.3

Technique 18.3 Kneading of pectoralis major in a sidelying position

Patient

- Sidelying with the front of the body near to the side of the table that you are standing.
- The head is resting on a pillow or folded towel.
- The trunk should remain perpendicular to the table.
- The forearm the patient is lying on is flexed at the elbow and rests against the front of their chest.
- The uppermost arm is abducted.

Therapist

- Stand at the head of the table, near to the side the patient is facing.
- Grasp the patient's uppermost arm with your cephalad hand or drape it over your arm.
- The patient's arm is abducted.
- Press into the muscle with your applicator.

Applicator

- Thumb, pisiform or heel of your caudad hand.

Tissue tension

- Take up the primary tissue tension with compression and add a transverse force by pushing from medial to lateral across the muscle with your applicator.
- Take up the longitudinal tension by abducting, extending, externally rotating and adding traction to the patient's arm with your cephalad hand.
- To increase longitudinal tension further a pillow may be placed under the patient's rib cage to sidebend their spine towards the table.

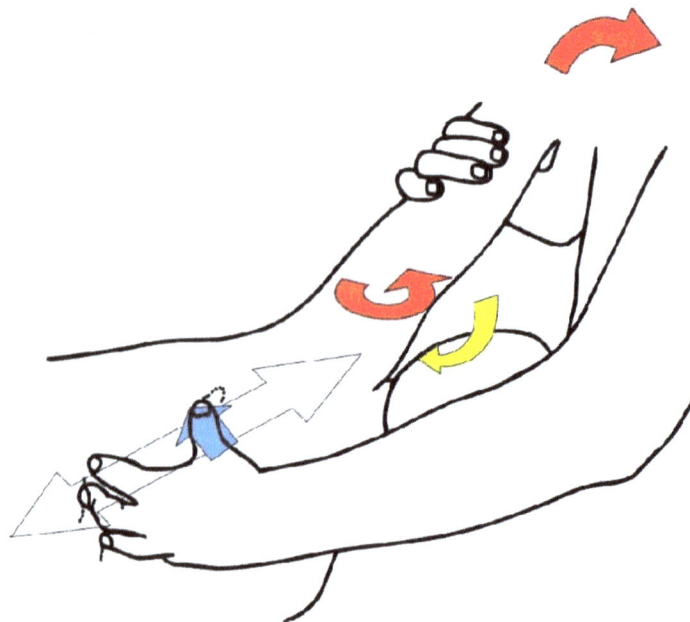

Figure 18.4

Muscle Fibres	⇕	Primary Force	⬇	Secondary Force	↺	Stretch Force	⬇	Contraction Force	⬇

Kneading

- Apply a rhythmical cycle of primary and longitudinal forces.
- Circumduct the patient's shoulder and when the muscle is at an optimal level of longitudinal tension increase the compression and transverse pressure.
- Apply cross fibre kneading from medial to lateral.
- Your pressure should be just short of discomfort.
- To relax the muscle, work with the patient's breathing cycle, about 15 breaths per minute.
- To stimulate, increase your speed to about 40 cycles per minute.

Active component

- Ask the patient to take a deep breath and hold it in.
- Ask the patient to try to bring their arm forwards and down towards their feet (extension) or rotate their arm so their thumb points down towards their feet (internal rotation) for 3 to 5 seconds using a 20% effort. The pectoralis major will contract.
- Resist their effort and maintain tissue lockup throughout the technique.
- Ask the patient to exhale and to relax their muscle contraction.
- As soon as you feel that the patient has relaxed their muscle completely (about 1-3 seconds), take up the tissue slack by increasing the primary and longitudinal tension.
- Take up the slack after each contraction and during exhalation.
- Repeat 2 or 3 times, or as required.

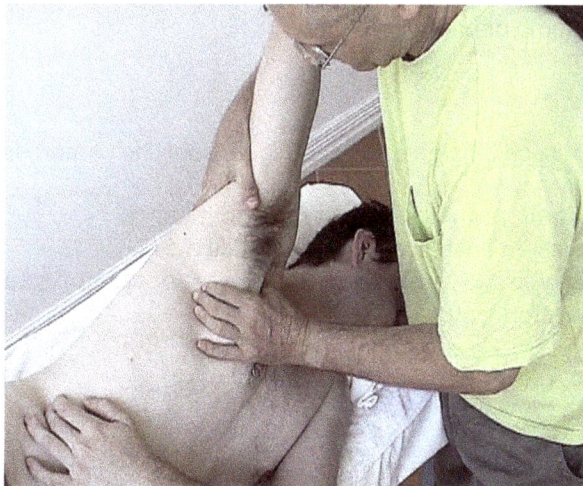

Picture 18.4

Technique 18.4 Kneading of pectoralis major with latissimus dorsi in a seated position

Patient

- Seated at the end of the table with legs hanging over the side of the table.
- Both arms hang at the side and the hands rest on their lap.

Therapist

- Stands at the head of the table, at the patient's side and facing the patient.
- Place the body of your sternum against the patient's shoulder.
- Ask the patient to slightly abduct the arm, which is furthest from you.
- Reach in front of the patient's chest and grasp their pectoralis major.
- Reach behind the patient's back and grasp their latissimus dorsi.
- Your fingers should sit high up in the axilla and the pads of your thumbs rest outside the axilla on the respective muscles.
- With both hands lift the shoulder and support its weight.
- The patient's trunk is pulled towards and sandwiched between your sternum and hands for stability.

Applicator

- The fingertips and thumb of one hand.

Tissue tension

- Take up the primary tissue tension with your fingers applying compression and a transverse force on the muscle.
- Pull up and then towards you with the fingers of both hands.
- Use latissimus dorsi as an anchor to treat pectoralis major.
- Take up the secondary tissue tension with your thumb applying a rotation force (torsion).
- Push down and away from you.

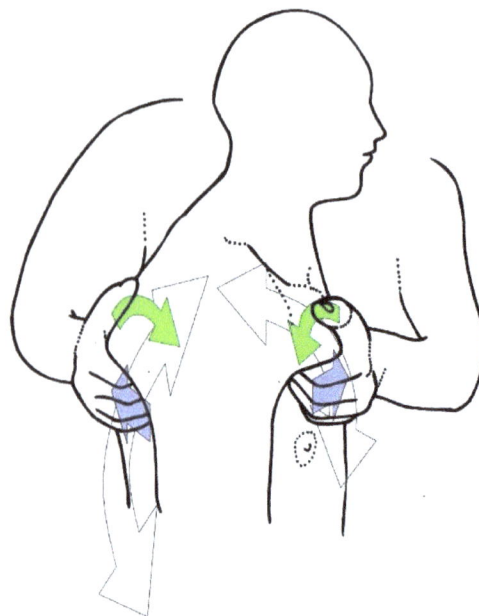

Figure 18.5

Muscle Fibres	⇕	Primary Force	⬇	Secondary Force	↻	Stretch Force	⬇	Contraction Force	⬇

164

Kneading

- Apply a rhythmical cycle of primary and secondary forces with your fingertips and thumb.
- When the muscle is at an optimal longitudinal tension increase the primary and secondary forces.
- Alternatively make a circle with the patient's shoulder girdle while maintaining primary and secondary pressure with your applicator.
- Your pressure should be just short of discomfort.
- To relax the muscle, work with the patient's breathing cycle, about 15 breaths per minute.
- To stimulate, increase your speed to about 40 cycles per minute.

Active component

- Ask the patient to take a deep breath and hold it in.
- Ask the patient to pull their shoulder down towards the floor (depress their shoulder) and pull their arm into the side of their body (adduct their shoulder) for 3 to 5 seconds using a 10% effort. Pectoralis major will contract.
- Resist the patient's effort.
- Maintain tissue lockup throughout inhalation.
- Ask the patient to exhale and to relax their muscle contraction.
- As soon as you feel that the patient has relaxed their muscle completely (1-3 seconds), take up the tissue slack by increasing the primary and secondary tension.
- Take up the slack after each contraction and during exhalation.
- Repeat 2 or 3 times, or as required.

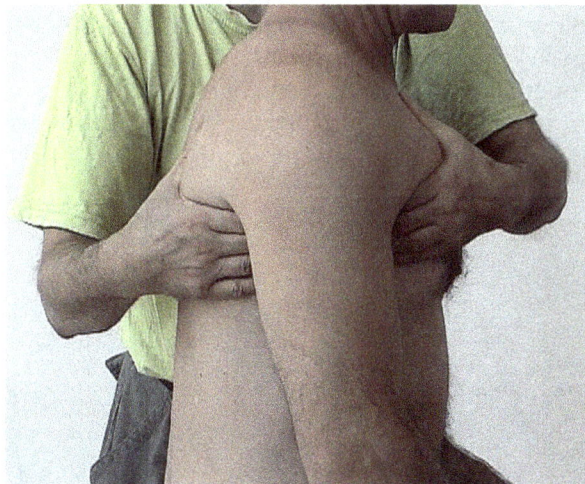

Picture 18.5

Technique 18.5 Kneading of pectoralis major

Patient

- The patient should lie supine, close to the side of the table that you are standing, with their head rotated away from you.

Therapist

- Stand at the side of the table, level with the patient's rib cage and facing the patient's head.
- Grasp the patient's wrist with your cephalad hand.
- The patient's forearm is flexed to 90 degrees and the arm is abducted and externally rotated.
- Fully flex your caudad forearm and internally rotate your arm.
- Reach over the patient's chest with your elbow.
- Your elbow points towards the patient's head and your thumb points back at yourself.
- Make contact on the muscle with your applicator.

Applicator

- The pad and lateral side of your thumb, the pisiform or heel of your hand.

Tissue tension

- Take up the primary tissue tension with compression and a transverse force.
- The muscle runs from medial to lateral across the chest in an oblique direction.
- Start medially and push your applicator in an inferior and lateral direction.
- Your force is always perpendicular to that of the muscle fibre.
- Horizontal extension and external rotation increases longitudinal tension for all fibres of pectoralis major.

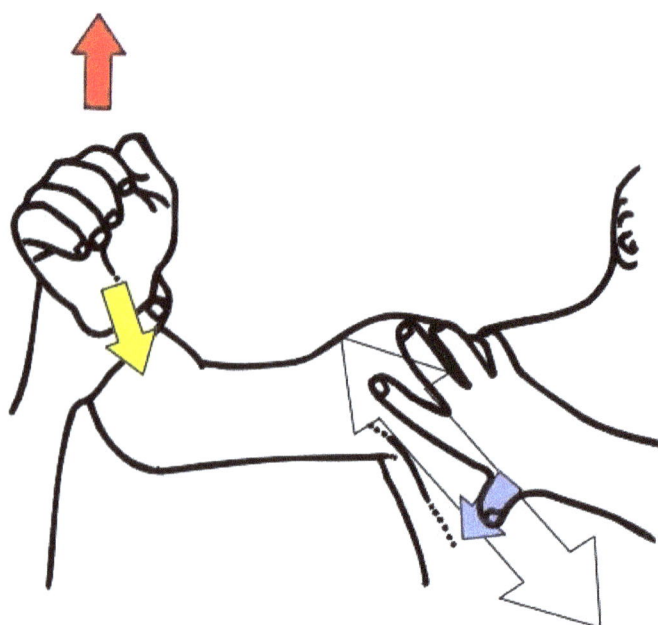

Figure 18.6

Muscle Fibres	⇕	Primary Force	⬇	Secondary Force	↺	Stretch Force	⬇	Contraction Force	⬇

166

- Take the patient's wrist and forearm away from you and towards the floor to induce extension and external rotation at the shoulder.
- The optimum position for increased longitudinal tension varies according to which part of the muscle you are manipulating - clavicular or sternal.
- When treating the clavicular fibres emphasis shoulder adduction.
- When treating the sternocostal fibres emphasis shoulder abduction.

Kneading

- Apply a rhythmical cycle of primary and longitudinal forces.
- The primary tension includes compression and a transverse force.
- Circumduct the shoulder using a combination of the longitudinal forces flexion and extension, adduction and abduction, internal and external rotation.
- Maintain your applicator pressure on the muscle throughout the technique but increase it when the muscle is at an optimal longitudinal tension.
- Mainly utilise shoulder external rotation.
- Your pressure should be just short of discomfort.
- To relax pectoralis major, work with the patients breathing cycle, which is about 15 breaths per minute.
- To stimulate, the muscle increase your speed to about 40 cycles per minute.

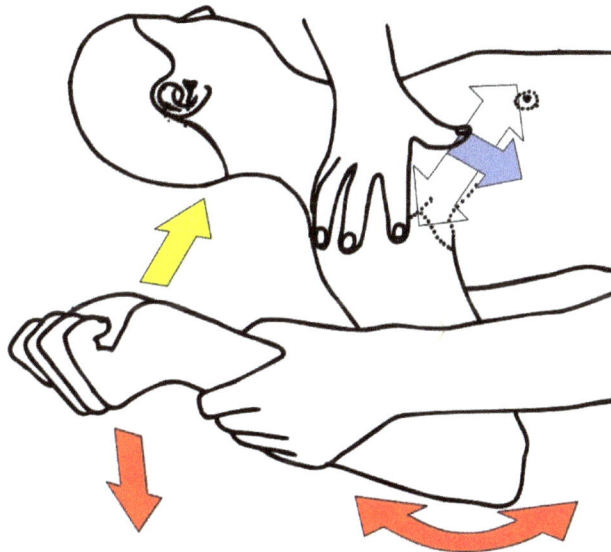

Figure 18.7

Muscle Fibres	⇕	Primary Force	⬇	Secondary Force	↻	Stretch Force	⬇	Contraction Force	⬇

Active component

- Ask the patient to take a deep breath and hold it in.
- Ask the patient to attempt to push their wrist up to the ceiling and down to their feet in an arc (internal rotation) for 3 to 5 seconds using 10% of full contraction of the muscle.
- Resist their effort and maintain tissue lockup throughout inhalation.
- Ask the patient to exhale and to relax their muscle contraction.
- As soon as you feel that the patient has relaxed their muscle completely (about 1-3 seconds), take up the tissue slack by increasing the primary and longitudinal tension.
- Take up the slack after each contraction and during exhalation.
- Repeat 2 or 3 times, or as required.

Note: If the therapist is unable to internally rotate their shoulder sufficiently, this technique may be done by the therapist standing at the head of the table.

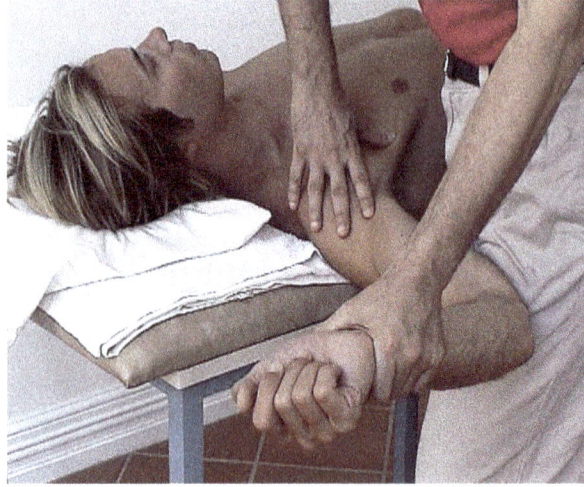

Picture 18.6

19. Pectoralis minor

Anatomy

Pectoralis minor is a thin muscle best palpated with the arm relaxed and using resisted protraction. The muscle arises from the upper margins and outer surface of ribs 3 to 5, near the costochondral junction and from fascia covering the external intercostals. The fibres run superiorly and laterally to attach on the medial border of the coracoid process. Some tendon fibres or all of the pectoralis minor tendon may bypass the coracoid process and attach on the acromion or humerus. Sometimes the muscle arises from ribs 1 or 2 and goes as far inferiorly as rib 4. The muscle is deep to pectoralis major. It lies over the upper ribs, external intercostals, and serratus anterior and forms the posterior part of the anterior axillary fold.

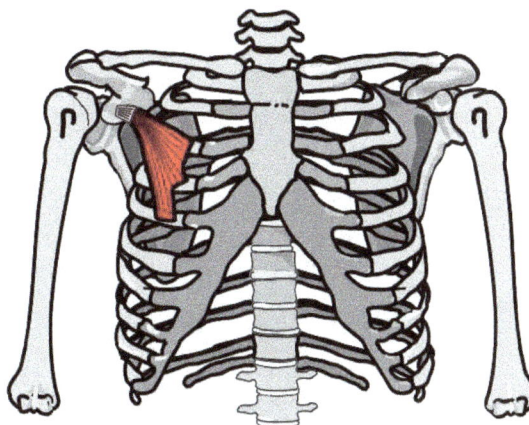

Action: Draws scapula down & forward around the chest.
Clinical considerations: The brachial plexus passes between pectoralis minor and rib 1. This muscle is the major cause of postural distortion in the upper body since it pulls the shoulder forward. A hypertonic pectoralis minor muscle may compress the neurovascular structures that lie deep to it resulting in symptoms of numbness and tingling in the hand. The symptoms are made worse when the patient fully abducts and extends the arm and hence stretches pectoralis minor. This muscle is frequently found short and tender because of the prevalent slumping posture patterns existing in our society.
Nerve supply: medial and lateral pectoral nerves C6, **7** and 8.

Technique 19.1 Kneading or inhibition of pectoralis minor

Patient

- Supine with their head rotated away from the side you are standing.
- The patient should lie close to the edge of the table near to the side you are standing so the inferior angle of the scapula rests on the table, but the tip of the shoulder hangs off it.
- A small pillow or rolled up towel may be placed under the patient's scapula as a fulcrum.

Therapist

- Stand at the side of the table near to the head end.
- Grasp the patient's shoulder at the distal end of the clavicle with your caudad hand.
- Place the heel of your hand or pad of your thumb on the coracoid process.
- Abduct the patient's arm slightly to have better access to pectoralis minor.
- Make contact on the muscle with your applicator.
- Work in the axilla under pectoralis major

Applicator

- The fingertips of you cephalad hand or interdigitating fingers of both hands.

Tissue tension

- Take up the primary tissue tension with your applicator applying compression and transverse pressure on the muscle.
- Take up the longitudinal tension by pushing the coracoid process of the scapula upwards and backwards with your caudad hand (scapula elevation and upwards rotation).

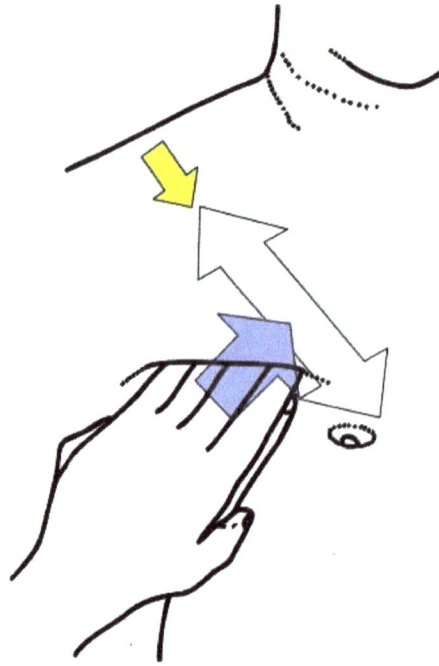

Figure 19.1

Muscle Fibres	⇕	Primary Force	⬇	Secondary Force	↻	Stretch Force	⬇	Contraction Force	⬇

Kneading

- Apply a rhythmical cycle of primary and longitudinal forces.
- When the muscle is at an optimal longitudinal tension increase the primary forces.
- Your pressure should be just short of discomfort. The axilla contains sensitive neurovascular structures.
- To relax the muscle work with the patients breathing cycle, about 15 breaths per minute.
- To stimulate increase your speed to about 40 cycles per minute.

Active component

- Ask the patient to take a deep breath and hold it in.
- Ask the patient to attempt to push their shoulder towards their naval for 3 to 5 seconds using a 10% effort. Pectoralis minor will contract.
- Resist their effort and maintain tissue lockup throughout inhalation.
- Ask the patient to exhale and to relax their muscle contraction.

170

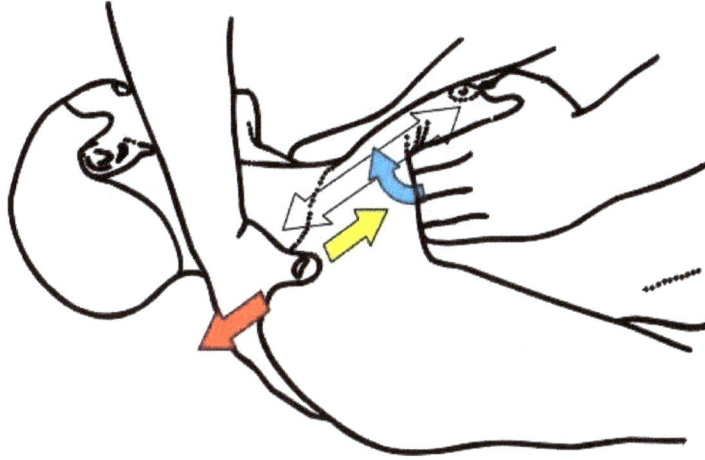

Figure 19.2

Muscle Fibres	⇕	Primary Force	⬇	Secondary Force	↻	Stretch Force	⬇	Contraction Force	⬇

- As soon as you feel that the patient has relaxed their muscle completely (about 1-3 seconds) take up the tissue slack by increasing the primary and longitudinal tension.
- Take up the slack after each contraction and during exhalation.
- Repeat 2 or 3 times or as required.

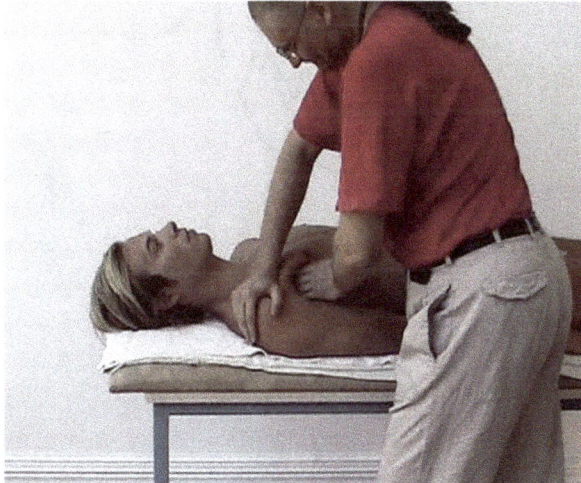

Picture 19.1

Technique 19.2 Stretch for pectoralis minor

Patient

- Supine with their arms at the side of their body.

Therapist

- Stand at the side of the table near to the head end.
- Grasp the patient's shoulder at the distal end of the clavicle with your cephalad hand.
- Abduct the patient's arm slightly.
- Lift the patient's shoulder off the table.
- Reach your caudad hand between the patient's arm and rib cage and slide it between the patient's scapula and the table.
- The inferior angle of the scapula sits in the palm of the hand.
- Make contact on the coracoid process with the heel of your cephalad hand.

Applicator

- The heel of your cephalad hand.

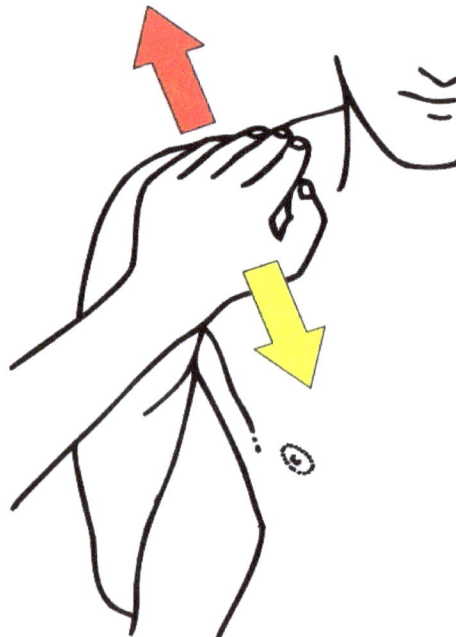

Figure 19.3

Muscle Fibres	⇕	Primary Force	⬇	Secondary Force	↻	Stretch Force	⬇	Contraction Force	⬇

Tissue tension

- Take up the longitudinal tension by pushing the shoulder upwards and backwards posteriorly with your cephalad hand (elevation and upwards rotation).

Stretching

- Apply a slow rhythmical cycle of longitudinal force.

Active component

- Ask the patient to take a deep breath and hold it in.
- Ask the patient to attempt to push their shoulder towards their naval for 3 to 5 seconds using a 10% effort. Pectoralis minor will contract.
- Resist their effort throughout inhalation.
- Ask the patient to exhale and to relax their muscle contraction.
- As soon as you feel that the patient has relaxed their muscle completely (about 1-3 seconds) take up the tissue slack by increasing the longitudinal tension.
- Take up the slack after each contraction and during exhalation.
- Repeat 2 or 3 times or as required.

Alternative

The inferior angle of the patient's scapula rests on the table or over a rolled up towel and the tip of the shoulder hangs just over the edge of the table.

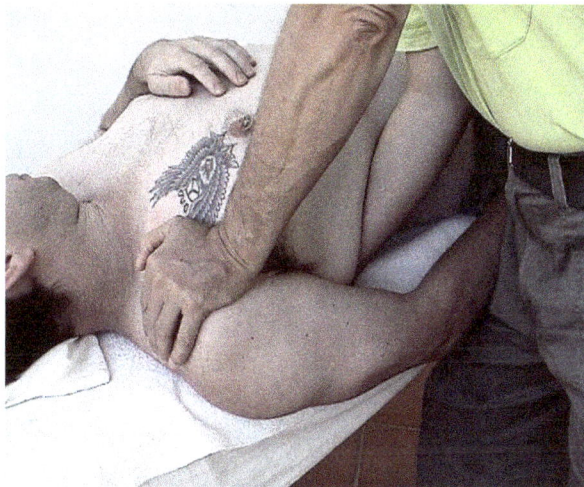

Picture 19.2

20. Serratus anterior

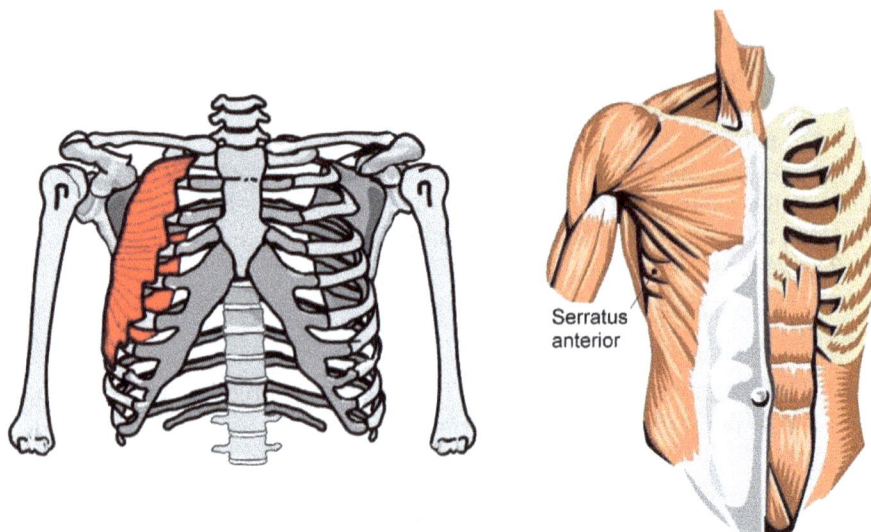

Serratus
anterior

Anatomy

The muscle arises from interdigitations on ribs 1 to 8 (sometimes 10). It runs back and around the thoracic as a muscular sheet, passing under the scapula to attach along the medial border of scapula. The lower four or five digitations are more powerful. They attach on the inferior angle of the scapula and act in upward rotation.

Action: Protraction and upward rotation of scapula. Reaching or pushing and taking the arm above the head.
Clinical indications: Frozen shoulder syndrome and rotator cuff strains causing compensation.
Nerve supply: Long thoracic nerve (C5, 6 and 7). Damage leads to weakness of serratus anterior and winging of scapula.

Technique 20.1 Kneading of serratus anterior in a seated position

Patient

- Seated at the head of the table with legs hanging over the side of the table.
- Places the hand on the opposite side to the therapist behind their neck.

Therapist

- Stands at the head of the table and at the patient's side.
- Place the body of your sternum against the patient's shoulder.
- Reach in front of the patient's chest and grasp their opposite side elbow.
- Reach behind the patient's back and grasp their serratus anterior.
- Your fingers should sit high up in the axilla.
- The patient's trunk is pulled towards and sandwiched between your sternum and hands.

Applicator

- The hooked fingertips.

Tissue tension

- Take up the primary tissue tension with compression and a transverse force by raking across the muscle fibres in an inferior direction with your fingertips.
- Take up the longitudinal tension by pushing against the patient's elbow. The force is transmitted through the arm to the scapula.
- Guide the scapula medially into retraction and downward rotation.

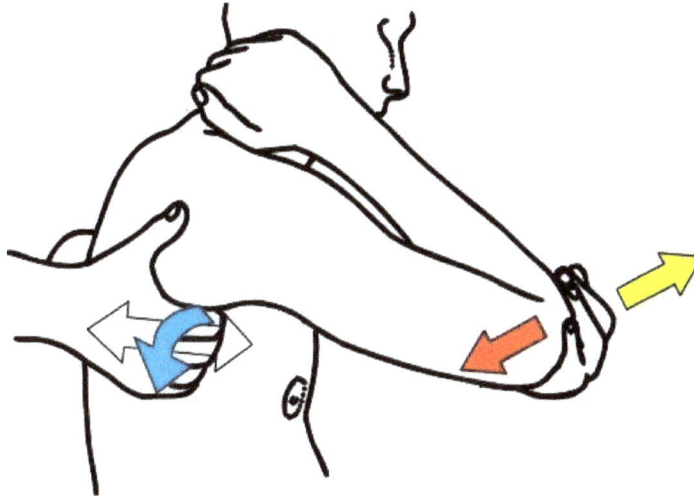

Figure 20.1

Muscle Fibres	⇕	Primary Force	⬇	Secondary Force	↻	Stretch Force	⬇	Contraction Force	⬇

Kneading

- Apply a rhythmical cycle of primary and longitudinal forces.
- Move the patient's elbow in a circle and maintain primary pressure with your applicator.
- When the muscle is at an optimal longitudinal tension increase the forces.
- Your pressure should be just short of discomfort.
- To relax the muscle work with the patients breathing cycle, about 15 breaths per minute.
- To stimulate increase your speed to about 40 cycles per minute.

Active component

- Ask the patient to take a deep breath and hold it in.
- Ask the patient to push their elbow forward away from their body or up towards the ceiling for 3 to 5 seconds using a 10% effort. Serratus anterior will contract.
- Resist their effort.
- Maintain tissue lockup throughout inhalation.
- Ask the patient to exhale and to relax their muscle contraction.
- As soon as you feel that the patient has relaxed their muscle completely (1-3 seconds) take up the tissue slack by increasing the primary and longitudinal tension.
- Take up the slack after each contraction and during exhalation.
- Repeat 2 or 3 times or as required

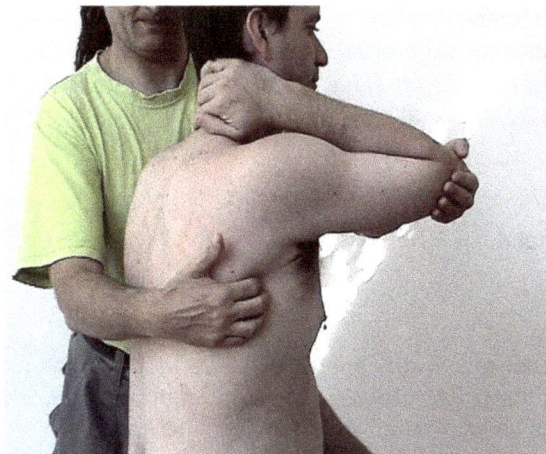

Picture 20.1

Technique 20.2 Kneading of serratus anterior in a sidelying position

Patient

- Sidelying with the front of the body near to the side of the table that you are standing.
- The head is resting on a pillow or folded towel.
- The shoulder the patient is lying on is positioned so that the trunk remains perpendicular to the table. The arm will lie under the patient or in front of the patient. Pillow may be used to prop up the patient.
- The uppermost arm is flexed to 90 degrees.
- The forearm is flexed so the patient's hand rests on the side of their head.

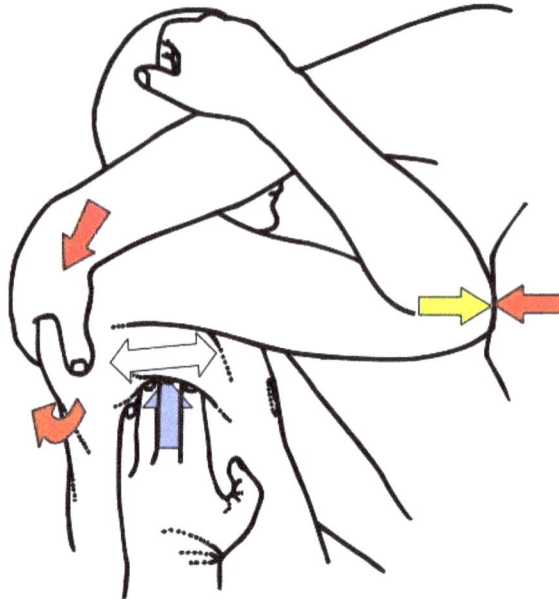

Figure 20.2

Muscle Fibres	⇕	Primary Force	⬇	Secondary Force	↻	Stretch Force	⬇	Contraction Force	⬇

Therapist

- Stand by the side of the table facing the patient and level with their shoulders.
- Reach under the patient's uppermost forearm with your cephalad hand and grasp the patient's scapula.
- Your fingertips contact the rib angles.
- Place the patient's elbow on your sternum.
- Place the palm of your caudad hand flat on the patient's lateral rib cage.
- The fingertips of your hand are at right angles to the fibres of serratus anterior.

Applicator

- All fingertips of one hand.

Contact

- Start at the lower border of serratus anterior and work up into the axilla.
- Alternatively start on the upper fibres of serratus anterior and work down and across the ribs and muscle fibres using a rake like action with the fingers.
- The scapula and pectoralis muscles restrict access to parts of serratus.

- Follow the lateral border of the scapula.
- Work the tendon at the inferior angle of the scapula.
- Work down to rib eight and as far anteriorly as the mid clavicular line.
- As you move down the rib cage more of serratus anterior will become accessible.

Tissue tension

- Take up the transverse tissue tension by pushing up superiorly or raking across the muscle fibres inferiorly with your fingertips. The upper fibres are roughly parallel but the lower fibres of the muscle diverge.
- Take up the longitudinal tension by pushing against the patient's elbow. The force is transmitted through the arm to the scapula.
- With your cephalad hand guide the scapula medially into retraction.
- Take up the longitudinal tension on the lower fibres of serratus anterior by guiding the scapular into retraction and downward rotation.

Kneading

- Apply a rhythmical cycle of transverse and longitudinal force.
- When the muscle is at an optimal longitudinal tension increase the transverse pressure.
- Your pressure should be just short of discomfort.
- To relax the muscle, work with the patients breathing cycle, about 15 breaths per minute.
- To stimulate increase your speed to about 40 cycles per minute.

Active component

- Ask the patient to take a deep breath and hold it in.
- Ask the patient to attempt to push their elbow away and into your chest for 3 to 5 seconds using a 10% effort. The serratus anterior will contract.
- Resist their effort and maintain tissue lockup including scapula stabilisation throughout the technique.
- Ask the patient to exhale and to relax their muscle contraction.
- As soon as you feel that the patient has relaxed their muscle completely (about 1-3 seconds) take up the tissue slack by increasing the primary and longitudinal tension.
- Take up the slack after each contraction and during exhalation.
- Repeat 2 or 3 times or as required.

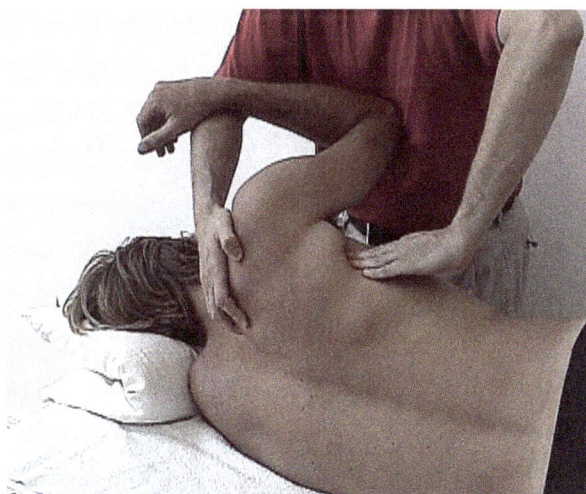

Picture 20.2

21. Latissimus dorsi

Anatomy

This triangular muscle arises as thoracolumbar fascia from the sacrum, iliac crest and spinous processes of thoracic vertebrae T6 to T12 and all lumbar vertebrae. Between T6 and T12 it is deep to trapezius.

It arises directly as muscle from ribs 9 to 12, the iliac crest and usually from the inferior angle of the scapula. The muscle fibres run superiorly and laterally. They pass over the lower part of teres major posteriorly and then twist around it so that the anterior surface faces backwards and is in contact with the anterior surface of teres major. Together they form the posterior axillary fold. The tendon attaches on a lower part intertubercular sulcus/bicipital groove of humerus. The highest midline fibres form the lowest tendon attachment and the lowest midline fibres form the highest tendon attachment on the humerus.

Actions: Latissimus dorsi extends, adducts and medially rotates the humerus. It depresses shoulder as in climbing. It is active in forced exhalation as in coughing. Fibres that arise from the inferior angle of the scapula contribute towards stabilisation of the scapula.

Nerve supply: Thoracodorsal nerve (C**6**, **7** and 8) from brachial plexus descends over medial wall of axilla to enter muscle in the axilla.

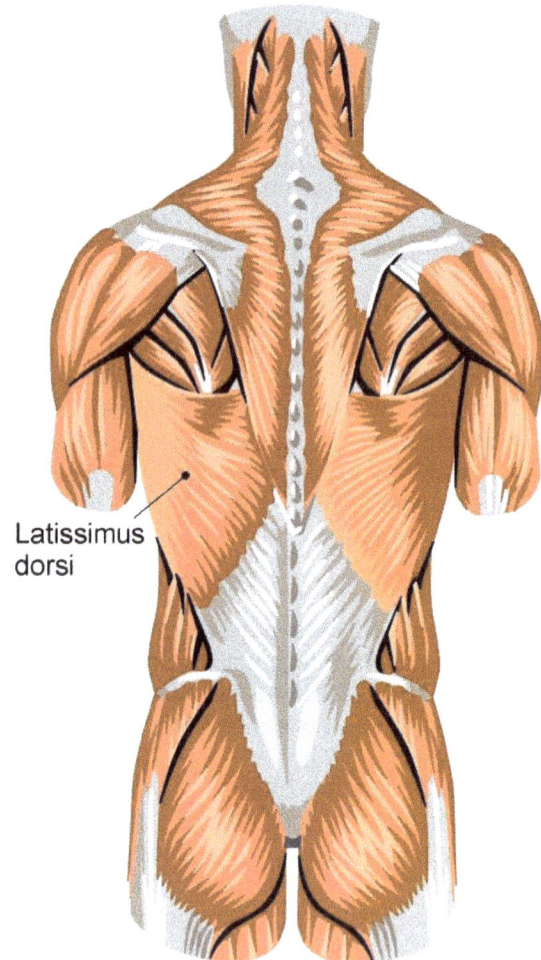

Latissimus dorsi

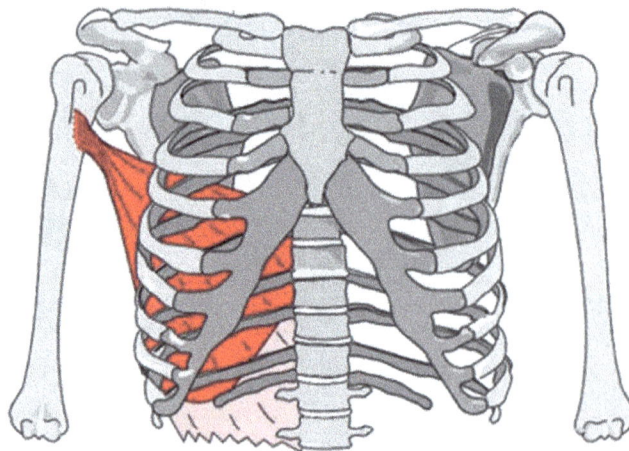

Technique 21.1 Kneading of latissimus dorsi in a prone position

Patient

- Prone with the head rotated away from the side you are standing.
- The patient should lie close to the side of the table that you are standing.

Therapist

- Stand at the side of the table level with the patient's ribs and facing the patient's head.
- Reach over and around the patient's arm that is nearest you and grasp their triceps with your cephalad hand.
- Abduct the patient's arm ninety degrees and then externally rotate their arm.
- Fully flex your caudad forearm and internally rotate your arm.
- Reach over the patient's chest with your elbow.
- Your elbow points towards the patient's head and your thumb points back at yourself.
- Make contact on the muscle with your applicator.

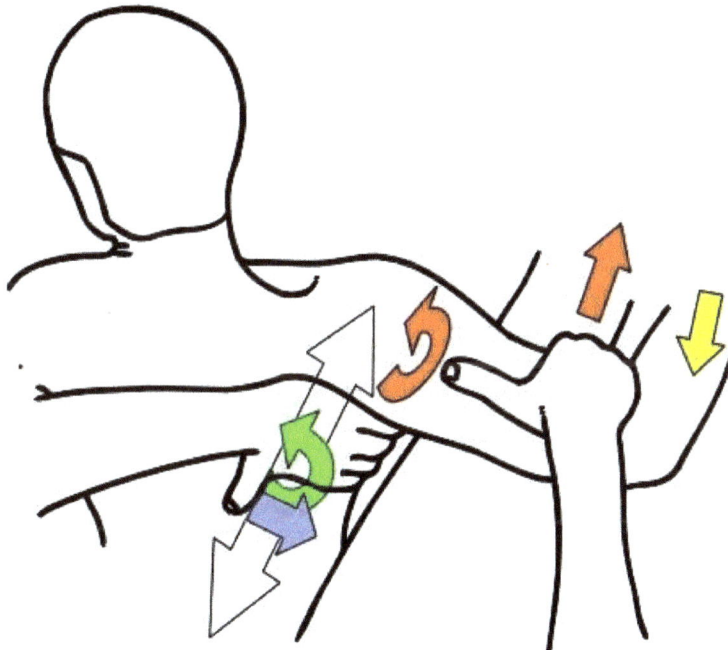

Figure 21.1

Muscle Fibres	⇕	Primary Force	⬇	Secondary Force	↺	Stretch Force	⬇	Contraction Force	⬇

If you are unable to perform this manoeuvre the technique may be performed from a position nearer to the head of the table. The fingertips become the primary applicator and the thumb the secondary applicator (Figure 21.2). Alternatively, the technique may be performed from the head of the table with the cephalad hand as the applicator.

Applicator

- The pad and lateral side of your thumb, the pisiform or heel of your caudad hand.

Tissue tension

- Take up the primary tissue tension with compression and a transverse force.
- The muscle runs superiorly from medial to lateral across the back in an oblique direction.
- Start medially and push your applicator in an inferior and lateral direction.
- Your force is always perpendicular to that of the muscle fibre.
- Take up the longitudinal tension by increasing shoulder abduction and external rotation.

Kneading

- Apply a rhythmical cycle of primary and longitudinal forces.
- The primary tension includes compression and a transverse force.
- Circumduct the shoulder using a combination of the longitudinal forces flexion and extension, adduction and abduction, internal and external rotation.
- Maintain your applicator pressure on the muscle throughout the technique but increase it when the muscle is at an optimal longitudinal tension.
- Your pressure should be just short of discomfort.
- To relax latissimus dorsi work with the patients breathing cycle, which is about 15 breaths per minute.
- To stimulate the muscle, increase your speed to about 40 cycles per minute.
- Apply cross fibre kneading by pressing into the muscle, working from medial to lateral with your applicator

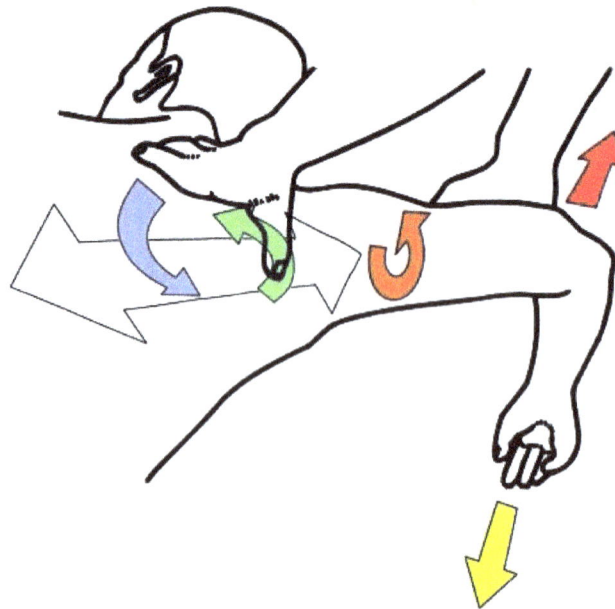

Figure 21.2

Muscle Fibres	⇕	Primary Force	⬇	Secondary Force	↻	Stretch Force	⬇	Contraction Force	⬇

Active component

- Ask the patient to take a deep breath and hold it in.
- Ask the patient to attempt to push their wrist down to the floor and down to their feet in an arc (internal rotation) for 3 to 5 seconds using 10% of full contraction of the muscle.
- Resist their effort and maintain tissue lockup throughout inhalation.
- Ask the patient to exhale and to relax their muscle contraction.

- As soon as you feel that the patient has relaxed their muscle completely (about 1-3 seconds) take up the tissue slack by increasing the primary and longitudinal tension.
- Take up the slack after each contraction and during exhalation.
- Repeat 2 or 3 times or as required.

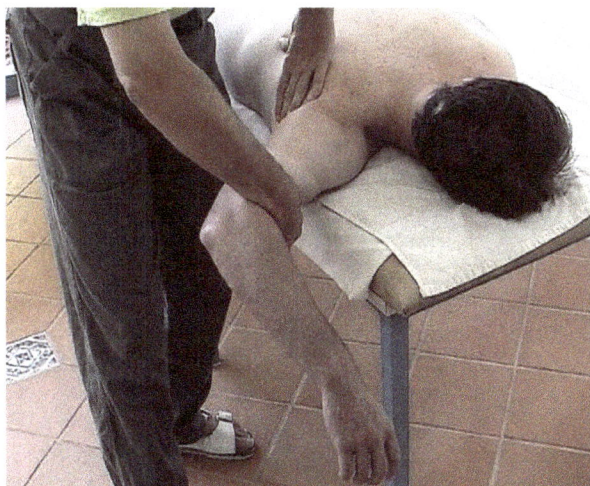

Picture 21.1

Technique 21.2 Kneading of latissimus dorsi in a sidelying position

Patient

- Sidelying with the back of the body near to the edge of the table.
- The head resting on a pillow or folded towel.
- The trunk should remain perpendicular to the table.
- The forearm the patient is lying on is flexed at the elbow and rests against the front of their chest.
- The uppermost arm is abducted.

Therapist

- Stand at the head of the table near to the side the patient's back is facing.
- Grasp the patient's uppermost arm with your cephalad hand or drape it over your arm.
- Press into the muscle with your applicator.

Applicator

- Thumb, pisiform or heel of your caudad hand.

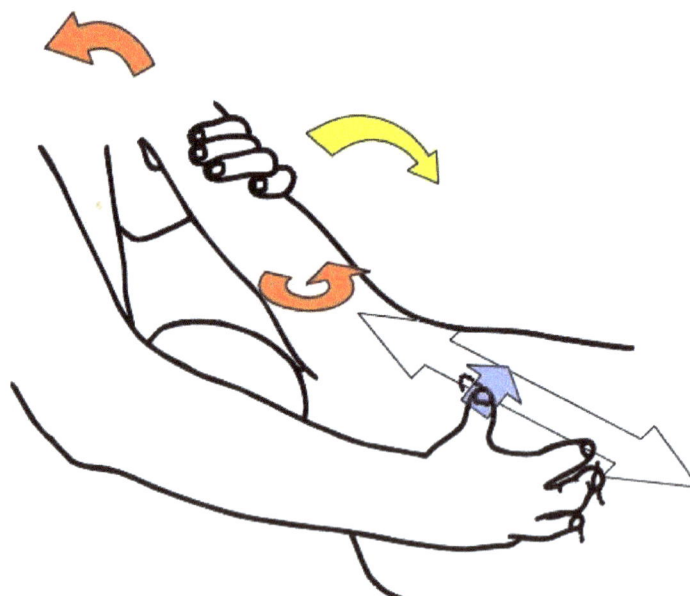

Figure 21.3

Muscle Fibres	⇅	Primary Force	⬇	Secondary Force	↺	Stretch Force	⬇	Contraction Force	⬇

Tissue tension

- Take up the primary tissue tension with compression and add a transverse force by pushing across the muscle from medial to lateral with your applicator.
- Take up the longitudinal tension by abducting, externally rotating and adding traction to the patient's arm with your cephalad hand.
- To increase longitudinal tension further a pillow may be placed under the patient's rib cage to sidebend their spine towards the table

Kneading

- Apply a rhythmical cycle of primary and longitudinal forces.
- Circumduct the patients shoulder and when the muscle is at an optimal level of longitudinal tension increase the compression and transverse pressure.
- Alternatively, circumduct the shoulder while maintaining a constant applicator pressure on the muscle.
- Apply cross fibre kneading from medial to lateral.
- Your pressure should be just short of discomfort.
- To relax the muscle, work with the patients breathing cycle, about 15 breaths per minute.
- To stimulate increase your speed to about 40 cycles per minute.

Active component

- Ask the patient to take a deep breath and hold it in.
- Ask the patient to try to bring their arm forwards and down towards their feet (extension) or rotate their arm so their thumb points down towards their feet (internal rotation) for 3 to 5 seconds using a 20% effort. Latissimus dorsi will contract.
- Resist their effort and maintain tissue lockup throughout the technique.
- Ask the patient to exhale and to relax their muscle contraction.
- As soon as you feel that the patient has relaxed their muscle completely (about 1-3 seconds) take up the tissue slack by increasing the primary and longitudinal tension.
- Take up the slack after each contraction and during exhalation.
- Repeat 2 or 3 times or as required.

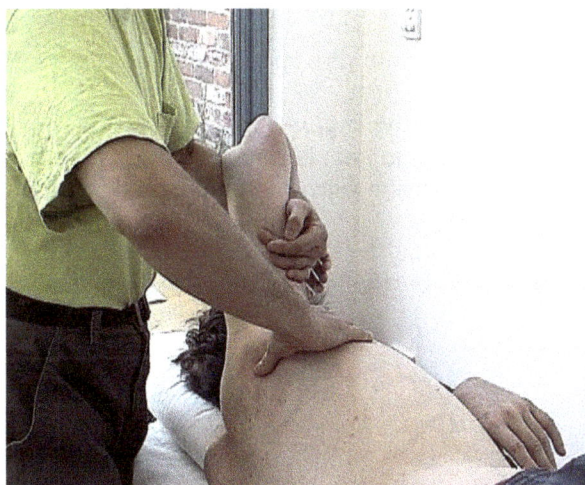

Picture 21.2

Technique 21.3 Kneading of latissimus dorsi in a seated position

Patient

- Seated at one end of the table with legs hanging over the side of the table.
- Places the hand on the opposite side to the therapist behind their neck.
- Grasps the elbow on the opposite side to the therapist with the hand nearest the therapist.

Therapist

- Stands at the head of the table and at the patient's side.
- Place the body of your sternum against the patient's shoulder.
- Ask the patient to slightly abduct the arm, which is furthest from you.
- Reach in front of the patient's chest and grasp their pectoralis major.
- Reach behind the patient's back and grasp their latissimus dorsi.
- Your fingers should sit high up in the axilla and the pads of your thumbs rest outside the axilla on the respective muscles.
- With both hands lift the shoulder and support its weight.
- The patient's trunk is pulled towards and sandwiched between your sternum and hands.

Applicator

- The fingers and thumbs of both hands.

Tissue tension

- Take up the primary tissue tension with your fingers applying compression and a transverse force on the muscle.
- Pull up and then towards you with the fingers of both hands.
- Use pectoralis major as an anchor to treat latissimus dorsi.
- Take up the secondary tissue tension with your thumb applying a rotation force (torsion). Push down and away from you.
- Grasp latissimus dorsi between your fingertips and thumbs.
- Take up the longitudinal tension by starting the technique with the patient's arm flexed.

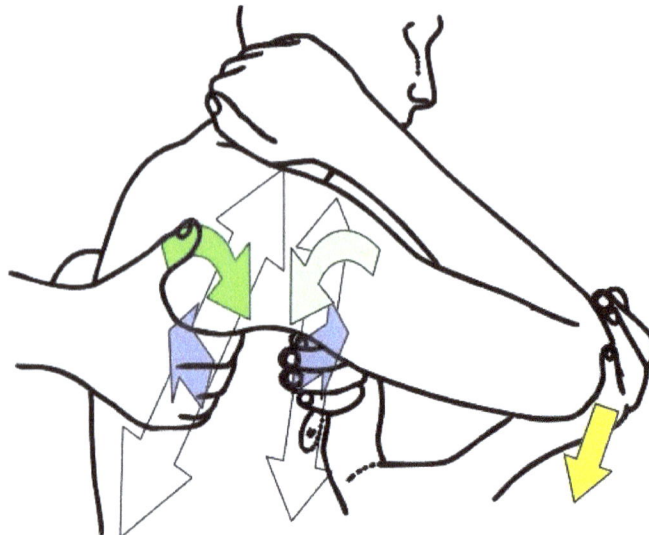

Figure 21.4

Muscle Fibres	⇕	Primary Force	⬇	Secondary Force	↻	Stretch Force	⬇	Contraction Force	⬇

Kneading

- Apply a rhythmical cycle of primary, secondary and longitudinal forces.
- Alternatively make a circle with the patient's shoulder girdle while maintaining primary and secondary pressure with your applicator.
- When the muscle is at an optimal longitudinal tension increase the primary and secondary forces.
- Your pressure should be just short of discomfort.
- To relax the muscle work with the patients breathing cycle, about 15 breaths per minute.
- To stimulate increase your speed to about 40 cycles per minute.

Active component

- Ask the patient to take a deep breath and hold it in.
- Ask the patient to push their elbow down to the floor and simultaneously push their hand forward and down against the back of their own neck for 3 to 5 seconds using a 10% effort. Latissimus dorsi will contract.
- The patient should resist his or her own effort.
- Alternatively, you may grasp the patient's elbow on the opposite side to which you are standing and offer resistance to the patient's effort.
- Maintain tissue lockup throughout inhalation.
- Ask the patient to exhale and to relax their muscle contraction.
- As soon as you feel that the patient has relaxed their muscle completely (1-3 seconds) take up the tissue slack by increasing the primary, secondary and longitudinal tension.
- Take up the slack after each contraction and during exhalation.
- Repeat 2 or 3 times or as required.

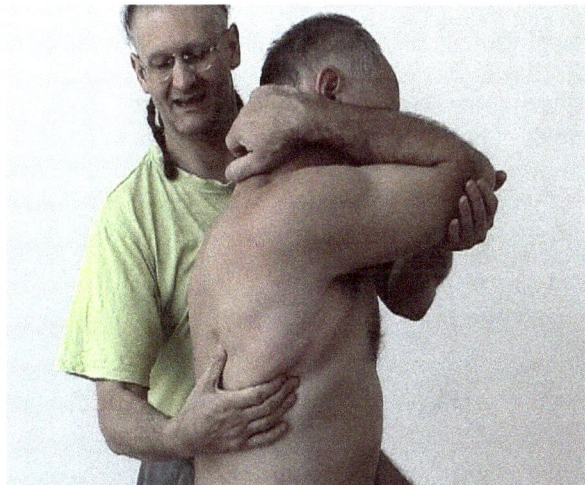

Picture 21.3

22. Teres major

Anatomy

Teres major arises as muscle from the inferior angle and posterior surface of the scapula and its flat tendon attaches on the crest of the lesser tubercle and medial lip of intertubercular sulcus (bicipital groove).
It is palpable as it passes laterally from under latissimus dorsi and acts as latissimus dorsi's 'little helper'.

Actions: It adducts, extends and medially rotates the humerus.
Nerve supply: Subscapular nerve C **6** and 7.

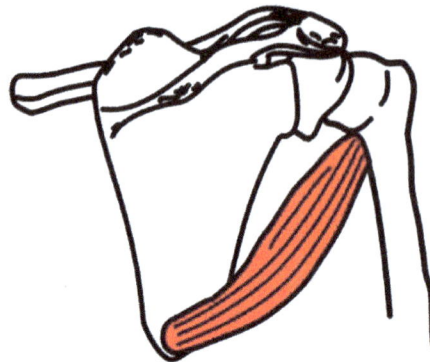

Technique 22.1 Kneading of teres major

Patient

- Prone with their head rotated away from the side you are standing.
- The patient should lie close to the side of the table that you are standing.

Therapist

- Stand at the side of the table at the level of the patient's rib cage and facing the patient's head.
- Reach over and around the patient's arm that is nearest you and grasp their triceps with your cephalad hand.
- Abduct the patient's arm ninety degrees and internally rotate their arm.
- Grasp the medial border of the scapula with your fingertips of you caudad hand.
- The applicator of your caudad hand makes contact on the muscle to be treated.

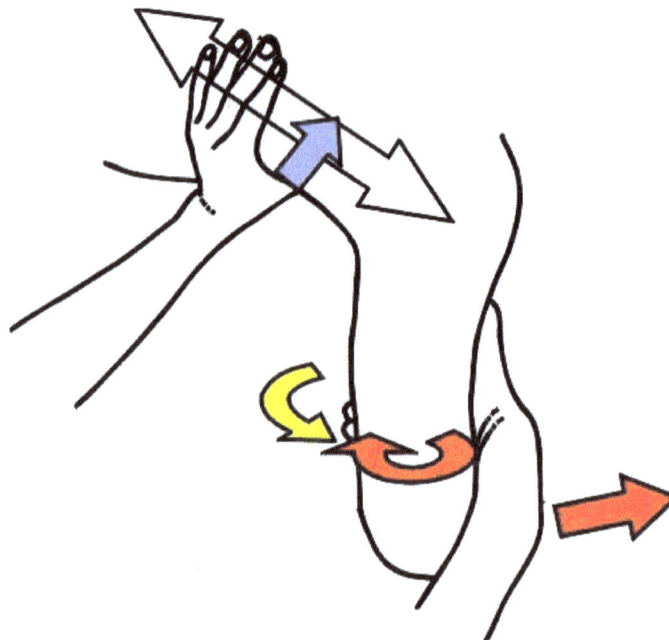

Figure 22.1

Muscle Fibres	⇕	Primary Force	⬇	Secondary Force	↻	Stretch Force	⬇	Contraction Force	⬇

Applicator

- The tip of the thumb of your caudad hand.

Tissue tension

- Take up the primary tissue tension with your applicator applying compression and transverse pressure on the muscle.
- The fingers of you caudad hand are firmly anchored to the medial border of the scapula and work in opposition with your thumb to increase pressure.
- Take up the longitudinal tension with external rotation and further abduction of the shoulder applied by the cephalad hand.

Kneading

- Apply a rhythmical cycle of primary and longitudinal forces.
- When the muscle is at an optimal longitudinal tension increase the primary forces.
- Your pressure should be just short of discomfort.
- To relax the muscle work with the patients breathing cycle, about 15 breaths per minute.
- To stimulate increase your speed to about 40 cycles per minute.

Active component

- Ask the patient to take a deep breath and hold it in.
- Ask the patient to attempt to rotate their arm and push their wrist down towards their feet (internal rotation) or bring their arm to their side (adduction) for 3 to 5 seconds using a 10% effort. The teres minor will contract.
- Resist their effort and maintain tissue lockup throughout inhalation.
- Ask the patient to exhale and to relax their muscle contraction.
- As soon as you feel that the patient has relaxed the muscle completely (about 1-3 seconds) take up the tissue slack by increasing the primary and longitudinal tension.
- Take up the slack after each contraction and during exhalation.
- Repeat 2 or 3 times or as required.

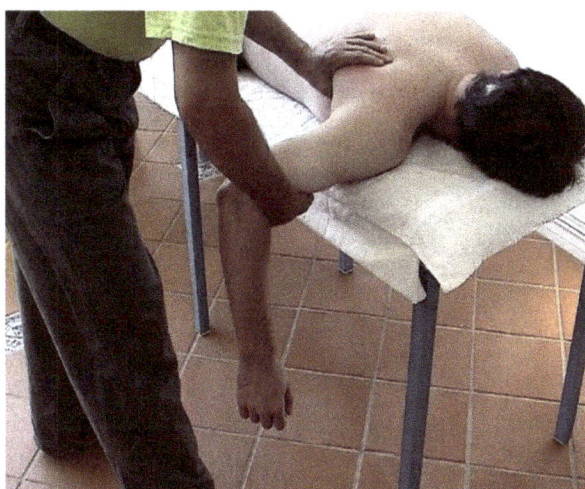

Picture 22.1

23. Triceps brachii

Anatomy

The tendon of the long head of **triceps brachii** arises from the infraglenoid tubercle of the scapula and from the capsule of the glenohumeral joint. The medial or deep head arises from the posterior shaft of the humerus, below the radial groove. The lateral head arises from an area on the posterior and lateral shaft of the humerus, above the radial groove. A common tendon inserts on the posterior and upper olecranon and blends with the antebrachial fascia of the forearm. Continuous with deep fascia overlying pectoralis major, deltoid and latissimus dorsi and the antebrachial fascia, the brachial fascia is thickest where it covers the triceps and epicondyles of the humerus. It attaches to the epicondyles and the olecranon process of the ulna. An olecranon bursa may be palpable when inflamed or thickened.

Action: Forearm extension is consistently produced by the medial head and by the long and lateral heads when acting against resistance. The power of the long head depends on the position of the shoulder. Triceps assists arm extension when the arm moves from a position of flexion.
Nerve supply: Radial nerve C6, **7** and **8**.

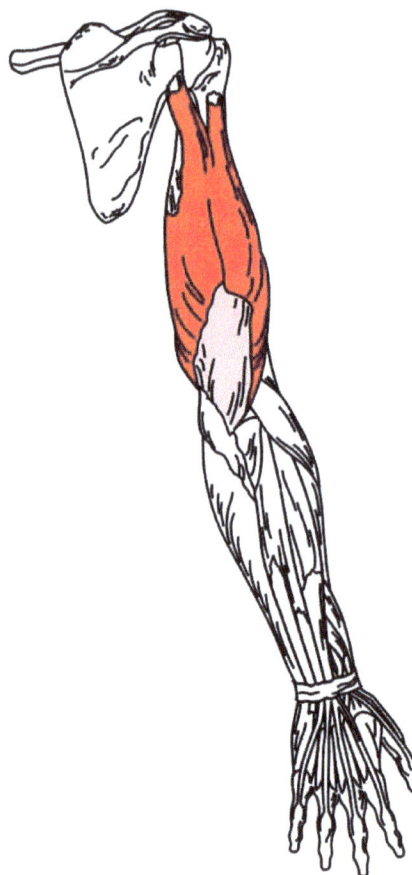

Technique 23.1 Kneading in a lateral direction of the medial, lateral and long head of triceps

This technique may also be done standing by the side of the table level with the patient's head and facing the patient's feet and kneading in a medial direction.

Patient

- Supine with the head resting on a pillow or folded towel.

Therapist

- Stand by the side of the table level with the patient's rib cage and facing the patient's head.
- Grasp the patients wrist in your cephalad hand.
- Abduct their arm to 90 degrees and flex their forearm to 90 degrees.
- The patient's elbow rests on the table or for better control rests on your thigh.
- Reach over the patient's arm and grasp one of the heads of triceps in your caudad hand.

Applicator

- The fingertips of your caudad hand. You may use your thumb to add secondary tension.

Tissue tension

- Take up the primary tissue tension with compression and a transverse force by flexing your fingers and pulling up (superiorly) with the fingertips of your caudad hand.
- Take up the secondary (torsion) tissue tension by pushing with your thumb. Take care not to pinch the skin.
- Secondary tension is also taken up by pushing the patient's wrist and forearm away from you and externally rotating their arm.
- Take up the longitudinal tissue tension by increasing flexion of the patient's forearm.

Kneading

- Apply a rhythmical cycle of primary, secondary and longitudinal forces.
- When the muscle is at an optimal longitudinal tension increase the primary and secondary forces.
- Your pressure should be just short of discomfort.
- To relax the triceps, work with the patients breathing cycle, which is about 15 breaths per minute.
- To stimulate the triceps, increase your speed to about 40 cycles per minute.

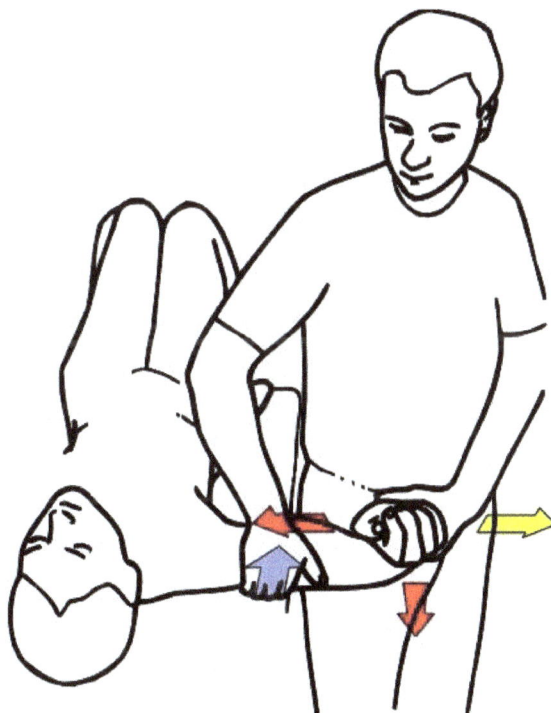

Figure 23.1

Muscle Fibres	⇕	Primary Force	⬇	Secondary Force	↺	Stretch Force	⬇	Contraction Force	⬇

Active component

- Ask the patient to take a deep breath and hold it in.
- Ask the patient to attempt to straighten (extend) their forearm for 3 to 5 seconds using 10% of full contraction of their triceps.
- Resist their effort and maintain tissue lockup throughout inhalation.
- Ask the patient to exhale and to relax their muscle contraction.
- As soon as you feel the patient has relaxed their triceps completely (about 1-3 seconds) take up the tissue slack by increasing the primary, secondary and longitudinal tension.

- Take up the slack after each contraction and during exhalation.
- Repeat 2 or 3 times or as required.

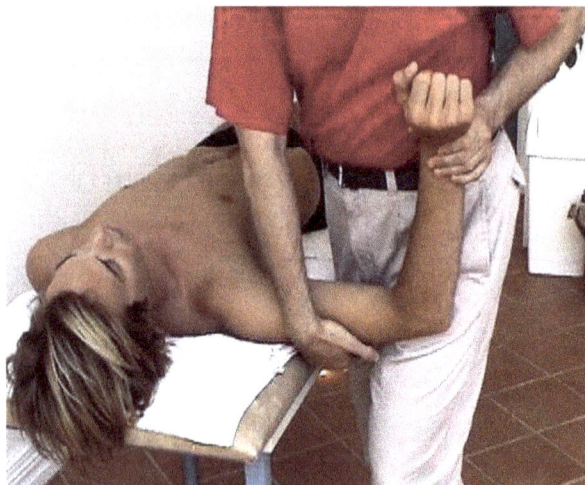

Picture 23.1

24. Deltoid

Anatomy

Deltoid gives the shoulder its rounded shape. It has three parts, anterior, posterior and middle or intermediate which are separates by deep fascia.

The anterior deltoid arises on the anterior superior border of the distal clavicle, the middle deltoid arises on the lateral margin of the superior acromion and the posterior deltoid arises on the lower border of the spine of the scapula. All insert on the deltoid tuberosity on the lateral shaft of the humerus via a short thick tendon. The anterior and posterior deltoid attach on the tendon directly whereas the middle deltoid attaches on the tendon via four intramuscular tendinous septa which makes it the strongest part of the muscle.

The tendon is usually joined with the tendon of pectoralis major and some fibres from the tendon merge with deep brachial fascia. Superficial and deep fasciae and platysma are superficial to the deltoid. The fascia is continuous with the pectoral, infraspinous and brachial fascia and attaches to the clavicle, acromion and spine of scapular. The muscle may unite with pectoralis major.

Actions: Anterior deltoid is an arm flexor and horizontal flexor; Middle deltoid is an arm abductor; Posterior deltoid is an arm extensor and horizontal extensor.
Clinical indications: Shoulder injuries such as to the rotator cuff tendon may result in compensatory changes in the muscle.
Nerve supply: Axillary nerve C**5** and 6.

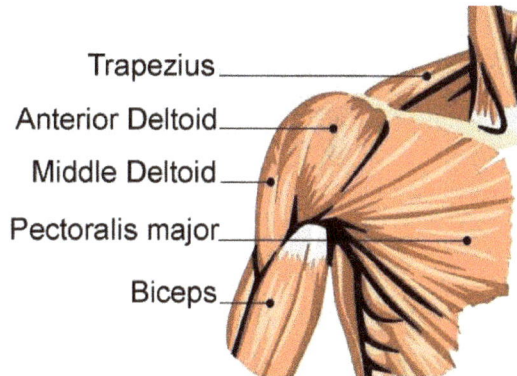

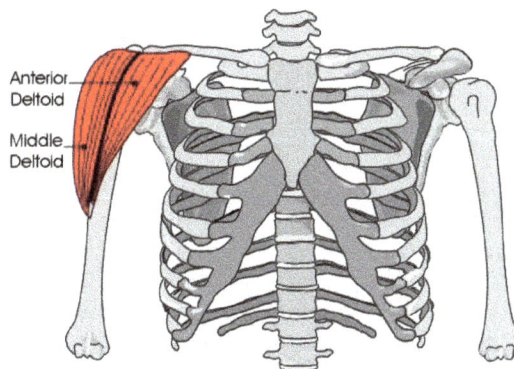

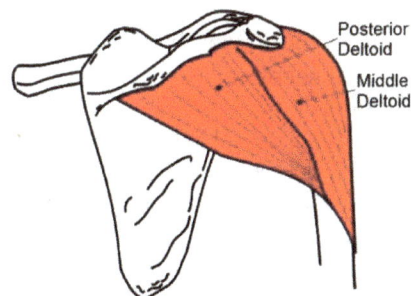

Trapezius
Anterior Deltoid
Middle Deltoid
Pectoralis major
Biceps

Anterior Deltoid
Middle Deltoid

Posterior Deltoid
Middle Deltoid

Technique 24.1 Kneading of anterior deltoid

Patient

- Supine with the head straight and resting on a pillow or folded towel.
- The patient lies near to the side of the table that you are standing.
- The principles of this technique may be applied to the posterior deltoid in the prone position.

Therapist

- Stand by the side of the table level with the patient's rib cage.
- Grasp the patients hand or wrist with your cephalad hand.
- Flex their forearm to 90 degrees, abduct their arm to 90 degrees and externally rotate their arm fully.
- The patient's elbow rests on your thigh.
- Place the applicator of your caudad hand on the patient's anterior deltoid muscle.

Applicator

- The heel of your caudad hand or the side of your thumb and fingertips of you caudad hand.

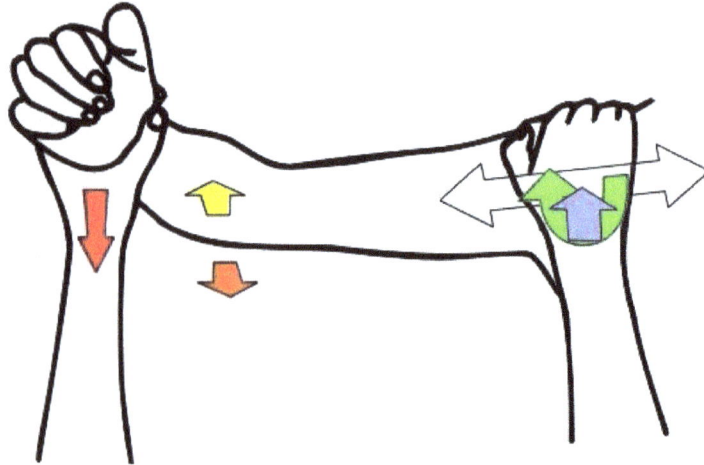

Figure 24.1

Muscle Fibres	↕	Primary Force	⬇	Secondary Force	↺	Stretch Force	⬇	Contraction Force	⬇

Tissue tension

- Take up the primary tissue tension with compression and a transverse force by pushing away (superiorly and posteriorly) with the heel of your hand or the side of your thumb.
- Take up the secondary tissue tension by sidebending your wrist into either abduction or adduction.
- If your thumb is the applicator the secondary tension may be taken up by flexing your fingers and pulling the fibres with your fingertips. Take care not to pinch the skin.
- Additional secondary tension may be taken up by pulling the patient's wrist towards you and internally rotating their arm.
- Take up longitudinal tissue tension with horizontal extension and by starting the technique with the arm in external rotation and abduction.
- Use your knee to control the patient's arm.

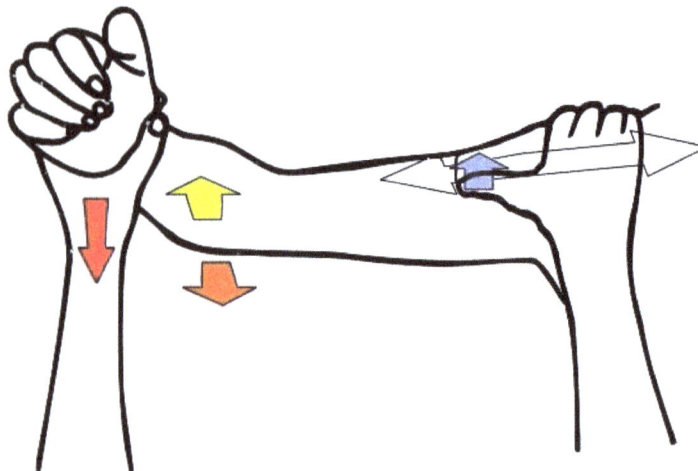

Figure 24.2

Muscle Fibres	↕	Primary Force	⬇	Secondary Force	↺	Stretch Force	⬇	Contraction Force	⬇

Kneading

- Apply a rhythmical cycle of primary, secondary and longitudinal forces.
- When the muscle is at an optimal longitudinal and secondary tension increase the primary forces.
- Your pressure should be just short of discomfort.
- To relax the deltoid work with the patients breathing cycle, which is about 15 breaths per minute.
- To stimulate the deltoid increase your speed to about 40 cycles per minute.

Active component

- Ask the patient to take a deep breath and hold it in.
- Ask the patient to: push their arm upward towards the ceiling (horizontal flexion) for 3 to 5 seconds using 10% of full contraction of their anterior deltoid.
- Resist their effort and maintain tissue lockup throughout inhalation.
- Ask the patient to exhale and to relax their muscle contraction.
- As soon as you feel that the patient has relaxed their anterior deltoid completely (about 1-3 seconds) take up the tissue slack by increasing the primary, secondary and longitudinal tension.
- Take up the slack after each contraction and during exhalation.
- Repeat 2 or 3 times or as required.

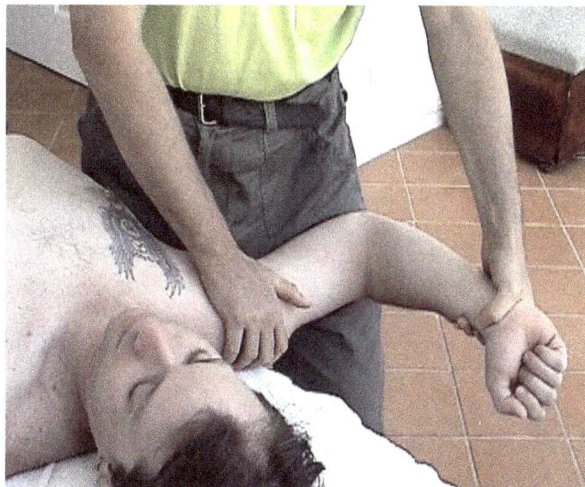

Picture 24.1

Technique 24.2 Kneading of posterior deltoid

Patient

- Supine with the head straight and resting on a pillow or folded towel.
- The patient lies near to the side of the table that you are standing.
- This technique may be applied to the anterior deltoid in the prone position.

Therapist

- Stand by the side of the table level with the patient's rib cage.
- Grasp the patients hand or wrist with your cephalad hand.
- Flex their forearm to 90 degrees, abduct their arm to 90 degrees and internally rotate their arm fully.
- The patient's elbow rests on your thigh.
- Place the applicator of your caudad hand on the patient's posterior deltoid muscle.

Applicator

- The fingertips of your caudad hand.

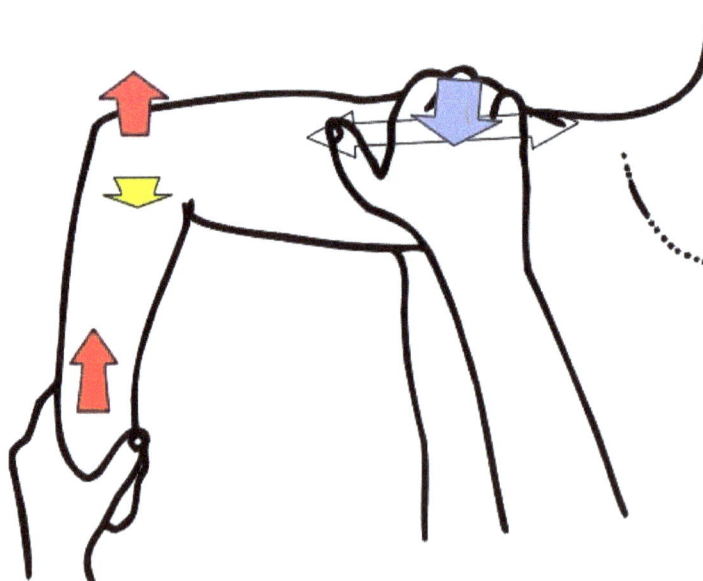

Figure 24.3

Muscle Fibres	⇕	Primary Force	⬇	Secondary Force	↻	Stretch Force	⬇	Contraction Force	⬇

Tissue tension

- Take up the primary tissue tension with compression and a transverse force by flexing your fingers and pulling (superiorly and anteriorly) with your fingertips.
- Take up the secondary tissue tension by taking the patient's wrist upwards and away from you and externally rotating their arm.
- Take up longitudinal tissue tension with horizontal flexion and by starting the technique with the arm in internal rotation and abduction.
- Use your knee to control the patient's arm.

Kneading

- Apply a rhythmical cycle of primary, secondary and longitudinal forces.
- When the muscle is at an optimal longitudinal and secondary tension increase the primary forces.
- Your pressure should be just short of discomfort.
- To relax the deltoid work with the patients breathing cycle, which is about 15 breaths per minute.
- To stimulate the deltoid, increase your speed to about 40 cycles per minute.

Active component

- Ask the patient to take a deep breath and hold it in.
- Ask the patient to push their arm down towards the floor (horizontal extension) for 3 to 5 seconds using 10% of full contraction of the posterior deltoid.
- Resist their effort and maintain tissue lockup throughout inhalation.
- Ask the patient to exhale and to relax their muscle contraction.
- As soon as you feel that the patient has relaxed their posterior deltoid completely (about 1-3 seconds) take up the tissue slack by increasing the primary, secondary and longitudinal tension.
- Take up the slack after each contraction and during exhalation.
- Repeat 2 or 3 times or as required.

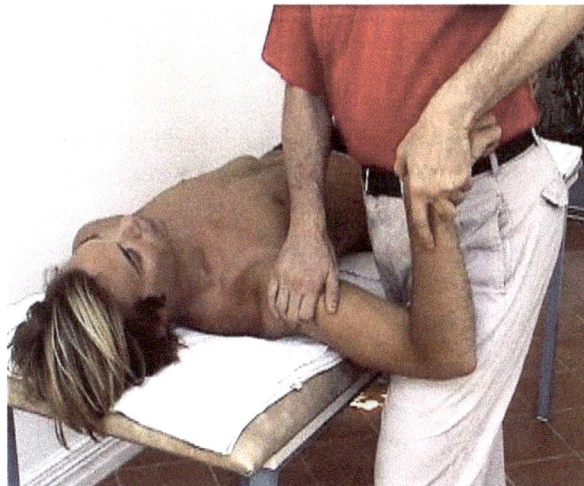

Picture 24.2

Technique 24.3 Kneading of middle deltoid

Patient

- Supine with the head straight and resting on a pillow or folded towel.
- The patient lies near to the side of the table that you are standing.

Therapist

- Stand by the side of the table level with the patient's rib cage.
- Reach across the patient's body with your caudad hand and grasp their hand or wrist on the opposite side to which you are standing.
- Flex their forearm to 90 degrees and internally rotate their arm until their forearm makes contact with the front of their body.
- Reach across the patient's body with your cephalad hand and place your applicator on the patient's middle deltoid muscle.

Applicator

- The fingertips of your cephalad hand.

Tissue tension

- Take up the primary tissue tension with compression and a transverse force by flexing your fingers and pulling (medially and anteriorly) with your fingertips.
- Take up the secondary tissue tension by taking the patient's wrist upwards and away from you and externally rotating their arm.
- The middle fibres are the strongest part of the deltoid and are under most tension when the arm is adducted. Take up longitudinal tissue tension by starting the technique with the arm in adduction.

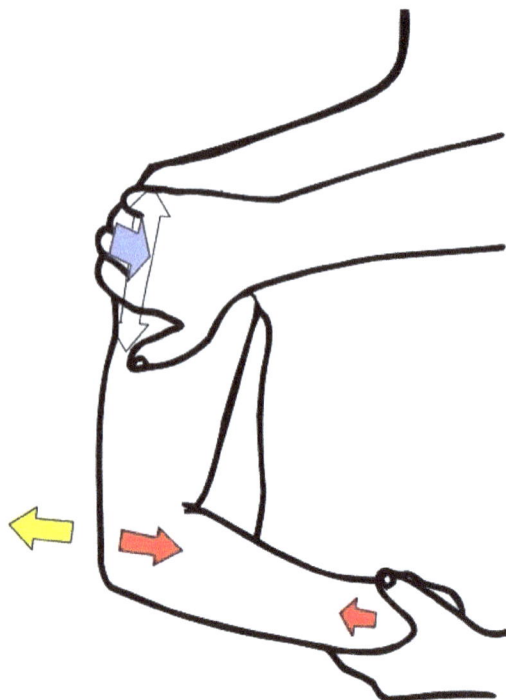

Figure 24.4

Muscle Fibres	⇕	Primary Force	⬇	Secondary Force	↺	Stretch Force	⬇	Contraction Force	⬇

Kneading

- Apply a rhythmical cycle of primary, secondary and longitudinal forces.
- When the muscle is at an optimal secondary tension increase the primary forces.
- Your pressure should be just short of discomfort.
- To relax the deltoid work with the patients breathing cycle, which is about 15 breaths per minute.
- To stimulate the deltoid, increase your speed to about 40 cycles per minute.

Active component

- Ask the patient to take a deep breath and hold it in.
- Ask the patient to push their arm away from the side of their body (abduction) for 3 to 5 seconds using 10% of full contraction of the middle deltoid.
- Resist their effort and maintain tissue lockup throughout inhalation.
- Ask the patient to exhale and to relax their muscle contraction.
- As soon as you feel that the patient has relaxed their middle deltoid completely (about 1-3 seconds) take up the tissue slack by increasing the primary, secondary and longitudinal tension.
- Take up the slack after each contraction and during exhalation.
- Repeat 2 or 3 times or as required.

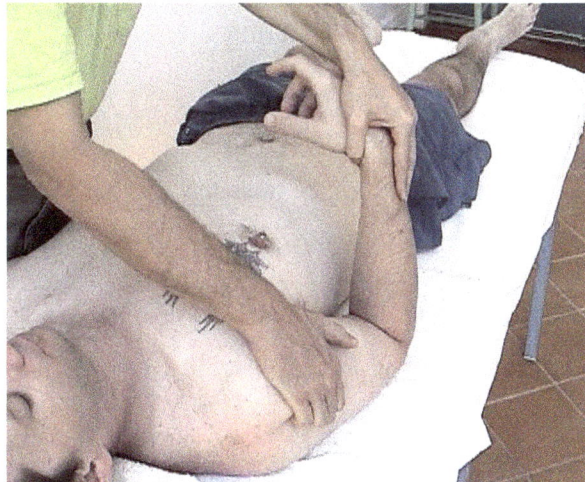

Picture 24.3

25. Coracobrachialis

Anatomy

Coracobrachialis arises from the apex of coracoid process where it shares a common tendon with the short head of biceps. The rope like muscle passes down the upper medial shaft of humerus and it can be palpated as a round ridge close to the brachial artery before it attaches to broad area halfway down the medial shaft of the humerus.

Actions: It is a flexor, horizontal flexor and adductor of the humerus, especially from a position of extension and acts as a stabiliser of the shoulder.
Nerve supply: Musculocutaneous nerve C5, **6** and 7.

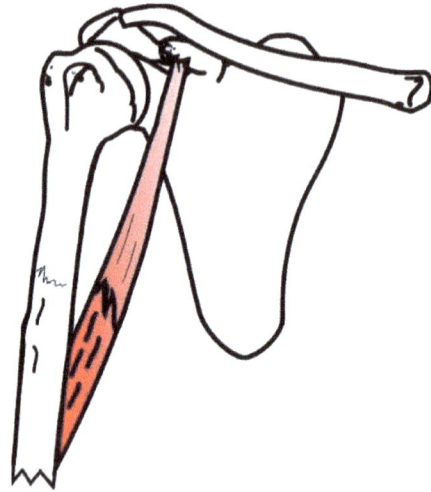

Technique 25.1 Kneading of coracobrachialis

Patient

- Supine with the head straight and resting on a folded towel.
- The patient should lie close to the side of the table that you are standing.

Therapist

- Stand by the side of the table near the head end.
- Grasp the patients wrist in your caudad hand.
- Flex their forearm to 90 degrees and abduct their arm to 45 degrees.
- The patient's elbow rests on your thigh.
- Hook the middle fingertip of your cephalad hand around the coracobrachialis.

Applicator

- The middle fingertip of your cephalad hand.

Tissue tension

- Take up the primary (transverse) tissue tension by pulling up on the muscle with the fingertip of your cephalad hand.
- Take up the longitudinal tissue tension by abducting, extending and horizontally extending the patient's arm.

Kneading

- Apply a rhythmical cycle of primary and longitudinal forces.
- When the muscle is at an optimal longitudinal tension increase the primary forces.
- Your pressure should be just short of discomfort. Be careful of sensitive neurovascular structures in the axilla and medial side of arm.
- To relax the coracobrachialis work with the patients breathing cycle, which is about 15 breaths per minute.
- To stimulate the muscle, increase your speed to about 40 cycles per minute.

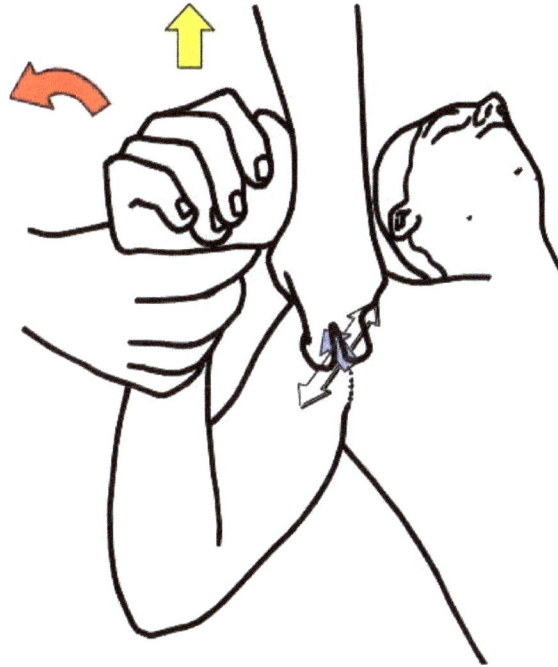

Figure 25.1

Muscle Fibres	⇕	Primary Force	⬇	Secondary Force	↺	Stretch Force	⬇	Contraction Force	⬇

Active component

- Ask the patient to take a deep breath and hold it in.
- Ask the patient to horizontally flex and adduct their arm for 3 to 5 seconds using 10% of full contraction.
- Resist their effort and maintain tissue lockup throughout inhalation.
- Ask the patient to exhale and to relax their muscle contraction.
- As soon as you feel that the patient has relaxed their muscle completely (about 1-3 seconds) take up the tissue slack by increasing the primary and longitudinal tension.
- Take up the slack after each contraction and during exhalation.
- Repeat 2 or 3 times or as required.

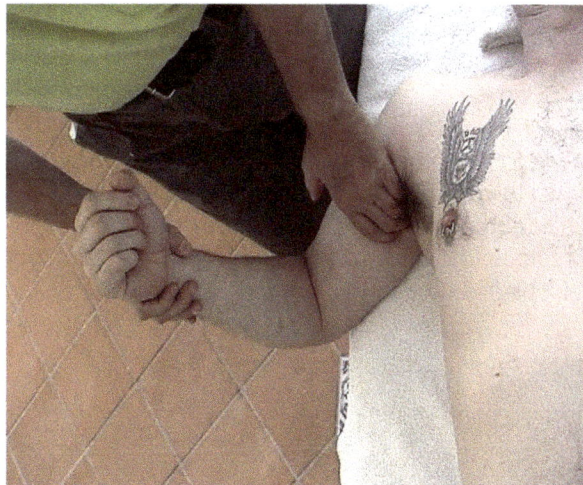

Picture 25.1

26. Biceps brachii

Anatomy

The short head of **biceps brachii** arises on the apex of the coracoid process. It shares a common tendon origin with coracobrachialis. The long head arises from within the capsule, on the glenoid labrum and the supraglenoid tubercle above the glenoid cavity. The long slender tendon passes down the bicipital groove /intertubercular sulcus of the humerus under cover of the transverse ligament and fibres of the pectoralis major tendon. The groove is palpable between the greater and lesser tuberosity.

The two fusiform muscles from each head join as a tendon that attaches on the posterior of the radial tuberosity and the bicipital aponeurosis. This aponeurosis is a broad fibrous expanse, which merges with the deep fascia of the flexor muscles of the forearm and attaches on the ulnar. It provides greater flexor pull and protects vessels and the median nerve in the cubital fossa. In 10% of the population a third head arises from the brachialis muscle and other heads may exist.

Actions: Forearm flexion and supination and arm flexion.
Clinical indications: Rupture of the muscle and tendonitis at the bicipital groove.
Nerve supply: Musculocutaneous C5 & **6**.

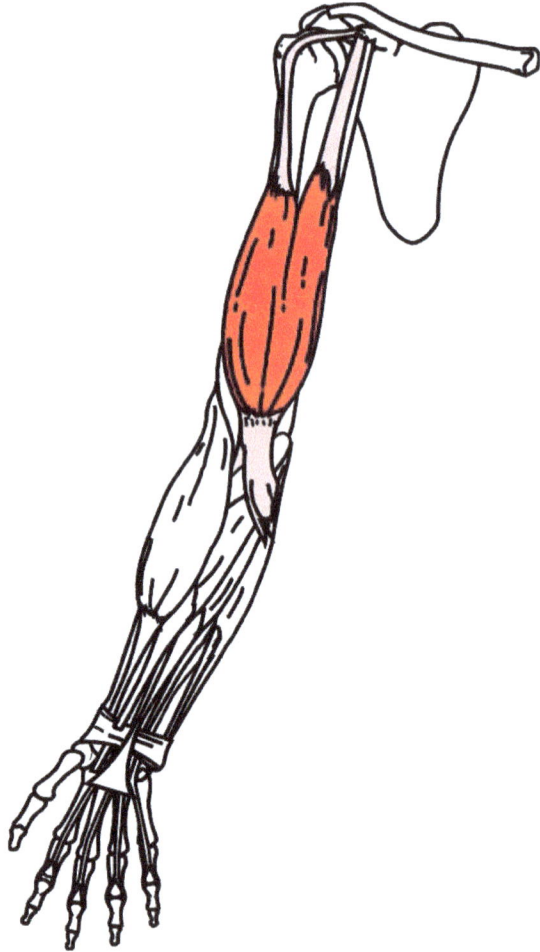

Technique 26.1 Kneading of biceps

Patient

- Supine with the head resting on a pillow or folded towel.

Therapist

- Stand by the side of the table at the level of the patient's rib cage.
- Grasp the patients wrist in your cephalad hand.
- Abduct their arm to 90 degrees and flex their forearm to 90 degrees.
- The patient's elbow rests on the table or for better control rests on your thigh.
- Grasp the patients biceps in your caudad hand.

Applicator

- Heel of hand and pisiform bone.

Tissue tension

- Take up the primary tissue tension with compression and a transverse force by pushing away with the heel of your caudad hand.

- Take up the secondary tissue tension by moving your pisiform about an axis passing through the hook of the hamate, in other words, abduction or radial deviation of the wrist.
- Further secondary tension is taken up by pulling the patient's wrist and forearm towards you and internally rotating their arm.
- Take up the longitudinal tissue tension by extending and pronating the patient's forearm.

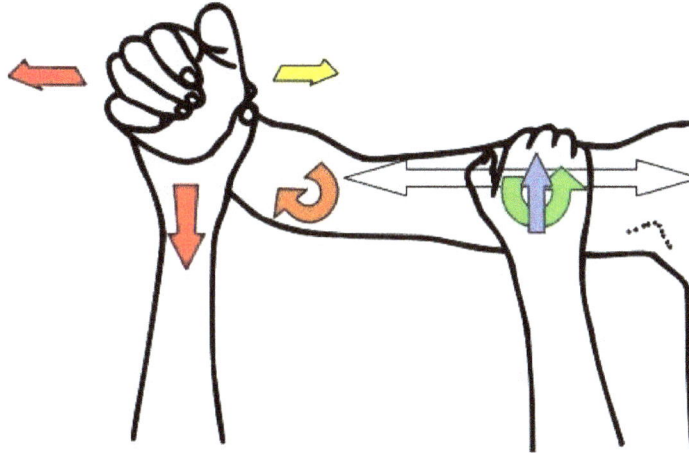

Figure 26.1

Muscle Fibres	⇕	Primary Force	⬇	Secondary Force	↻	Stretch Force	⬇	Contraction Force	⬇

Kneading

- Apply a rhythmical cycle of primary, secondary and longitudinal forces.
- When the muscle is at an optimal longitudinal tension increase the other forces.
- Your pressure should be just short of discomfort.
- Work with the patients breathing cycle, which is about 15 breaths per minute.
- To stimulate the biceps increase your speed to about 40 cycles per minute.

Active component

- Ask the patient to take a deep breath and hold it in.
- Ask the patient to flex their forearm for 3 to 5 seconds using 10% of full contraction.
- Resist their effort and maintain tissue lockup throughout inhalation.
- Ask the patient to exhale and to relax their muscle contraction.
- As soon as you feel that the patient has relaxed their biceps completely take up the tissue slack by increasing the primary, secondary and longitudinal tension.
- Take up the slack after each contraction and during exhalation and repeat as required.

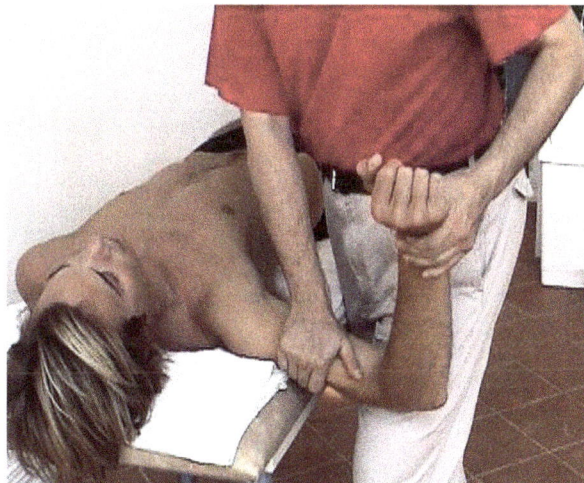

Picture 26.1

Technique 26.2 Kneading of biceps

Patient

- The technique is shown supine but may be done prone.

Therapist

- Stand by the side of the table at the level of the patient's rib cage.
- Grasp the patients wrist in your cephalad hand.
- Abduct their arm to 90 degrees and flex their forearm to 90 degrees.
- The patient's elbow rests on the table or for better control rests on your thigh.
- Grasp the patients biceps in your caudad hand.

Applicator

- The fingertips of your caudad hand.

Tissue tension

- Take up the primary tissue tension with compression and a transverse force by flexing your fingers and pulling back on the fibres with the fingertips of your caudad hand.
- Take up the secondary tissue tension by pushing the patient's wrist away from you and externally rotating their arm.
- Take up the longitudinal tissue tension by extending and pronating the patient's forearm.

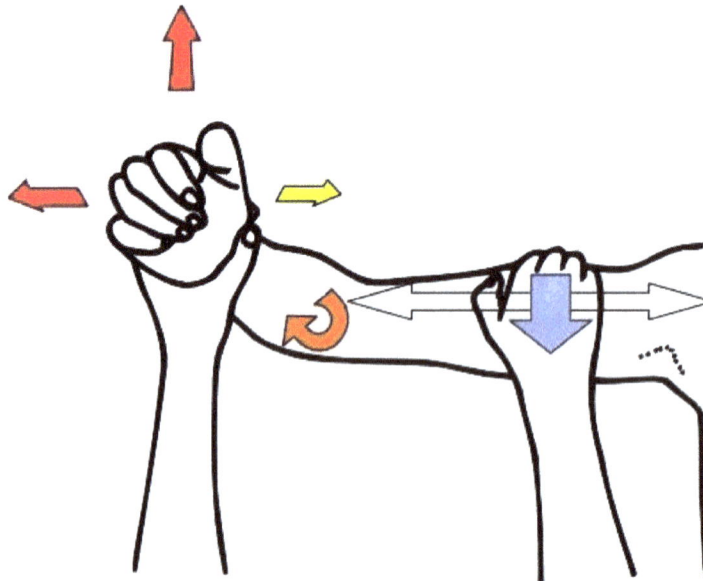

Figure 26.2

Muscle Fibres	⇕	Primary Force	⬇	Secondary Force	↺	Stretch Force	⬇	Contraction Force	⬇

Kneading

- Apply a rhythmical cycle of primary, secondary and longitudinal forces.
- When the muscle is at an optimal longitudinal and secondary tension increase the primary forces.
- Your pressure should be just short of discomfort.
- To relax the biceps, work with the patients breathing cycle, which is about 15 breaths per minute.
- To stimulate the biceps, increase your speed to about 40 cycles per minute.

Active component

- Ask the patient to take a deep breath and hold it in.
- Ask the patient to flex their forearm for 3 to 5 seconds using 10% of full contraction of their biceps.
- Resist their effort and maintain tissue lockup throughout inhalation.
- Ask the patient to exhale and to relax their muscle contraction.
- As soon as you feel that the patient has relaxed their biceps completely (about 1-3 seconds) take up the tissue slack by increasing the primary, secondary and longitudinal tension.
- Take up the slack after each contraction and during exhalation.
- Repeat 2 or 3 times or as required.

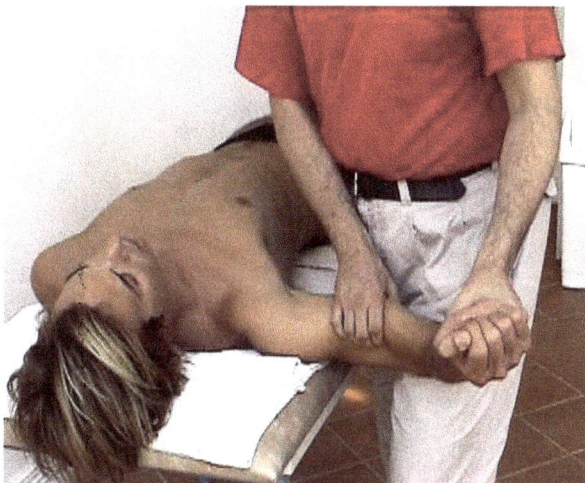

Picture 26.2

27. The biceps tendon

Anatomy

The distal biceps tendon runs from the two heads of the biceps muscle to the posterior of the radial tuberosity and the bicipital aponeurosis. This aponeurosis is a broad fibrous expanse, which merges with the deep fascia of the flexor muscles of the forearm and attaches on the ulnar.

Clinical indications: tendon strain and tendonitis.
See 'Technique' page 6 for more information on the treatment of tendonitis.

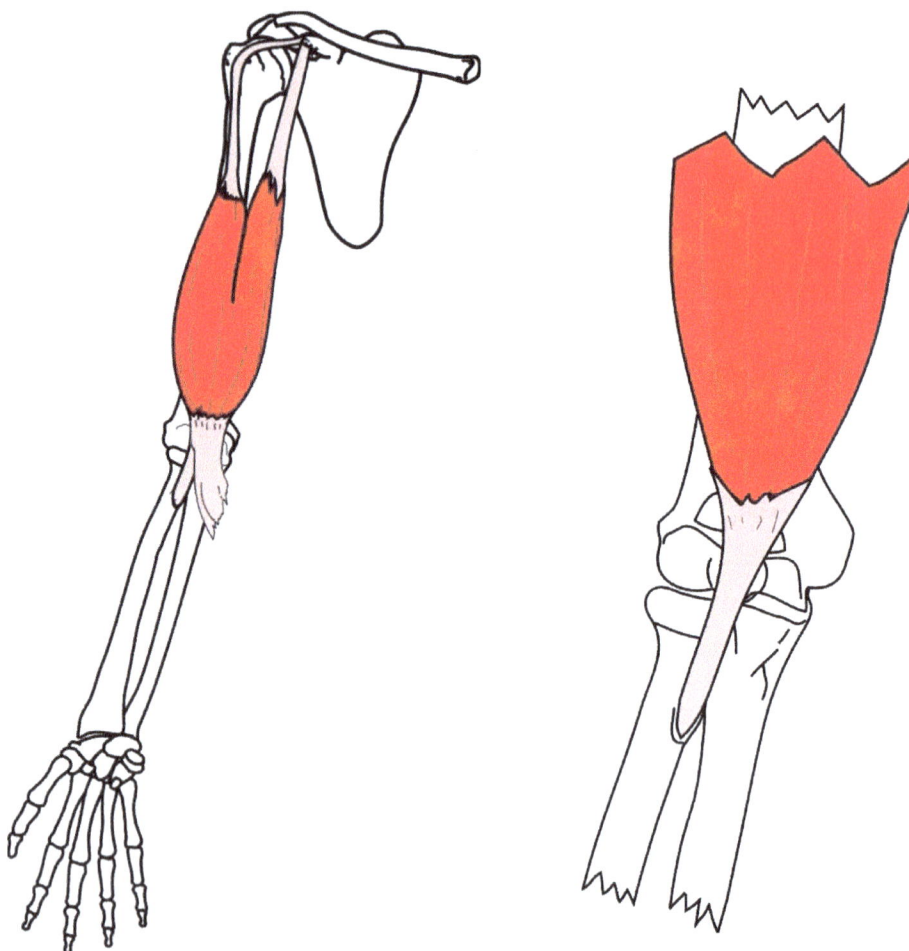

Muscle, tendon and aponeurosis   Biceps tendon with aponeurosis removed

Technique 27.1 Friction over the biceps tendon

Patient

- Supine with the head on a pillow or folded towel.

Therapist

- Stand at the side of the table level with the patient's elbow.
- Grasp the patient's hand with your cephalad hand and flex their elbow to 90 degrees.
- Place your applicator on the biceps tendon.

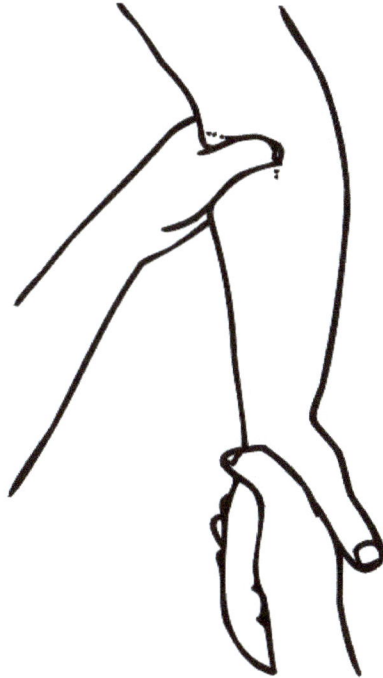

Figure 27.1

Applicator

The tip of the thumb of your cephalad hand.

Transverse Friction

Take up the tissue tension by gradually increasing your thumb pressure on the tendon.
Work across the biceps tendon with transverse friction.
Apply firm pressure over a small area.

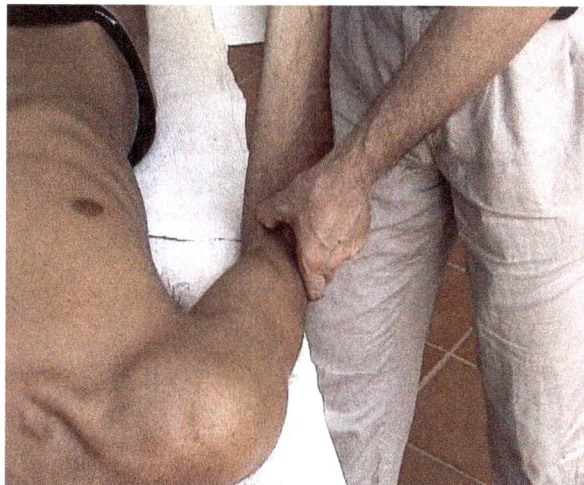

Picture 27.1

28. Elbow medial and lateral collateral ligaments

Anatomy

The **medial or ulnar collateral ligament** is a strong thick ligament. The apex of this triangular shaped ligament arises from the medial epicondyle of the humerus and the base attaches on the olecranon process and the medial border of the coronoid process and the area between. The ligament is not directly palpable.

The **lateral or radial collateral ligament** is short and fibrous. It arises on a distal area of the lateral epicondyle of the humerus and attaches on the lateral ulna and merges with the annular ligament. The annular ligament is not directly palpable, surrounds the head of the radius and articulates with it.

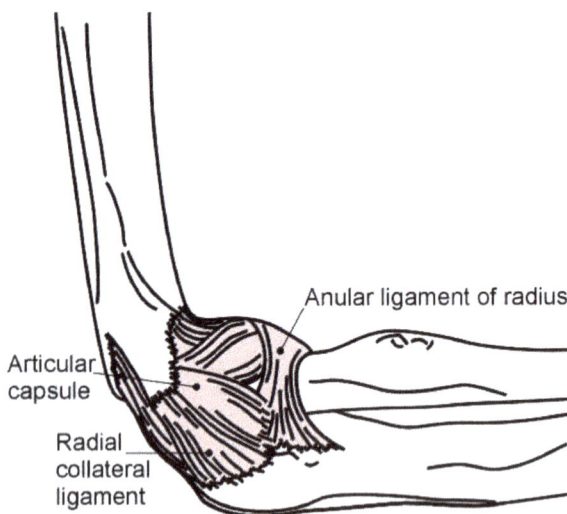

Anular ligament of radius

Articular capsule

Radial collateral ligament

Technique 28.1 Friction over the collateral ligaments

Patient

- Supine with the head on a pillow or folded towel.

Therapist

- Stand at the side of the table level with the patient's forearm.
- Grasp the patient's hand in your caudad hand.

Applicator

- The tip of the index finger or thumb of your cephalad hand.

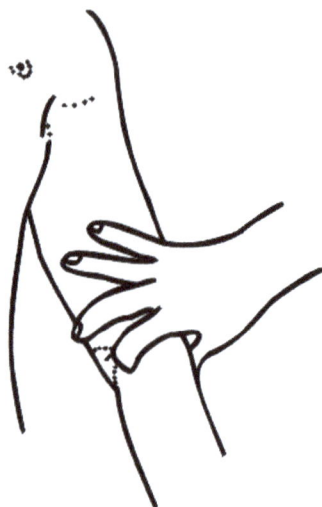

Figure 28.1 Medial ligament

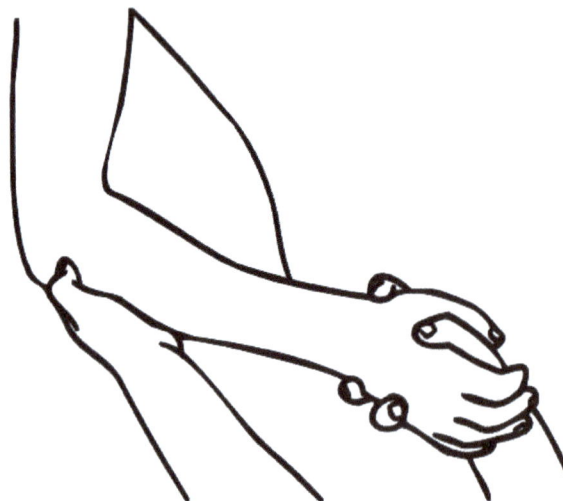

Figure 28.2 Lateral ligament

Tissue tension

- Find the joint line. You may need to flex the elbow.
- Place your applicator on the ligament.
- The ligament runs in a general inferior to superior direction.
- Take up the tissue tension by gradually increasing your pressure on the ligament.

Transverse Friction

- Work across the ligament with transverse friction.
- Apply firm pressure over a small area.

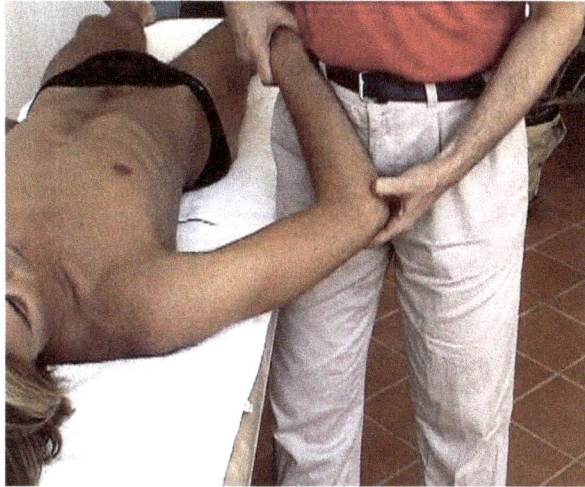

Picture 28.1

29. Medial forearm (flexor) muscles

Anatomy

<u>Superficial flexor group</u>
Flexor carpi radialis arises from the medial epicondyle as the common flexor tendon. Its long tendon starts about half-way along the forearm and attaches to the base of the second metacarpal, with slips to the third metacarpal. It is palpable. It may be absent or have additional slips to biceps tendon or aponeurosis, coronoid process, radius, flexor retinaculum, trapezium, or fourth metacarpal.
Actions: Wrist flexion and hand abduction.
Nerve supply: The median nerve C6 and **7**.

Palmaris longus arises on the medial epicondyle of the humerus as the common flexor tendon. It lies between flexor carpi radialis and flexor carpi ulnaris runs superficial to the flexor retinaculum. Its long tendon bisects the wrist and attaches on the palmar aponeurosis. It exhibits variation in its attachments and form. It may attach on adjacent muscles or antebrachial fascia, carpal ligaments or carpal bones. It may be double or its tendon devoid of muscle fibres. It may be absent unilaterally or bilaterally.
Actions: It flexes the hand and tenses the palmar fascia.
Nerve supply: The median nerve C7 and 8.

Flexor carpi ulnaris arises as a small head on the medial epicondyle of the humerus as the common flexor tendon and a larger head on medial olecranon and the proximal two-thirds of the posterior border of the ulna. It attaches on the pisiform bone. It also attaches on adjacent forearm and thenar muscles, the flexor retinaculum, and to the hamate and fifth metacarpal bone via carpal ligaments.

Actions: Wrist flexion and wrist adduction (when acting with extensor carpi ulnaris). Stabilisation of the wrist during thumb abduction and movement of the little finger.
Nerve supply: The ulnar nerve C7 and **8.**

Flexor digitorum superficialis is the largest muscle and lies deep to brachioradialis, pronator teres and the other muscles in the superficial flexor group. It has two heads. One head arises from the medial epicondyle of the humerus as the common flexor tendon, the medial collateral ligament and medial side of the coronoid process of ulna. The radial head arises as a thin sheet of muscle from an oblique line running from the radial tuberosity to a point about halfway down the anterior radius. The muscle separates into deep and superficial layers and gives rise to four tendons, which diverge after passing under the flexor retinaculum. Over the digits the tendons pass through fibrous sheaths lined by synovial membrane. At the level of the proximal phalanx each tendon splits to form a channel for the passage of the flexor digitorum profundus tendon

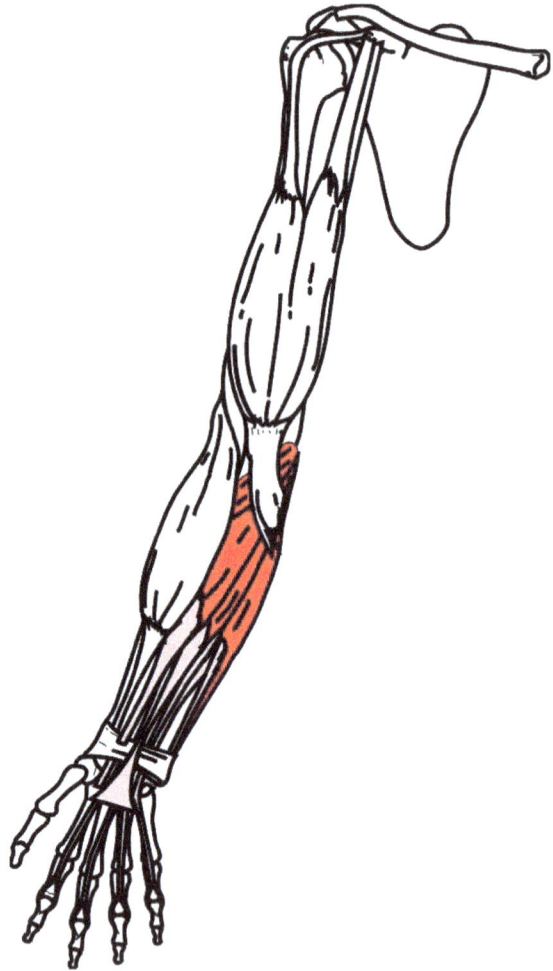

to the distal phalanx. The two tendon slips then insert on either side of the middle phalanx of all four fingers. The tendons may exhibit variation in number and form. The radial head may be absent.

Actions: Flexion of the middle and then proximal phalange. Fast and resisted finger flexion.
Nerve supply: The median nerve C7, **8** and T1.

<u>Deep flexor group</u>
Flexor digitorum profundus arises on the proximal three quarters of the anterior and medial ulna, the posterior ulna and on the anterior side of the medial half of the interosseous membrane. The muscle and its four tendons lie deep to flexor digitorum superficialis and its tendons. The tendons pass under the flexor retinaculum and then diverge. Over the digits the tendons pass through fibrous sheaths lined by synovial membrane. At the level of the proximal phalanges the individual tendons pass through a groove formed by a split in the flexor digitorum superficialis tendon. They attach on the anterior surface of the base of the distal phalanges. The muscle exhibits variations in its attachments. It may have fibres arising on the medial epicondyle, coronoid process, radius, flexor digitorum superficialis or flexor pollicis longus.

Actions: Flexion of the distal phalanges and wrist. Gentle unresisted finger flexion.
Nerve supply: The ulnar nerve for the medial muscle. The median nerve C8 and T1 for the lateral muscle.

Flexor pollicis longus arises on the anterior two-thirds of the shaft of the radius and interosseous membrane just distal to the radial tuberosity. The tendon passes under the flexor retinaculum and attaches on the base of distal phalanx of the thumb. Fibres may arise from the coronoid process, the medial epicondyle of the humerus, pronator teres, flexor digitorum superficialis or profundus. The muscle may be completely absent or may not have an interosseous attachment.

Action: Flexion of the distal phalanx of the thumb. It assists with flexion and adduction of the first metacarpal and flexion of the wrist.
Nerve supply: The median nerve C8 and T1.

Pronator teres forms the medial border of the cubital fossa. It has two heads. The larger head arises from the medial epicondyle of the humerus as the common flexor tendon and from antebrachial fascia and an intermuscular septum attached on flexor carpi radialis. The head is palpable between the medial epicondyle and biceps tendon. The other head arises on the medial side of coronoid process of ulna. The muscle runs diagonally across the anterior forearm and attaches about halfway down the lateral side of the radius. The ulnar head may be absent. In addition, fibres may attach on the biceps and brachialis or the medial intermuscular septum in the arm.

Actions: Resisted and rapid pronation of the forearm. A weak flexor of the forearm.
Nerve supply: The median nerve C6 and **7**.

Pronator quadratus
Deep to all the long forearm flexor tendons this flat rectangular muscle arises on a line running diagonally across the distal quarter of the anterior shaft of the ulna and attaches on a broad area on the distal quarter of the anterior shaft of the radius. The muscle is not palpable. Treat using muscle energy technique and stretching.

Actions: This is the main pronator of the forearm.
Nerve supply: The median nerve C8 and T1.

Deep fascia, the **antebrachial fascia** covers the muscles of the forearm, and its internal surface serves as attachment for some of these muscles. It is attached to the olecranon and posterior ulna. It gives off transverse septa, which separate the deep and superficial layers of muscle. It is continuous with the brachial fascia and strengthened by fibres extending from the biceps and triceps. At the wrist it has two thickenings the flexor and extensor retinacula.

Technique 29.1 Kneading of flexor carpi radialis, palmaris longus, flexor carpi ulnaris, flexor digitorum superficialis, flexor digitorum profundus, flexor pollicis longus and pronator teres

Patient

- Supine with the arm resting on the table by the side of the body.

Therapist

- Stand at the side of the table level with the patient's abdomen.
- Grasp the patient's hand with your either your caudad or cephalad hand, abduct their arm to about 30 degrees and flex their forearm to 90 degrees.
- The 'handshake' grip (Figure 29.1) enables the therapist to have better control over wrist flexion and extension but the 'non-handshake' grip where the fingers pass over the web spacing between the index finger and thumb is better for firm control of supination and pronation.
- Extend the patient's wrist.
- Reach around the front of the patient's forearm with the fingers of your other hand and hook your fingertips around the muscle that you are treating.
- Your thumb rests as an anchor on the posterior border of patient's ulna to enable the fingers to grip the appropriate muscle fibres firmly.

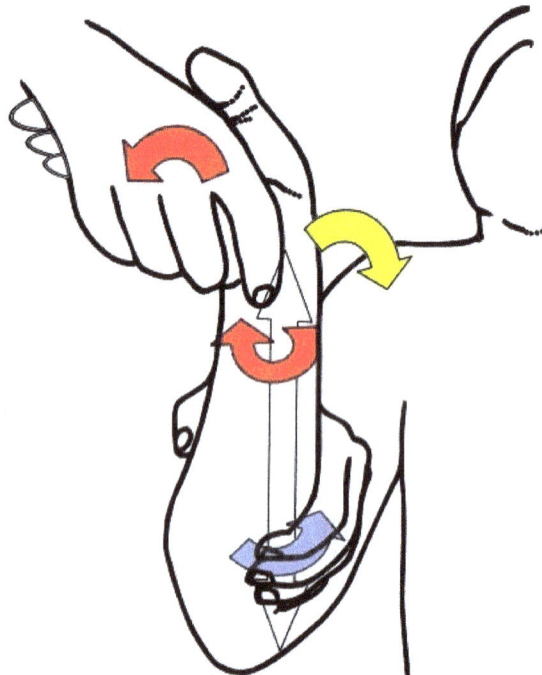

Figure 29.1

Muscle Fibres	⇕	Primary Force	⬇	Secondary Force	↻	Stretch Force	⬇	Contraction Force	⬇

Applicator

- The fingertips of your cephalad hand working across the muscle in a lateral direction or the fingertips of your caudad hand working across the muscle in a medial direction.
- Your fingertips should be together.

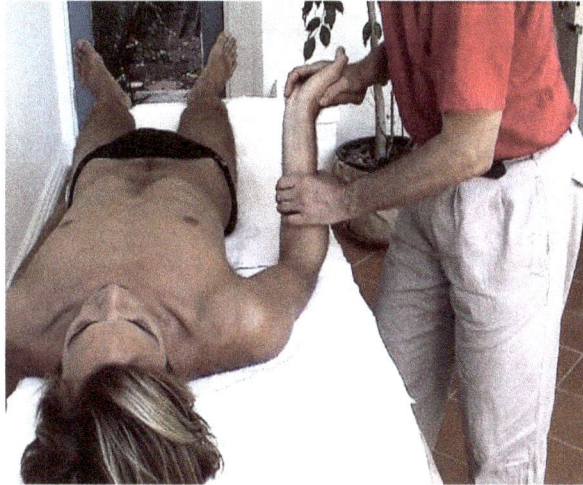

Picture 29.1

Tissue tension

- Take up the primary tissue tension with compression and a transverse force by flexing your fingertips.
- Keep your thumb anchored to the patient's ulna.
- Your force is perpendicular to the muscle fibres.
- Longitudinal tension is taken up by extending the patient's wrist and for flexor pollicis longus also extending the patient's thumb.
- Secondary tension is taken up by rotating the patient's forearm in the opposite direction to your primary force. Supinate when using your caudad hand as the applicator and pronate when using your cephalad hand as the applicator.

Kneading

- With the fingertips of one hand apply a rhythmical cycle of primary, secondary and longitudinal forces.
- Your hooked fingertips pull back on the muscle as you pronate or supinate and extend the wrist.
- For flexor pollicis longus also extend the patient's thumb.
- When the muscle is at an optimum longitudinal and secondary tension increase the primary force.
- Your pressure should be just short of discomfort.
- Start at the proximal attachment of the muscle and work your way down the forearm.
- To relax the muscle work with the patients breathing cycle, about 15 breaths per minute.
- To stimulate increase your speed to about 40 cycles per minute.

Active component

- For the wrist flexor muscles ask the patient to straighten (flex) their wrist.
- For the finger flexor muscles ask the patient to squeeze your hand (flex the fingers).
- For flexor pollicis longus ask the patient to flex their thumb.
- For pronator teres ask the patient to rotate (pronate) their forearm inwards.

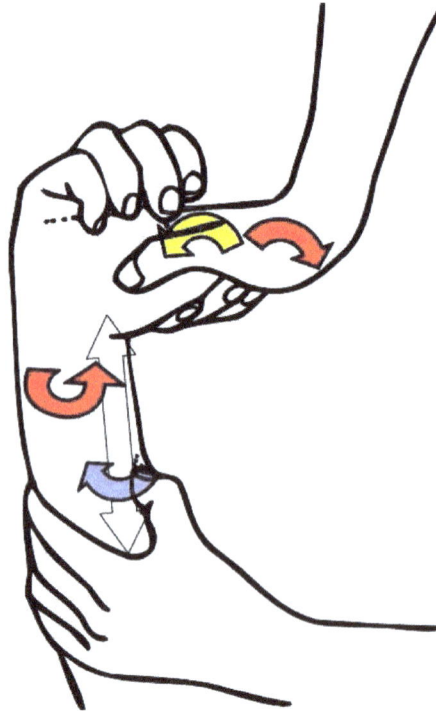

Figure 29.2

Muscle Fibres	↕	Primary Force	⬇	Secondary Force	↻	Stretch Force	⬇	Contraction Force	⬇

- Contract the muscles for 3 to 5 seconds using a 10% effort.
- Resist the patient's effort and maintain tissue lockup throughout the technique.
- Ask the patient to exhale and to relax their muscle contraction.
- When you feel that the patient has relaxed their muscles completely (about 1-3 seconds) take up the tissue slack by increasing the primary, secondary and longitudinal tension.
- Take up the slack after each contraction and during exhalation.
- Repeat 2 or 3 times or as required.

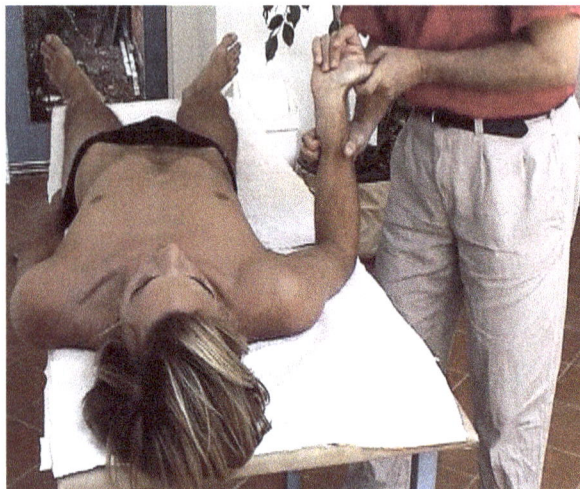

Picture 29.2

30. Lateral forearm (extensor) muscles

Anatomy

Brachioradialis is the most lateral and most superficial muscle of the group. It arises on the lateral supracondylar ridge and lateral intermuscular septum and attaches on the lateral side of the distal radius near the styloid process. It is more easily observed with resisted elbow flexion halfway between pronation and supination.
Actions: It is a forearm flexor, pronator or supinator depending on its position.
Nerve supply: Radial nerve C5, **6** and 7.

Extensor carpi ulnaris is the most medial of the extensor muscles. It arises on the lateral epicondyle by the common extensor tendon, from antebrachial fascia and aponeurosis attached to the posterior ulna and attaches on to the base of the fifth metacarpal bone.
Actions: hand extension and adduction.
Posterior interosseous nerve C7 and **8**.

Extensor carpi radialis longus arises on the lateral supracondylar ridge of humerus and lateral intermuscular septum and attaches on the posterior base of the second metacarpal. It may send slips to the first and third metacarpal bone.
Actions: hand extension and abduction.
Nerve supply: Radial nerve C6 and 7.

Extensor carpi radialis brevis arises on the lateral epicondyle of humerus by the common extensor tendon and from an intermuscular septum and the lateral collateral ligament of the elbow and attaches on the posterior base of the third metacarpal bone.
Actions: hand extension and abduction.
Nerve supply: Posterior interosseous nerve C**7** and 8. (Radial nerve)

Extensor digitorum (communis) arises on the lateral epicondyle of the humerus by the common extensor tendon and from an intermuscular septum and from antebrachial fascia and attaches on the base of the second and third phalanges of all fingers.
Action: extension of hand and fingers.
Nerve supply to extensors: Posterior interosseous nerve C**7** and 8. (Radial nerve)

Supinator is a deep muscle and forms the lateral floor of the cubital fossa. It arises on the lateral epicondyle of humerus, the lateral collateral ligament and annular ligament and on the ulna below the radial notch, and winds around the radius anteriorly to insert on the lateral surface of the proximal third of the radius.
Action: supination of the forearm.
Posterior interosseous nerve C5 and **6**. (Radial nerve)
Clinical indications of the extensors: Strain and overuse including tennis elbow.

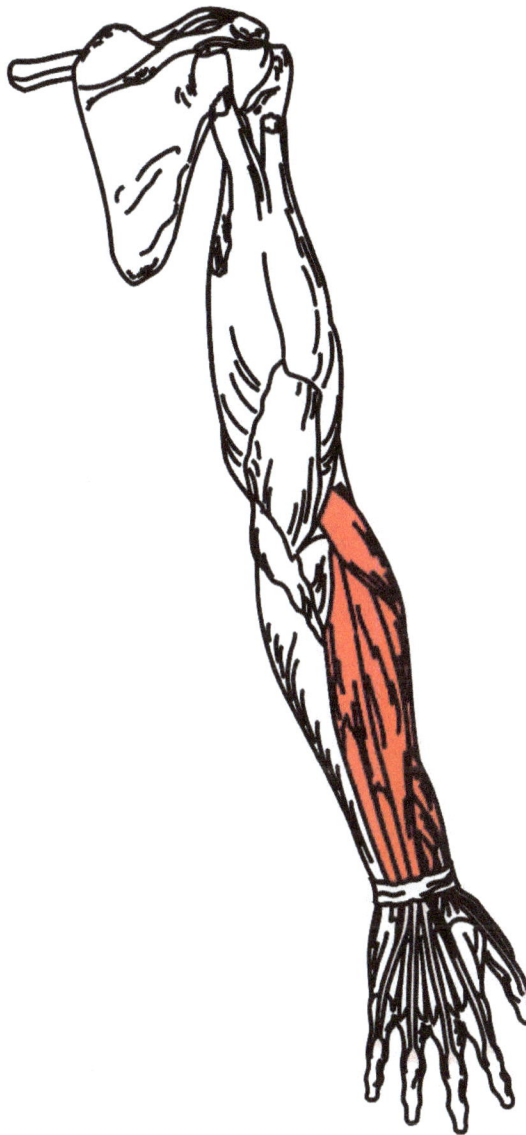

Technique 30.1 Kneading of brachioradialis, extensor carpi ulnaris, extensor carpi radialis longus and brevis, extensor digitorum and supinator

Patient

- Supine with the arm resting on the table by the side of the body.

Therapist

- Stand at the side of the table level with the patient's abdomen.
- Grasp the patient's hand with your caudad or cephalad hand and flex their wrist.
- Abduct their arm to about 30 degrees and flex their forearm to 90 degrees.
- Reach around the patient's forearm with your other hand and hook your fingertips around the muscle you are treating.
- Your thumb rests as an anchor on the posterior border of patient's ulna to enable the fingers to grip the appropriate muscle fibres firmly.

Applicator

- The fingertips of your cephalad hand work across the muscle in a lateral direction.
- Alternatively work the fingertips of your caudad hand in a medial direction.
- You fingertips should be together.

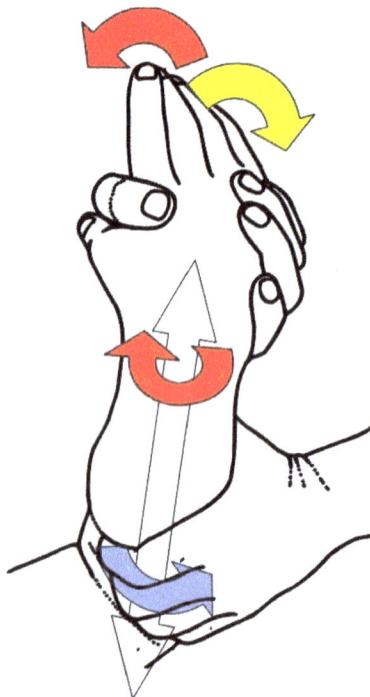

Figure 30.1

Muscle Fibres	⇕	Primary Force	⬇	Secondary Force	↻	Stretch Force	⬇	Contraction Force	⬇

Tissue tension

- Keep your wrist anchored to the patient's ulna.
- Take up the primary tissue tension with compression and a transverse force achieved by flexing your fingertips.

214

- Your force is perpendicular to the muscle.
- Longitudinal tension is taken up by flexing the patient's wrist.
- Secondary tension is taken up by rotating the patient's forearm in the opposite direction to your primary force. Supinate when using your caudad hand as the applicator and pronate when using your cephalad hand as the applicator.

Kneading

- With the fingertips of one hand apply a rhythmical cycle of primary, secondary and longitudinal forces.
- Your hooked fingertips pull back on the muscle as you pronate or supinate and flex the wrist.
- When the muscle is at an optimum longitudinal and secondary tension increase the primary force.
- Your pressure should be just short of discomfort.
- Start at the proximal attachment of the muscle and work your way down the forearm.
- To relax the muscle, work with the patients breathing cycle, about 15 breaths per minute.
- To stimulate increase your speed to about 40 cycles per minute.

Active component

- For the wrist and finger extensor muscles ask the patient to straighten (extend) their wrist.
- For brachioradialis ask the patient to flex their forearm.
- For supinator ask the patient to rotate (supinate) their forearm outwards.
- Contract the muscles for 3 to 5 seconds using a 10% effort.
- Resist the patient's effort and maintain tissue lockup throughout the technique.
- Ask the patient to exhale and to relax their muscle contraction.
- When you feel that the patient has relaxed their muscles completely (about 1-3 seconds) take up the tissue slack by increasing the primary, secondary and longitudinal tension.
- Take up the slack after each contraction and during exhalation.
- Repeat 2 or 3 times or as required.

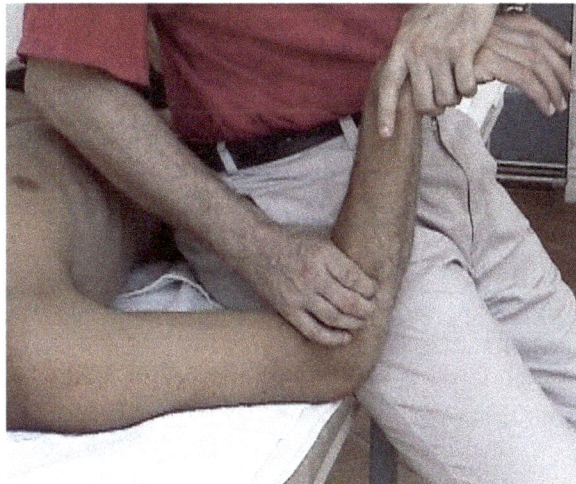

Picture 30.1

31. Forearm extensor tendons

Anatomy

On the lateral aspect is the radial styloid process and adjacent groove for abductor pollicis longus and extensor pollicis brevis tendons. On the medial aspect is the ulnar styloid process and the adjacent groove for the extensor carpi ulnaris tendon. Three synovial sheaths prevent friction as finger tendons act around angles. Six osseofascial dorsal tunnels are formed by extensor retinaculum over bone. Retinacula and transverse ligaments hold the extensor tendons in place. They support tendons of:

From lateral to medial

1) **Extensor pollicis brevis** arises on the posterior radius and interosseous membrane and attaches to the base of the first phalanx of the thumb. The most dorsal muscle and may be absent. **Abductor pollicis longus** arises on the lateral posterior ulna, interosseous membrane and posterior radius and attaches to the lateral side of the base of the first metacarpal bone. The tendon forms the radial border of the anatomical snuffbox.

2) **Extensor carpi radialis longus** arises on the lateral supracondylar ridge of the humerus and attaches to the posterior base of the second metacarpal bone and **Extensor carpi radialis brevis** arises on the lateral epicondyle of the humerus and attaches to the posterior base of the third metacarpal bone. The tendon passes over the wrist on the radial side of the radial tubercle and is prominent when the fist clenched.

3) **Extensor pollicis longus** arises in the lateral posterior ulna and attaches to the base of the distal phalanx of the thumb. The tendon makes a 45-degree turn at the radial tubercle and forms the ulnar border of the anatomical snuffbox.

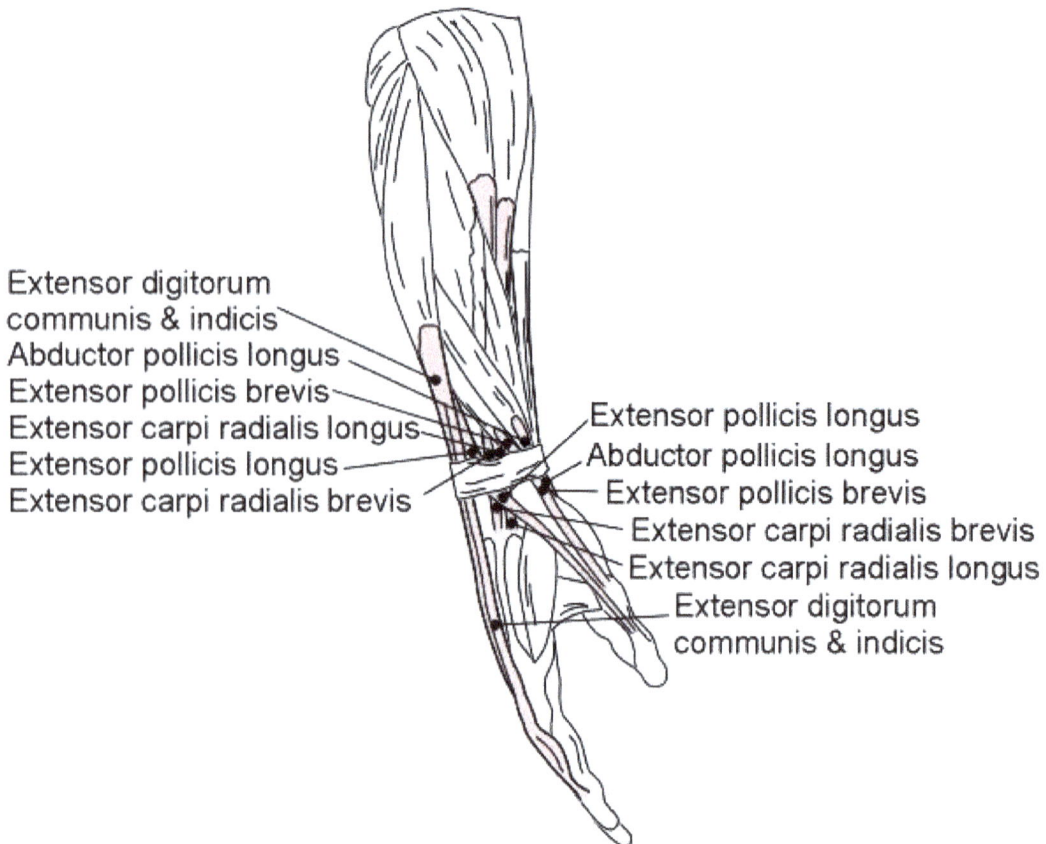

Extensor digitorum
communis & indicis
Abductor pollicis longus
Extensor pollicis brevis
Extensor carpi radialis longus
Extensor pollicis longus
Extensor carpi radialis brevis

Extensor pollicis longus
Abductor pollicis longus
Extensor pollicis brevis
Extensor carpi radialis brevis
Extensor carpi radialis longus
Extensor digitorum
communis & indicis

4) **Extensor digitorum communis** arises on the lateral epicondyle of the humerus and attaches to the base of the second and third phalanx of each finger and **Extensor indicis proprius** arises on the posterior ulna and interosseous membrane and attaches to the tendon of extensor digitorum communis on the index finger. The tendon is situated ulnar to extensor pollicis longus and is radial to the radioulnar joint. It is prominent when extending the index finger.

5) **Extensor digiti minimi** arises on the lateral epicondyle and attaches to the posterior aspect of first phalanx of the little finger. The tendon is situated radial to the ulnar styloid process and overlying the radioulnar joint.

6) **Extensor carpi ulnaris** arises on the lateral epicondyle and posterior ulna and attaches to the fifth metacarpal base. The tendon is situated along ulnar border of the wrist between the ulnar head and the styloid process.

Clinical indications: Rheumatoid arthritis, tendonitis and tenosynovitis.

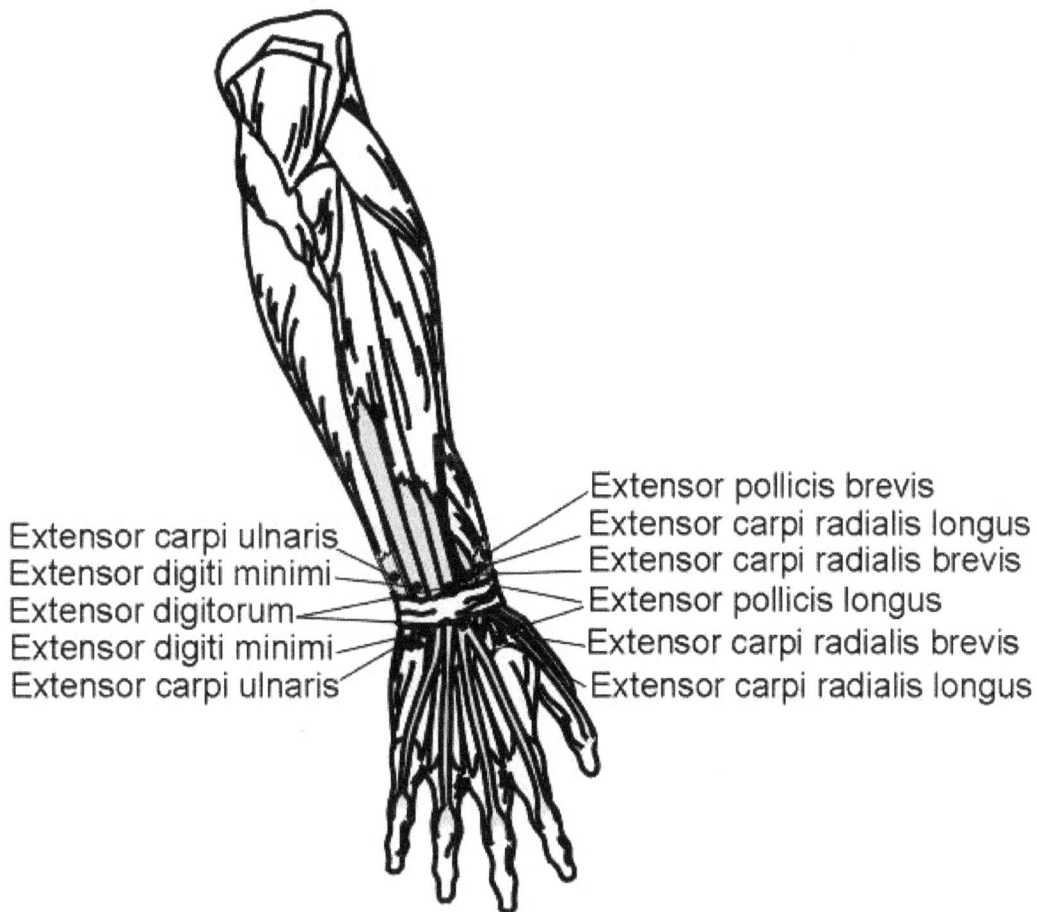

Extensor carpi ulnaris
Extensor digiti minimi
Extensor digitorum
Extensor digiti minimi
Extensor carpi ulnaris

Extensor pollicis brevis
Extensor carpi radialis longus
Extensor carpi radialis brevis
Extensor pollicis longus
Extensor carpi radialis brevis
Extensor carpi radialis longus

Technique 31.1 Transverse friction on the extensor tendons or tendon sheath

Patient

- Seated or supine with the head on a pillow or folded towel.

Therapist

- Stand at the side of the table level with the patient's forearm.
- Grasp the patient's forearm and flex it to about 45 degrees.
- Flex the wrist slightly so that the tendons are fixed but their sheaths free to move.

Applicator

- The tip of your thumb.

Tissue tension

- Find the tendon or sheath.
- Place your thumb on the tendon and take up the tissue tension by gradually increasing your thumb pressure on the tendon.

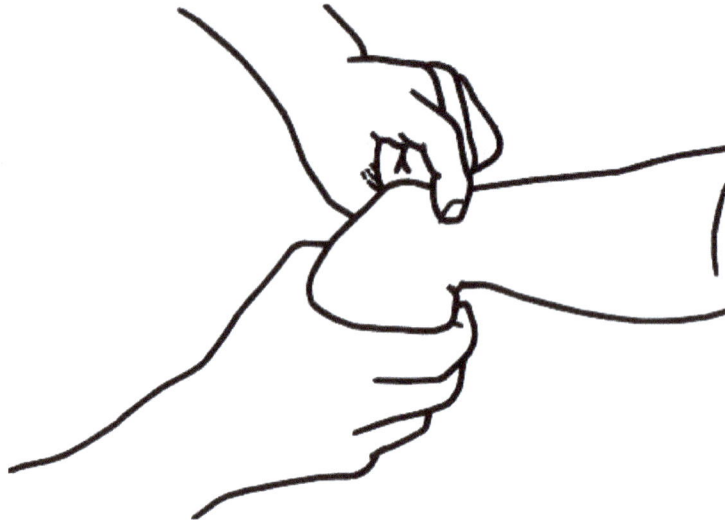

Transverse Friction

- Apply firm pressure over a small area.
- Apply transverse friction on the appropriate tendon or tendon sheath.

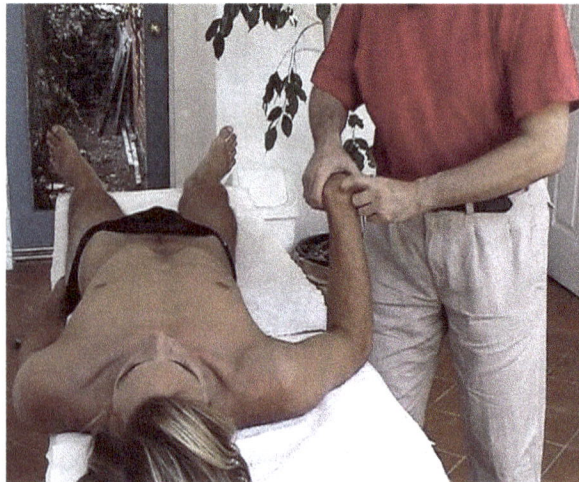

Picture 31.1

32. Muscles of the hand

Anatomy

Thenar eminence
Abductor pollicis brevis arises on the flexor retinaculum, scaphoid and trapezium and attaches to the lateral base of the first phalanx. It is the most superficial muscle of the group.

Opponens pollicis arises on the flexor retinaculum and trapezium and attaches to the lateral side of the first metacarpal bone.

Flexor pollicis brevis arises on the flexor retinaculum and trapezium and attaches to the medial and lateral sides of the base of the first phalanx. It is deep to the other muscles.

Adductor pollicis arises on the capitate, second and third metacarpal and attaches to the medial side of the base of the first phalanx. It is deep to the other muscles.

Actions: Abduction, opposition, flexion and adduction of the thumb.
Nerve supply: Median nerve C8 and T1 except adductor pollicis and the deep head of flexor pollicis brevis are supplied by the Ulnar nerve.

Hypothenar eminence
Abductor digiti minimi, Opponens digiti minimi and **Flexor digiti minimi** arise on the flexor retinaculum, pisiform and hamate and attach on the first phalanx and metacarpal of the little finger.

Actions: Abduction, opposition and flexion of the little finger.
Nerve supply: Ulnar nerve C8 and T1.

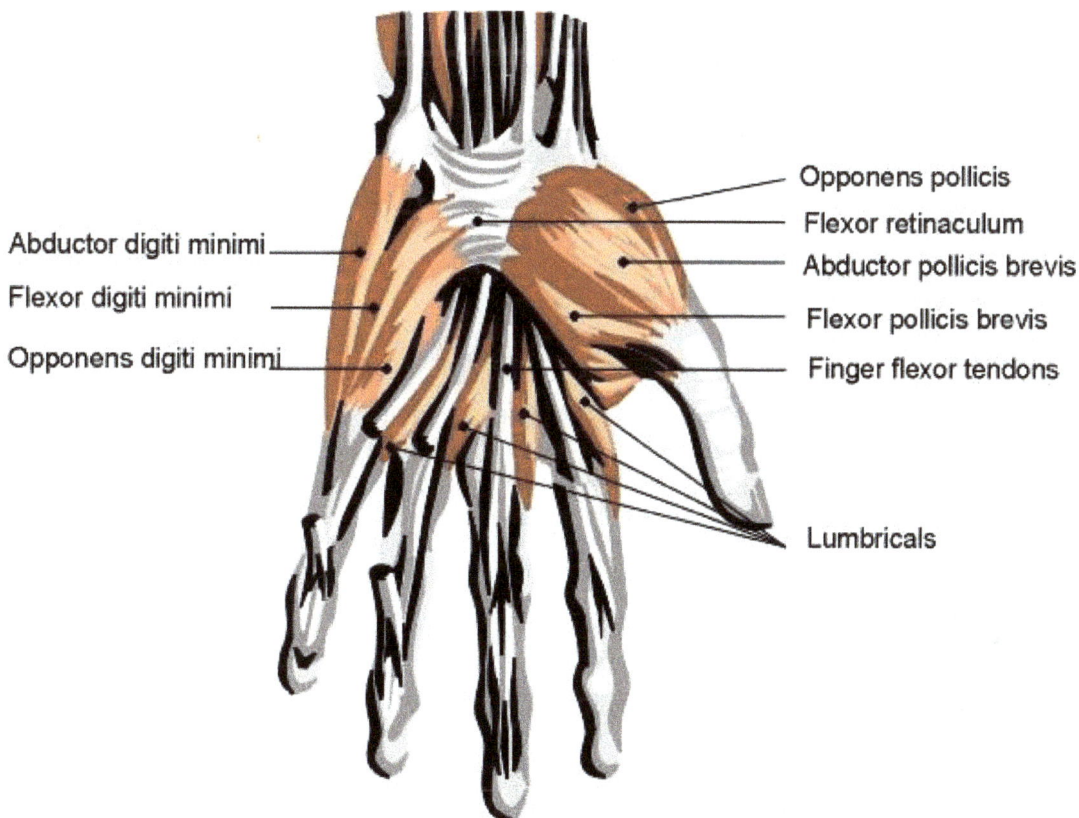

219

Other structures in the hand

The **skin** on the palmar creases of the hand is fixed to fascia, which binds it to the structures beneath. This fixation allows for objects to be held securely in the hand. The skin of the fingers is fixed to the lateral and medial sides of the carpal bones via septa and small ligaments. The skin on the dorsum of the hand is loose to permit the making of a fist.

On the palmar surface of the metacarpophalangeal joints are fleshy mounds containing **neurovascular bundles** which supply the fingers. The valleys are where the flexor tendons cross the joint.

A **palmar aponeurosis** covers the metacarpal bones, finger flexor tendons, lumbrical muscles and interosseous muscles and superficial and deep palmar arches.

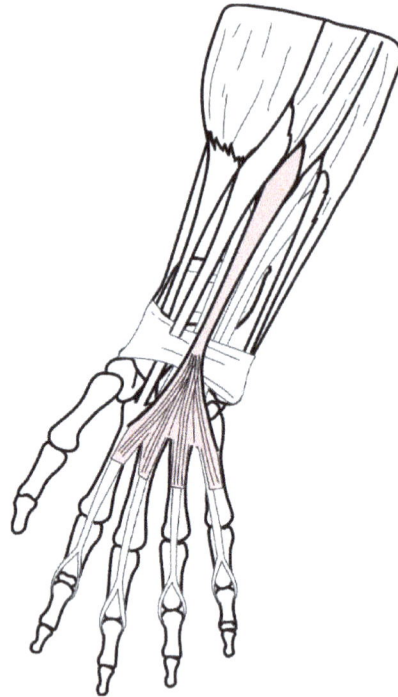

Technique 32.1 Kneading the muscles of the thenar or hypothenar eminence

Patient

- Supine with the head straight and resting on a folded towel or pillow.
- The arm rests on the table and at the side of the body.

Therapist

- Stand at the side of the table level with the patient's hips.
- Grasp the patient's hand and flex the forearm.
- Extend the patient's thumb with your cephalad hand.
- Place your applicator on the muscle.

Applicator

- The tip of the thumb of your caudad hand.

Tissue tension

- Take up the primary tissue tension with compression and a transverse force achieved by flexing and extending your thumb.
- Your force is perpendicular to the muscle.
- Longitudinal tension is taken up by extending and externally rotating the patient's thumb. It is not necessary to extend their wrist.
- For abductor pollicis brevis also adduct the thumb.

Kneading

- Apply a rhythmical cycle of primary and longitudinal forces.
- Circumduct the patient's thumb.
- When the muscle is at an optimal longitudinal tension increase the primary forces.
- With the tip of your hooked thumb push or pull on the muscle.
- Your pressure should be just short of discomfort.
- Start at the proximal attachment of the muscle and work your way to the base of the proximal phalanx.

- To relax the muscle, work with the patients breathing cycle, about 15 breaths per minute.
- To stimulate increase your speed to about 40 cycles per minute.

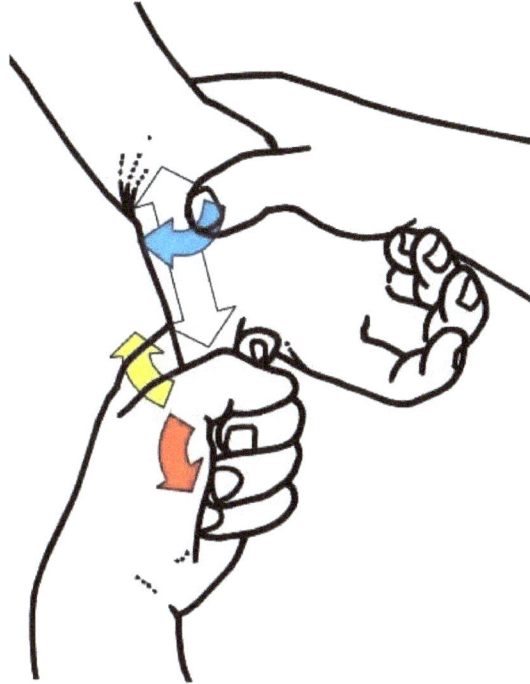

Figure 32.1

Muscle Fibres	⇕	Primary Force	⬇	Secondary Force	↻	Stretch Force	⬇	Contraction Force	⬇

Active component

- Ask the patient to take a deep breath and hold it in.
- Ask the patient to attempt to flex their thumb for 3 to 5 seconds using a 10% effort. The thenar muscles will contract.
- Resist their effort and maintain tissue lockup throughout inhalation.
- Ask the patient to exhale and to relax their muscle contraction.
- As soon as you feel that the patient has relaxed their muscles completely (about 1-3 seconds) take up the tissue slack by increasing the primary and longitudinal tension.
- Take up the slack after each contraction and during exhalation.
- Repeat 2 or 3 times or as required.

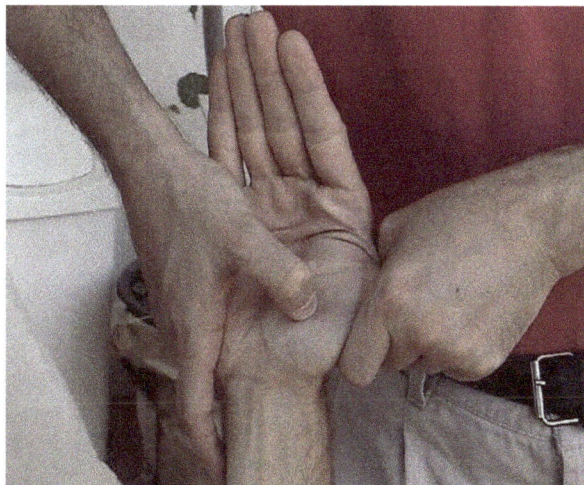

Picture 32.1

Technique 32.2 Kneading the muscles of the thenar and hypothenar eminence

Patient

- Supine with the head straight and resting on a folded towel or pillow.
- The arm rests on the table and at the side of the body and the forearm is pronated.

Therapist

- Stand at the side of the table level with the patient's hips.
- Grasp the patient's hand with both your hands and flex the forearm to 45 degrees.
- The palm of the patient's hand faces towards the floor.
- Place your thumbs together over the dorsum of the wrist.
- Reach around both sides of the patient's hand with your fingers and place your fingertips in the middle of the patient's palm with the fingernails touching each other.

Applicator

- The fingertips of both hands.

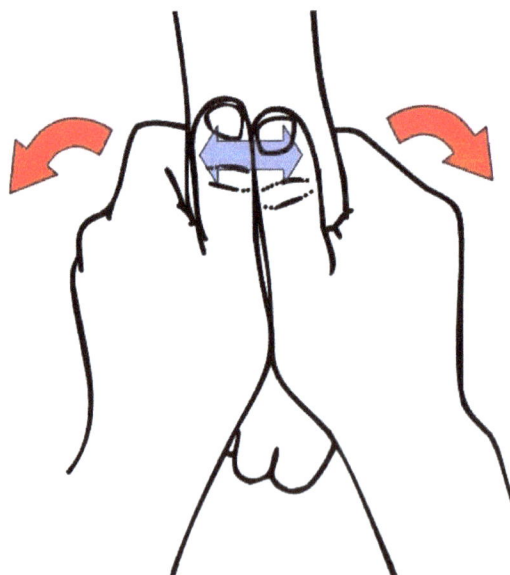

Figure 32.2

Muscle Fibres	⇕	Primary Force	⬇	Secondary Force	↺	Stretch Force	⬇	Contraction Force	⬇

Tissue tension

- Take up the primary tissue tension with compression and a transverse force achieved by flexing the fingers of both your hands while supinating both your forearms.
- Your force is perpendicular to the muscle.
- Finger pressure is countered by pressure on the dorsum of the wrist by the thumbs.

Kneading

- Apply a rhythmical cycle of primary forces.
- The patient's wrist remains in neutral.
- There is no longitudinal tension.
- This technique relies on a strong repeated grasping action with both hands.

- Your pressure should be just short of discomfort.
- Start at the proximal attachment of the muscles and work distally.
- To relax the muscle, work with the patients breathing cycle, about 15 breaths per minute.
- To stimulate increase your speed to about 40 cycles per minute.

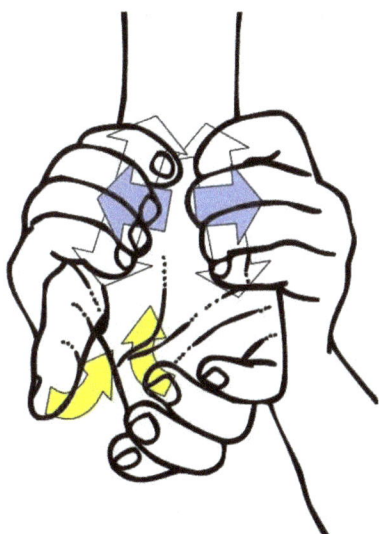 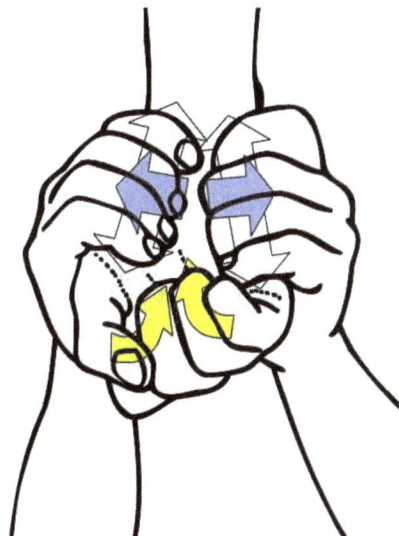

Figure 32.3   Figure 32.4

Muscle Fibres	⇕	Primary Force	⬇	Secondary Force	↻	Stretch Force	⬇	Contraction Force	⬇

Active component

- Ask the patient to take a deep breath and hold it in.
- Ask the patient to attempt to clench their fist for 3 to 5 seconds using a 10% effort. The thenar and hypothenar muscles will contract.
- Resist their effort and maintain tissue lockup throughout inhalation.
- Ask the patient to exhale and to relax their muscle contraction.
- As soon as you feel that the patient has relaxed their muscles completely (about 1-3 seconds) take up the tissue slack by increasing the primary tension.
- Take up the slack after each contraction and during exhalation.
- Repeat 2 or 3 times or as required

This technique may be used to treat carpal tunnel syndrome. The carpal tunnel is defined by the pisiform, tubercle of scaphoid, hook of hamate and tubercle of the trapezium. Attached on all four bones is the transverse carpal ligament or flexor retinaculum, which bridges the tunnel. It contains the median nerve and finger flexor tendons.

The pisiform lies within flexor carpi ulnaris tendon. The hook of the hamate is deep to the muscles of the hypothenar eminence. The tubercle of the trapezium lies under the thenar eminence. The scaphoid is just palpable anteriorly under the skin crease of the wrist.

Inflammation within the tunnel and narrowing of the tunnel may result in median nerve compression, thenar atrophy and possible restricted flexion.

In treatment the point of applicator contact is at either end of the flexor retinaculum and medial to the proximal attachments of the thenar and hypothenar muscles.

Technique 32.3 Kneading of the thenar and hypothenar muscles

Patient

- Supine with the head straight and resting on a folded towel or pillow.
- The arm rests on the table and at the side of the body and the forearm is supinated.

Therapist

- Stand at the side of the table level with the patient's hips.
- Flex the patient's elbow to 45 degrees
- Grasp the patient's hand with both your hands.
- The patient's wrist faces towards the ceiling.
- Feed the ring and little finger of your caudad hand between the patient's little and ring finger and ring and middle finger respectively.
- Feed the ring and little finger of your cephalad hand between the patient's and index finger and thumb and index and middle finger respectively.
- Place your fingertips on the dorsum of the patient's hand and extend the patients fingers and thumb.
- Place both your thumbs in the middle of the patient's palm and next to each other.

Applicator

- The pads and tips of both thumbs.

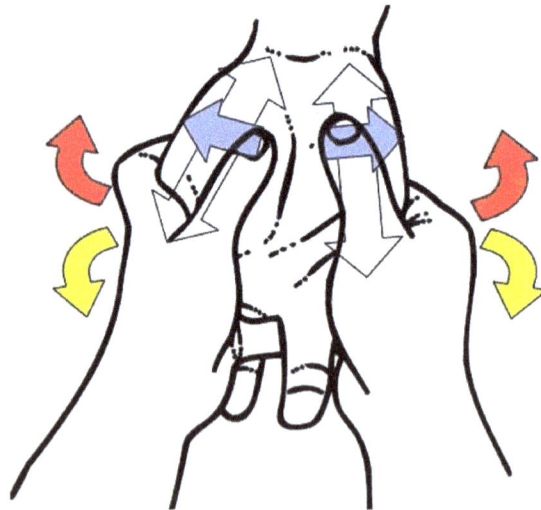

Figure 32.5

Muscle Fibres	⇕	Primary Force	⬇	Secondary Force	↻	Stretch Force	⬇	Contraction Force	⬇

Tissue tension

- Take up the primary tissue tension with compression and a transverse force by flexing both your thumbs.
- Your force is perpendicular to the muscles you are treating.
- Thumb pressure is counteracted by finger pressure on the dorsum of the hand.
- Longitudinal tension is produced by pulling back the fingers and thumb. Your fingertips act as pivots.

Kneading

- Apply a rhythmical cycle of primary and longitudinal forces.
- This technique relies on a coordinated extension of the patient's fingers and thumb with a kneading action of the therapist's thumbs.
- Your pressure should be just short of discomfort.
- Start at the proximal attachment of the muscles and work distally.
- To relax the muscle, work with the patients breathing cycle, about 15 breaths per minute.
- To stimulate increase your speed to about 40 cycles per minute.

Active component

- Ask the patient to take a deep breath and hold it in.
- Ask the patient to attempt to clench their fist for 3 to 5 seconds using a 10% effort. Their thenar and hypothenar muscles will contract.
- Resist their effort and maintain tissue lockup throughout inhalation.
- Ask the patient to exhale and to relax their muscle contraction.
- As soon as you feel that the patient has relaxed their muscles completely (about 1-3 seconds) take up the tissue slack by increasing the primary tension.
- Take up the slack after each contraction and during exhalation.
- Repeat 2 or 3 times or as required

Technique 32.4 Kneading and stretching of the palmar aponeurosis

Patient

- Supine with the head straight and resting on a folded towel or pillow.
- The arm rests on the table and at the side of the body and the forearm is pronated.

Therapist

- Stand at the side of the table level with the patient's hips.
- Flex the patient's elbow to 90 degrees
- Grasp the patient's hand with both your hands.
- Extend the patient's wrist so the palm of the patient's hand faces towards the ceiling.
- Feed the index finger and middle and little finger of your caudad hand between the patient's index and middle finger and index finger and thumb respectively.
- Feed the index and middle finger of your cephalad hand between the patient's ring and middle finger and ring finger and thumb respectively.
- Place your fingertips on the dorsum of the patient's hand and fully extend the patients fingers and thumb. The palmar aponeurosis becomes taught.
- Place both your thumbs in the middle of the patient's palm and next to each other.

Applicator

- The pads and tips of both thumbs.

Tissue tension

- Take up the primary tissue tension with compression and a transverse force by flexing both your thumbs.
- Your force is perpendicular to the muscle or fibres of the palmar aponeurosis.
- Thumb pressure is counteracted by finger pressure on the dorsum of the patient's hand.
- Longitudinal tension is produced by pulling back the fingers and thumb. Your fingertips act as pivots.

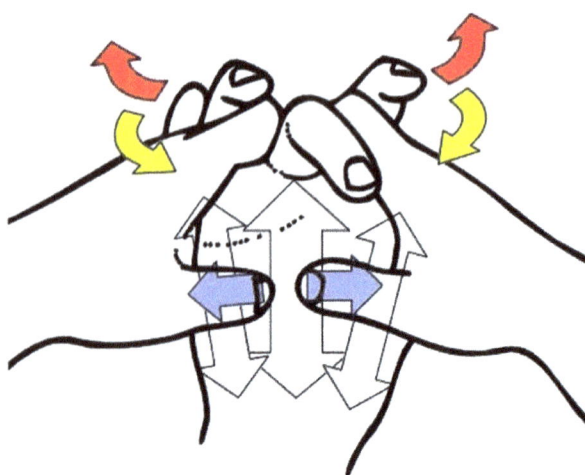

Figure 32.6

Muscle Fibres	⇕	Primary Force	⬇	Secondary Force	↺	Stretch Force	⬇	Contraction Force	⬇

Kneading

- Apply a rhythmical cycle of primary and longitudinal forces.
- The patient's wrist remains in extension.
- This technique relies on a coordinated extension of the patient's fingers with a kneading action of the therapist's thumbs.
- Your pressure should be just short of discomfort.
- Start at the proximal attachment of the muscles and work distally.
- To relax the muscle, work with the patients breathing cycle, about 15 breaths per minute.
- To stimulate increase your speed to about 40 cycles per minute.

Active component

- Ask the patient to take a deep breath and hold it in.
- Ask the patient to attempt to clench their fist for 3 to 5 seconds using a 10% effort. Their thenar and hypothenar muscles will contract and increase tension on the palmar aponeurosis.
- Resist their effort and maintain tissue lockup throughout inhalation.
- Ask the patient to exhale and to relax their muscle contraction.
- As soon as you feel that the patient has relaxed their muscles completely (about 1-3 seconds) take up the tissue slack by increasing the primary tension.
- Take up the slack after each contraction and during exhalation.
- Repeat 2 or 3 times or as required.

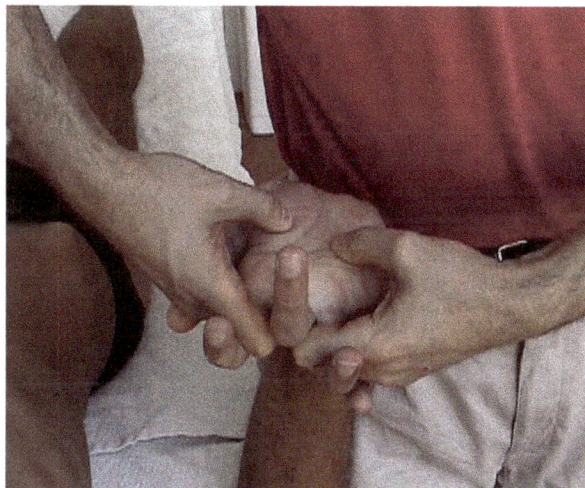

Picture 32.2

33. Iliacus and psoas major

Anatomy

Iliacus arises on the iliac fossa, iliac crest, anterior sacroiliac ligament and the base of the sacrum. Iliacus merges with the psoas tendon and directly attaches on the lesser trochanter of the femur. It is not directly palpable.
Actions: Iliacus flexes and laterally rotates the thigh.
Nerve supply: Femoral nerve L2 and L3.

Psoas major arises on the transverse processes and bodies of vertebrae L1 to L5 and intervertebral discs T12 to L5 and attaches on the lesser trochanter of the femur. It is not directly palpable. Iliac fascia covers the iliacus and psoas. It becomes thicker inferiorly. The tendon sits over a bursa, which may become inflamed.
Actions: Psoas flexes and laterally rotates the thigh. It flexes and sidebends the spine.
Nerve supply: L2 and L3.

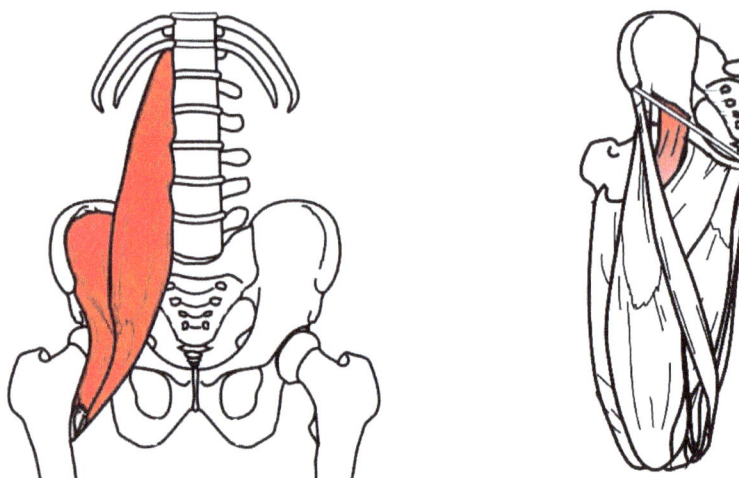

<u>Technique 33.1</u> Inhibition of psoas major

Patient

- Supine with hips and knees extended.

Therapist

- Stand at the side of the table level with the patient's abdomen.
- Place your caudad elbow against the patients thigh.
- Place the fingertips of your cephalad hand on the abdomen and push through the viscera until you feel you are on psoas major.
- There will be an increased sense of resistance felt when you are on the lumbar spine.
- Have the patient raise their right knee off the table about one centimetre.
- This action should cause a tightening of the psoas muscle, which will help the therapist to determine if the fingertips are correctly placed on the muscle.

Applicator

- Fingertips of one or both hands.

Tissue tension

- Take up tissue tension by gradually increasing your applicator pressure on the muscle.
- Extend the patient's hip to increase longitudinal tension.

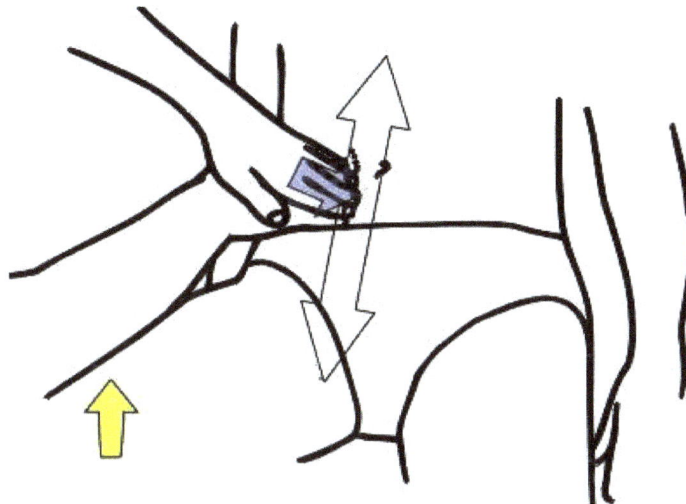

Figure 33.1

Inhibition

- Apply pressure on the psoas muscle through the abdominal wall and intestine.
- Follow a line along the lateral border of the rectus abdominis, the linea semilunaris.
- Increase compression during exhalation.
- Your pressure should be just short of discomfort. Ask the patient for feedback.
- To relax the muscle work with the patients breathing cycle, about 15 breaths per minute.
- Success of this technique depends on the build of the patient and their abdominal tone.

Active component

- Ask the patient to take a deep breath and hold it in.
- Ask the patient to attempt to lift the thigh on the side you are working, upward and off the table for 3 to 5 seconds using a 10% effort. The psoas and abdomen will contract.
- Maintain tissue compression.
- Ask the patient to exhale and to relax their muscle contraction. As soon as you feel that the patient has relaxed their muscles completely (about 3 seconds) take up the tissue slack by increasing your compression.
- Take up the slack after each contraction and during exhalation.
- Repeat 2 or 3 times or as required.

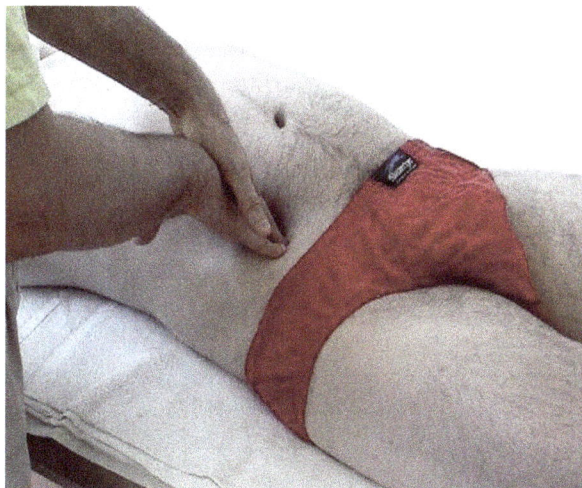

Picture 33.1

Technique 33.2 Kneading and friction over the iliopsoas muscle-tendon junction

Patient

- Supine with the head on a pillow or folded towel.

Therapist

- Stand at the side of the table level with the patient's thighs.
- Flex the patient's hip and knee that is nearest you.
- Place the patient's ankle above the knee of the other leg. The hip will abduct and externally rotate.
- Allow the patient's flexed knee to rest against your abdomen.
- Place your applicator in the depression between the patient's adductor longus and sartorius and below the inguinal ligament.
- Your fingertips rest against the upper lateral side of the femoral triangle.
- Fascia and muscles overly the iliopsoas.

Applicator

- The fingertips of both hands.

Tissue tension

- Abduct and adduct the patient's leg to find where the overlying fascia is least taught for best access for your applicator.
- Apply some compression by increasing your fingertip pressure.
- Add a transverse force to the muscle by flexing your fingers.
- Your force is perpendicular to the muscle.
- Work from medial to lateral to take the muscle away from the midline.

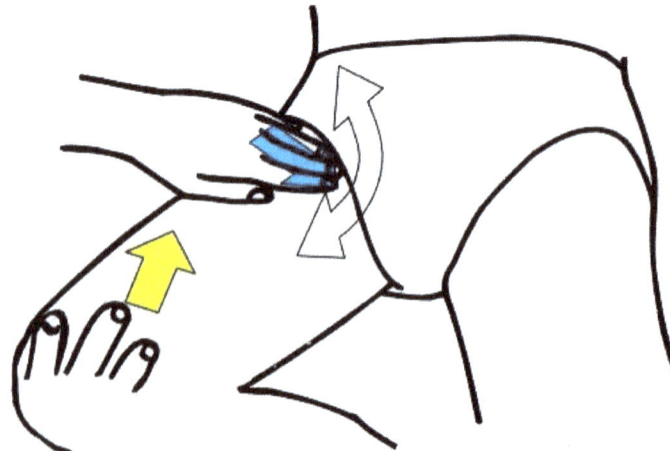

Figure 33.2

Muscle Fibres	⇕	Primary Force	⬇	Secondary Force	↻	Stretch Force	⬇	Contraction Force	⬇

230

Kneading

- With the fingertips of one hand apply a rhythmical cycle of transverse pressure.
- Start with a light 'kneading' pressure and build up to a firmer 'friction' pressure.
- Ask the patient for feedback.
- The femoral nerve, artery, vein and canal lie adjacent to the iliopsoas.
- Your pressure should be just short of discomfort.
- Work over a small surface area at one time.
- Cover the entire area.

Active component

- Ask the patient to take a deep breath in and hold it in.
- Ask the patient to contract their iliopsoas by attempting to lift their knee off the table and towards their abdomen for 3 to 5 seconds using a 10% effort.
- Resist the patient's effort and maintain tissue lockup throughout the technique.
- Ask the patient to exhale and to relax their muscle contraction.
- As soon as you feel that the patient has relaxed their muscles completely (about 1-3 seconds) take up the tissue slack by increasing the primary tension.
- Take up the slack after each contraction and during exhalation.
- Repeat 2 or 3 times or as required.

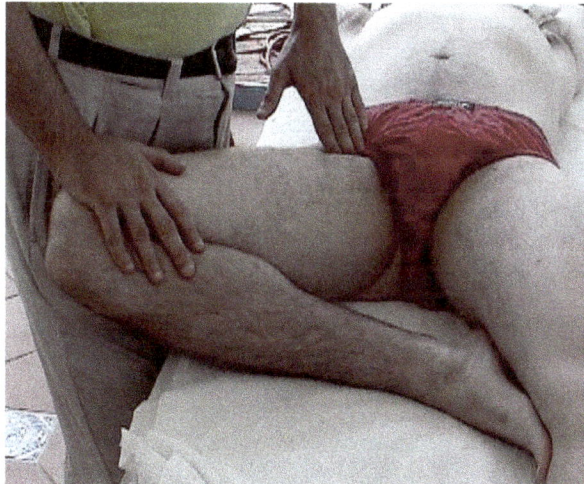

Picture 33.2

34. Gluteus minimus, gluteus medius, gluteus maximus, tensor fasciae latae and the iliotibial tract

Anatomy

Gluteus maximus arises from the aponeurosis of the erector spinae and the gluteus medius, from the posterior gluteal line of the ilium and a small area of the ilium just behind it, from the posterior surface of the inferior sacrum and from the side of the coccyx, and from the sacrospinous and sacrotuberous ligaments. Most of the muscle attaches on the iliotibial tract but the deeper fibres of the lower part of the muscle attach on the gluteal tuberosity. The muscle and adipose tissue define the characteristic roundness of the buttock.

Actions: The muscle is a hip extensor and lateral rotator. Its' upper fibres are involved in hip abduction. It adds tension to the iliotibial tract and helps balance the femur on the tibia when the quadriceps is relaxed. It is important in climbing and coming up from a flexed position. It is not active during standing.
Nerve supply: Inferior gluteal nerve L5, S**1** and **2**

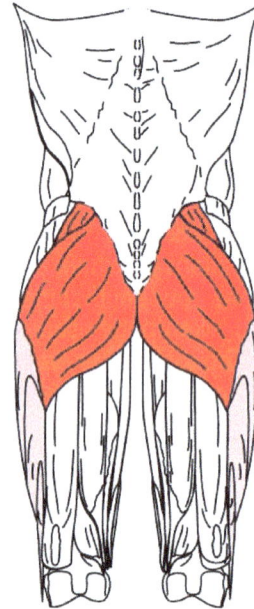

Gluteus minimus is deep to gluteus maximus and medius. It arises on the outer ilium between the anterior and inferior gluteal lines and attaches on the deep surface of an aponeurosis that ends on a tendon on the lateral side of the anterior surface of the greater trochanter. Some fibres attach on the joint capsule, and some may merge with the piriformis, gemellus superior and vastus lateralis.

Actions: Medial rotation and abduction of the hip. With gluteus medius it counters the tendency of the pelvis to drop when the foot is lifted off the ground such as in walking.
Nerve supply: Superior gluteal nerve L**5** and S1.

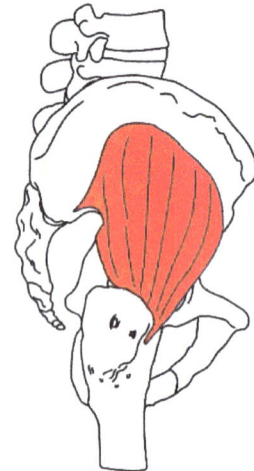

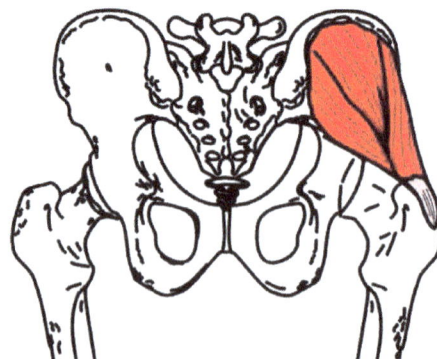

Gluteus medius arises on the outer ilium and crest and from deep fascia that covers it. It attaches on the lateral greater trochanter by a flat tendon. Its anterior two thirds is directly palpable below the iliac crest but its posterior third is covered by gluteus maximus.

Actions: The muscle is primarily a hip abductor. Its anterior fibres rotate the hip medially and its posterior fibres rotator it laterally. It is important in gait.
Nerve supply: Superior gluteal nerve L**5** and S1.

Tensor fasciae latae arises on the anterior iliac crest, anterior superior iliac spine and the surface of the fascia lata and attaches about one third of the way down the iliotibial tract. The iliotibial tract inserts on the lateral condyle of the tibia. The muscle and the iliotibial tract are palpable.

Actions: The muscle extends the knee and abducts and medially rotates the hip. It is most efficient when the knee is in extension. It works with gluteus maximus to help control posture. In the erect position it acts to stabilise the pelvis on the head of the femur and the condyles of the femur on the tibia. Nerve supply: The superior gluteal nerve L 4 and 5.

The **fascia lata** is the deep fascia of the thigh and although variable in thickness, surrounds the thigh like a stocking. It attaches on all the bones of the pelvis including the coccyx, the condyles of the femur and tibia and head of the fibula and to the linea aspera via two intermuscular septa. It attaches on the inguinal ligament and sacrotuberous ligament and serves as partial attachment for some muscles in the thigh. It splits into layers and envelops some muscles in the thigh.

On the lateral aspect of the thigh the fascia lata is thickened as the **Iliotibial tract**. It is thicker in the proximal thigh where gluteus maximus and tensor fascia lata attach and around the knee where biceps femoris, sartorius and quadriceps attach.

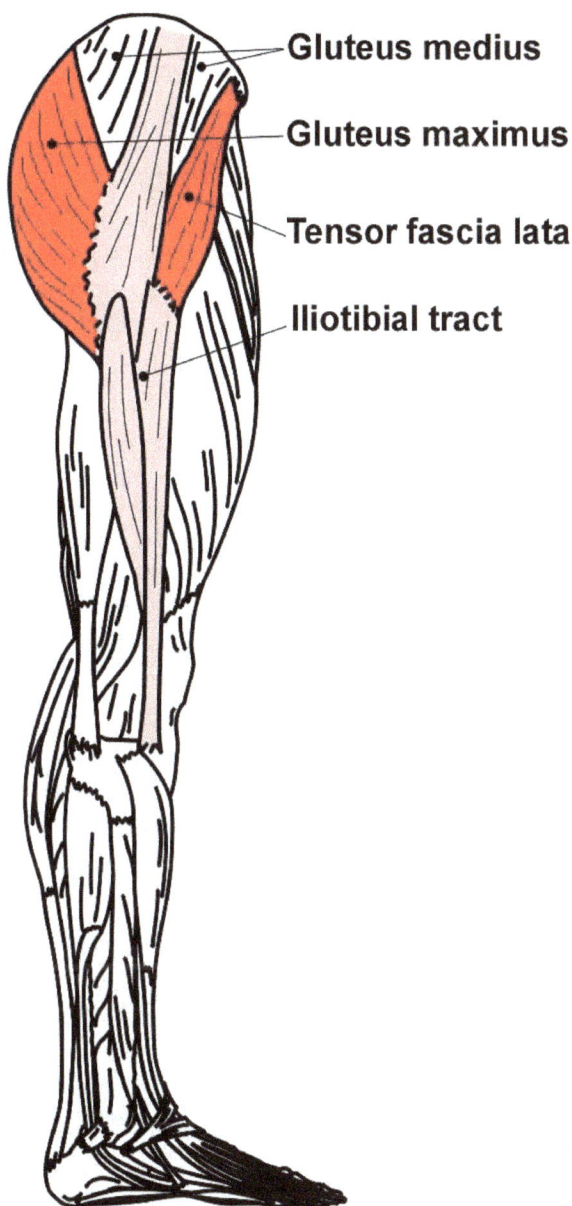

- Gluteus medius
- Gluteus maximus
- Tensor fascia lata
- Iliotibial tract

The iliotibial tract runs the length of the thigh and may function as a ligament and as a tendon. When the dense fascial sheet is taut it assist with the maintenance of an erect posture. It also acts as a shock absorber between the pelvis and the leg. When the muscle on one side becomes hypertonic its stabilising postural function becomes distorted. It may cause the pelvis to tilt anteriorly and inferiorly and increase a lumbar lordosis and create a functional short leg.

Technique 34.1 Kneading and inhibition of gluteus minimus, medius, maximus and tensor fasciae latae

Patient

- Prone with head straight or rotated.

Therapist

- Stand by the side of the table level with the patient's hips.
- Grasp the patient's ankle on the side nearest you with your caudad hand and flex their knee to 90 degrees.
- Your cephalad hand makes contact on the muscle to be treated.

Applicator

- The dorsal surface of the four proximal phalanges of the fingers of your caudad hand. This is the flat part on the back of the fingers clenched in a fist.
- Alternatives: knuckles of your index and middle finger, the pad and tip of your thumb, your pisiform bone, heel of hand or olecranon process.

Tissue tension

- Take up the primary tissue tension with compression by pushing into the muscle with your applicator.
- Take up the secondary (torsion) tissue tension by rotating your applicator. If this is a fist the axis of rotation passes through your forearm, in other words pronation and supination.

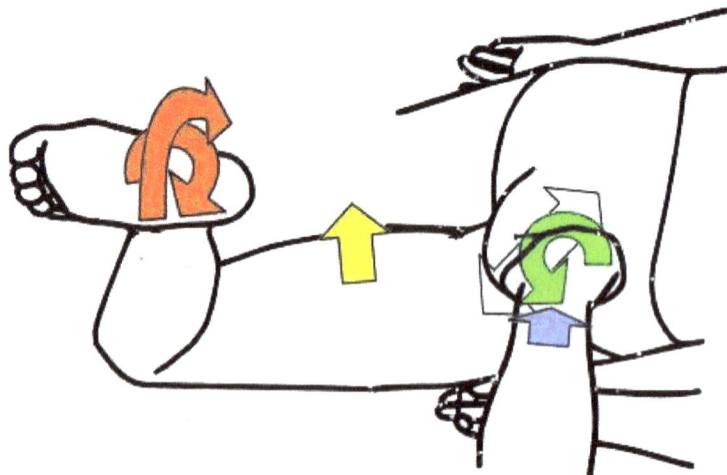

Figure 34.1

Muscle Fibres	↕	Primary Force	↓	Secondary Force	↻	Stretch Force	↓	Contraction Force	↓

Kneading

- Rotate the ankle in a circular motion thereby moving the hip through a cycle of internal and external rotation.
- Apply a rhythmical cycle of primary and secondary forces.
- When the muscle is at an optimal point in the rotation cycle increase the primary and secondary forces.

234

- The optimum point of tension depends on which fibres of the muscle you are treating. For gluteus minimus the optimum point to emphasis the pressure of your contact is in external rotation. For gluteus maximus and piriformis it is in internal rotation.
- Your pressure should be just short of discomfort.
- To relax the muscle work with the patient's breathing cycle, which is about 15 breaths per minute.
- To stimulate the muscle, increase your speed to about 40 cycles per minute.

Active component

- Ask the patient to take a deep breath and hold it in.
- Ask the patient to attempt to contract the muscle for 3 to 5 seconds using 10% of full contraction.
- For gluteus maximus ask them to lift their thigh off the table.
- For gluteus medius and tensor fascia lata ask them to push their thigh to the side.
- For gluteus minimus ask them to rotate their hip inwards.
- For the lateral rotator muscles ask them to rotate their hip outwards.
- Resist their effort and maintain tissue lockup throughout inhalation.
- Ask the patient to exhale and to relax their muscle contraction.
- As soon as you feel that the patient has relaxed their muscle completely (about 3 seconds) take up the tissue slack by increasing the primary and secondary tension.
- Take up the slack after each contraction and during exhalation.
- Repeat 2 or 3 times or as required.

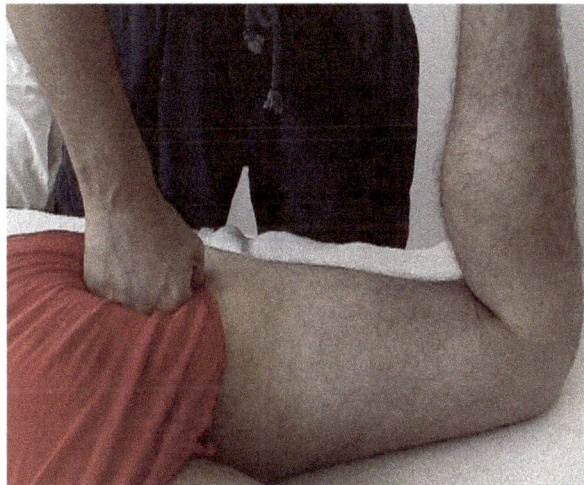

Picture 34.1

<u>Technique 34.2</u> Kneading of tensor fasciae latae and gluteal muscles and friction of the iliotibial tract

Patient

- Sidelying with the head on a pillow.
- The patient should lie diagonally across the table so that their legs are able to hang over the side of the table nearest you.
- The leg nearest the table is flexed to 90 degrees at the hip and flexed 90 degrees at the knee.

Therapist

- Stand at the side of the table behind the patient and at the level of their thigh.
- Fully flex your cephalad hip and knee.
- Place your cephalad thigh under the patient's upper thigh as close to their groin as possible.
- Your thigh acts as a fulcrum.
- You should be standing only on your caudad leg.
- Your cephalad hand makes contact on the patient's iliac crest.
- Your caudad hand grasps the patient's thigh just above the knee.
- Extend the patient's thigh until the leg is over the edge of the table.
- Adduct the thigh by lowering the leg over the side of the table towards the floor.
- Ask the patient to keep their knee straight (extended).

Applicator

- Side of thumb, pisiform bone, heel of hand, knuckles, ulna border of your forearm or olecranon process.

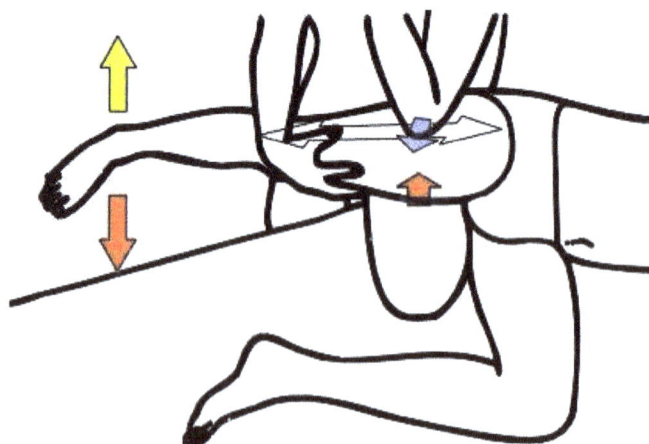

<u>Figure 34.2</u>

Muscle Fibres	⇕	Primary Force	⬇	Secondary Force	↻	Stretch Force	⬇	Contraction Force	⬇

Tissue tension

- Take up the tissue tension with your cephalad hand by applying compression and a transverse or oblique force with your applicator.
- Secondary tissue tension may be taken up with your applicator by applying a rotation force (torsion).
- Take up the longitudinal/stretch tension by adducting the patient's thigh with your caudad hand. Extend your caudad forearm and lower the leg over the side of the table.
- The thigh that you are using as a fulcrum may introduce traction at the hip.

Kneading

- Move the patient's hip through a cycle of adduction and abduction.
- Apply a rhythmical cycle of primary and secondary forces.
- When the muscle is at an optimal point in the cycle increase the forces.
- Your pressure should be just short of discomfort.
- To relax the muscle work with the patient's breathing cycle of 15 breaths per minute.
- To stimulate the muscle increase your speed to about 40 cycles per minute.

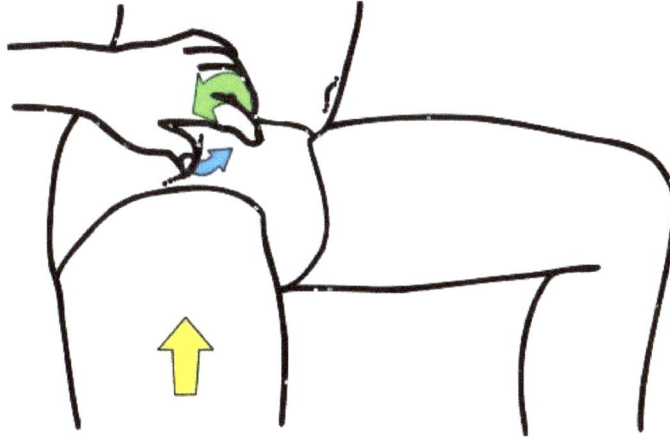

Figure 34.3

Muscle Fibres	⇕	Primary Force	⬇	Secondary Force	↺	Stretch Force	⬇	Contraction Force	⬇

Active component

- Ask the patient to take a deep breath and hold it in.
- Ask the patient to attempt to lift their thigh sideways off the table for 3 to 5 seconds using a 10% effort. The hip abductor muscles will contract.
- Resist their effort and maintain tissue lockup throughout inhalation.
- Ask the patient to exhale and to relax their muscle contraction.
- As soon as you feel that the patient has relaxed their muscles completely (about 1-3 seconds) take up the tissue slack by increasing the other tensions.
- Take up the slack after each contraction and during exhalation.
- Repeat 2 or 3 times or as required.

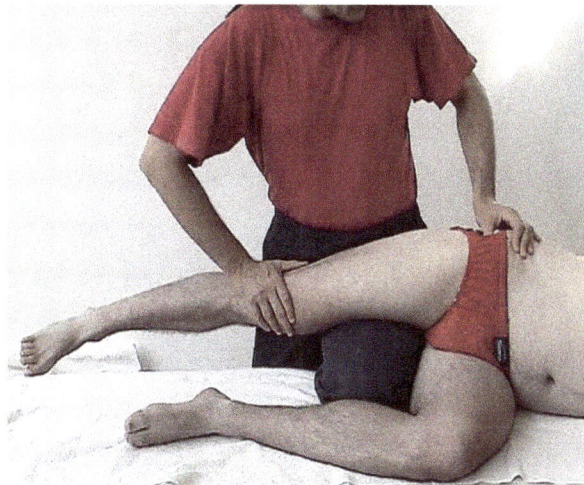

Picture 34.2

Transverse Friction

- If the iliotibial tract is dysfunctional there may be a palpable resistance and discomfort.
- Compare for symmetry but the problem may be bilateral.
- Work across the iliotibial tract with transverse friction.
- Apply firm pressure over a small area.

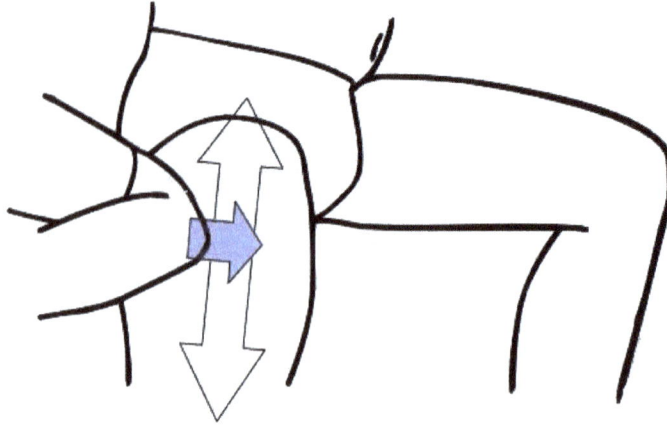

Figure 34.4

Muscle Fibres	⇕	Primary Force	⬇	Secondary Force	↻	Stretch Force	⬇	Contraction Force	⬇

- Move from the iliac crest towards its attachment on the lateral condyle of the tibia.
- It may be more appropriate to reduce longitudinal tension by allowing the patient's foot to rest on the table rather than to hang over the edge.

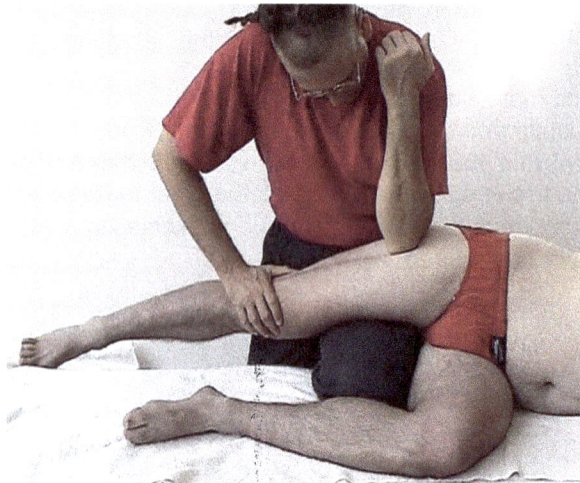

Picture 34.3

35. The posterior pelvic ligaments

Anatomy

The **sacrotuberous ligament** is a thick ligament that arises on the posterior iliac spine, lateral margin of the sacrum and upper coccyx. It runs inferiorly, laterally and anteriorly to attach on the ischial tuberosity. At the posterior iliac spine it merges with the sacroiliac ligament and at the sacrum it merges with the sacrospinous ligament. Its posterior border serves as an attachment for gluteus maximus and some of its superficial fibres merge with the tendon of the long head of biceps femoris.

The **sacrospinous ligament** arises on the lateral margin of the sacrum and coccyx just anterior to the sacrotuberous ligament. It runs inferiorly, laterally and anteriorly to attach on the ischial spine.

Actions: The sacrotuberous and sacrospinous ligaments passively oppose the forward tilting (nutation) of the sacrum on the ilium.

The **posterior sacroiliac ligaments** are long and short ligaments running between the sacrum and ilium. They are superficial to the stronger interosseous sacroiliac ligaments and the sacroiliac joints. The short posterior sacroiliac ligament arises on an inner lip of the dorsal iliac crest and attaches on an area on the superior posterior sacrum. The long posterior sacroiliac ligament arises on posterior superior iliac spine and attaches on the third and fourth segments of the lateral sacrum. They are easily palpable unless they are covered by a fibrolipoma. The ligaments may be strained from the lifting of heavy objects by unprepared or weak muscles.

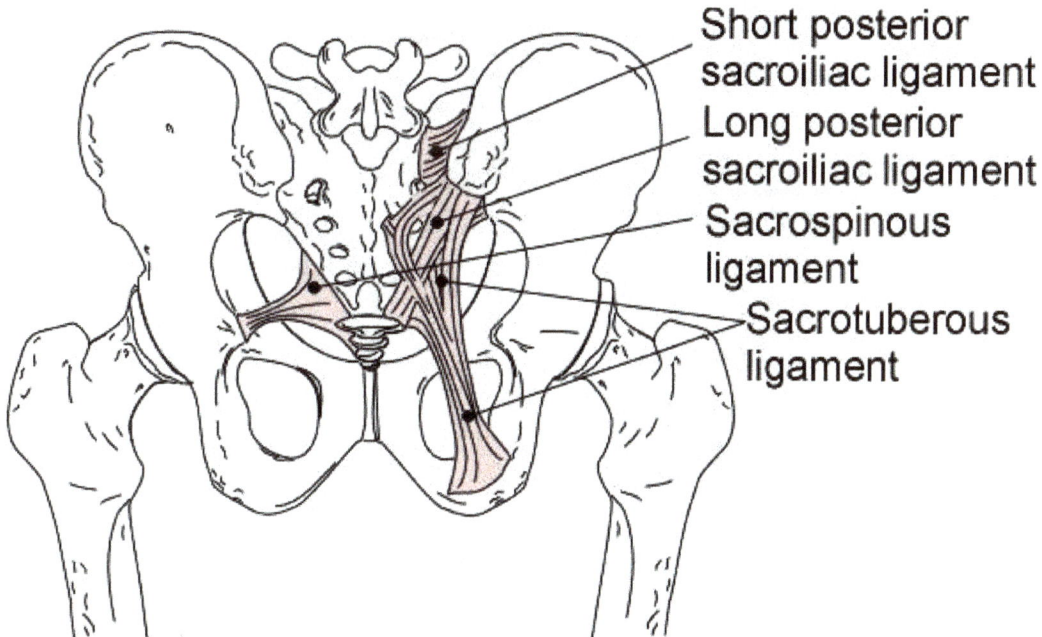

Short posterior sacroiliac ligament
Long posterior sacroiliac ligament
Sacrospinous ligament
Sacrotuberous ligament

Technique 35.1 Friction over the posterior sacroiliac ligament

Patient

- Prone with their head rotated or forward in face hole.

Therapist

- Stand at the side of the table level with the patient's lumbar spine.

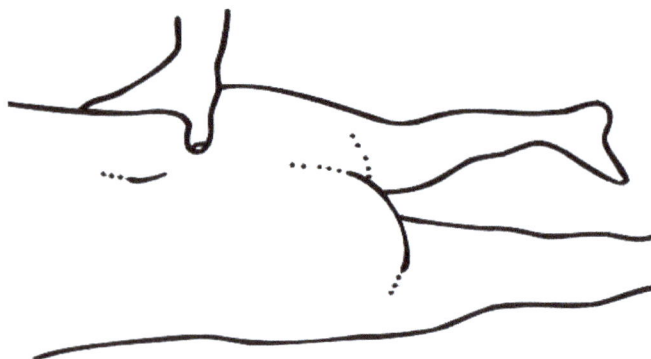

Figure 35.1

Applicator

- Tips of thumbs or a T bar.
- They are more accessible with the spine flexed over a pillow.

Transverse Friction

- Place the tips of both thumbs over the sacroiliac ligament.
- Apply transverse friction to the ligament.
- Apply firm pressure over a small area and perpendicular to the ligament.
- This is in a superior inferior direction.

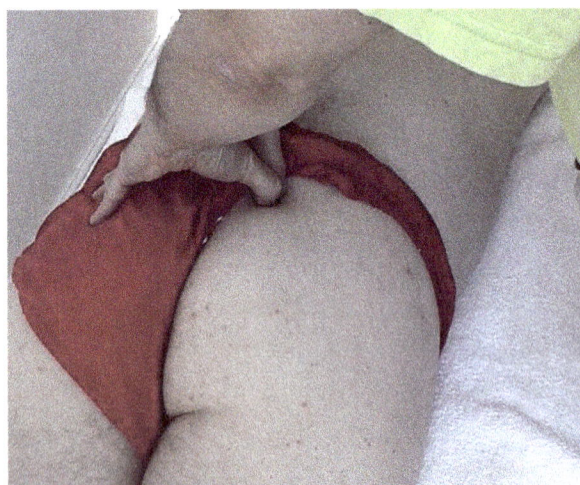

Picture 35.1

Technique 35.2 Friction over the sacrotuberous ligament

Patient

- Prone with their head rotated or forward in face hole.

Therapist

- Stand at the side of the table level with the patient's hips.

Applicator

- The tips of both thumbs.

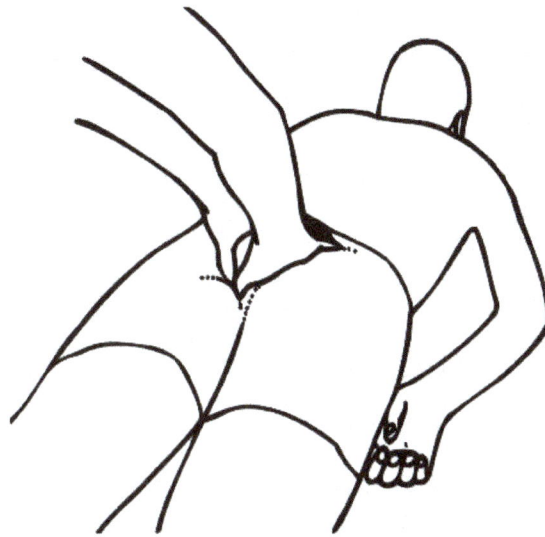

Figure 35.2

Tissue tension

- Place both thumbs on the ischial tuberosity. This is the inferior attachment of the sacrotuberous ligament.
- From here the ligament angles 45 degrees superiorly and medially toward the sacrum.
- Move about 2 inches (5 cm) towards the middle of the sacrotuberous ligament.
- Take up the tissue tension by gradually increasing your thumb pressure on the posterior aspect of the ligament.
- Press into the ligament through the gluteus maximus.
- If the gluteus maximus is hypertonic there will be a palpable resistance and discomfort. If there is sacral dysfunction one of both ligaments may be tight and tender. Compare for symmetry but the problem may be bilateral.

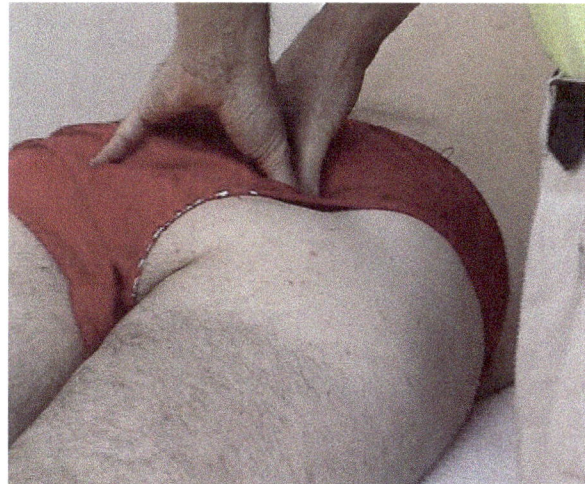

Picture 35.2

Transverse Friction

- Work across the ligament with transverse friction.
- Apply firm pressure over a small area.
- Move from the ischial tuberosity towards its attachment on the inferior lateral angle of the sacrum.

36. The ligaments and capsule of the hip joint

Anatomy

The **hip joint capsule** arises on the rim of the acetabulum, the acetabular labrum, transverse acetabular ligament and the edge of the obturator foramen. It attaches to the neck of the femur and to the trochanteric line anteriorly. It surrounds the acetabulum, the joint, the head and the neck of the femur. It has deep circular fibres that form a collar around the joint and longitudinal fibres. The capsule blends with and is strengthened by the iliofemoral ligament anteriorly and the ischiofemoral ligament and the pubofemoral ligament posteriorly.

The **iliofemoral ligament** is strong and situated anterior to the joint. It arises on the anterior inferior iliac spine, spirals around the joint and attaches on the tubercle and trochanteric line of the femur.

The **ischiofemoral ligament** is posterior to the joint. It arises on the ischium and attaches on the greater trochanter and the circular fibre of the joint capsule.

The **pubofemoral ligament** arises on the iliopectineal eminence, pubic ramus, and the obturator crest and membrane. It merges with the capsule and the iliofemoral ligament.

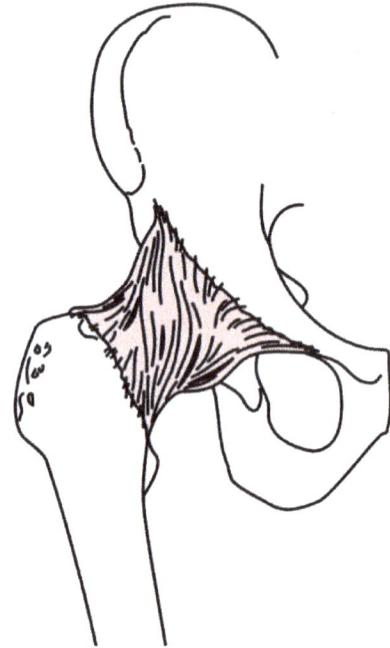

Actions: All limit hip extension.
Clinical indications: Osteoarthritis: rarely strain.

Technique 36.1 Friction over the ligaments and capsule of the hip joint

Patient

- Prone with their head rotated or forward in face hole.

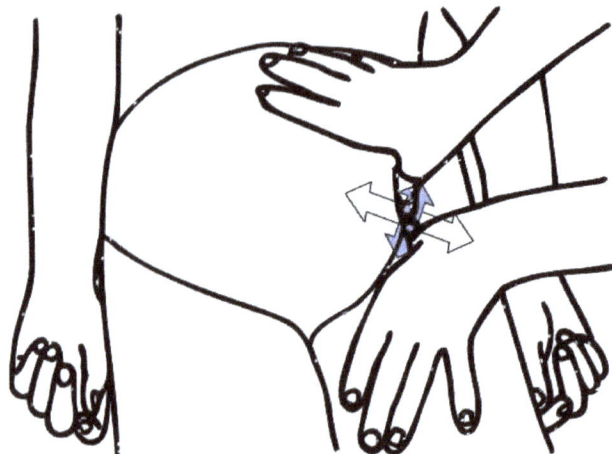

Figure 36.1

Muscle Fibres	⇕	Primary Force	⬇	Secondary Force	↻	Stretch Force	⬇	Contraction Force	⬇

Therapist

- Stand at the side of the table level with the patient's hips.

Applicator

- The tips of both thumbs.

Tissue tension

- Place the tips of both thumbs on a posterior point along the joint line.
- Take up the tissue tension by gradually increasing your thumb pressure on the ligament.
- Press into the ligament through the gluteus maximus.

Transverse Friction

- Work across the ligament with transverse friction. This is in a superior-inferior direction.
- Apply firm pressure over a small area.
- Start at the most inferior part of the joint and work superiorly and then follow the bony contour of the joint line as far as it is accessible anteriorly.

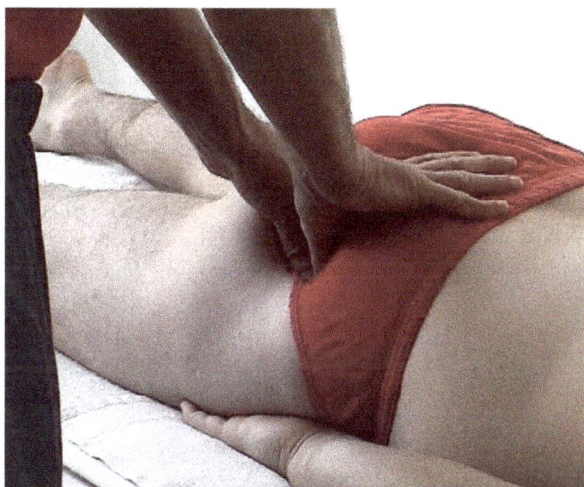

Picture 36.1

37. Inguinal ligament

Anatomy

The **inguinal ligament** arises from the aponeurotic border of the external oblique muscle. It runs from the anterior superior iliac spine to the pubic tubercle.

Clinical indications: strain, herniation and scared after surgery.

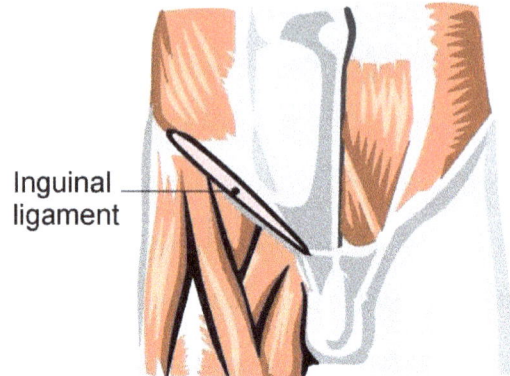

Inguinal ligament

Technique 37.1 Friction over the inguinal ligament

Patient

- Supine with the knee flexed and the hip flexed and abducted.
- Alternatively, the leg can remain straight and resting on the table.

Therapist

- Stand at the side of the table level with the patient's thighs.
- Support the weight of the patient's leg by resting their knee on your abdomen.

Applicator

- Tips of thumbs, fingers or a T bar.

Transverse Friction

- Place the applicator over the inguinal ligament.
- Apply transverse friction to the ligament.
- Apply firm pressure over a small area and perpendicular to the ligament.

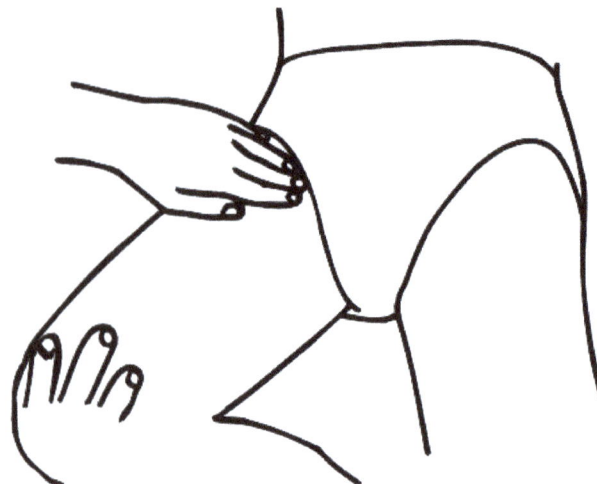

Figure 37.1

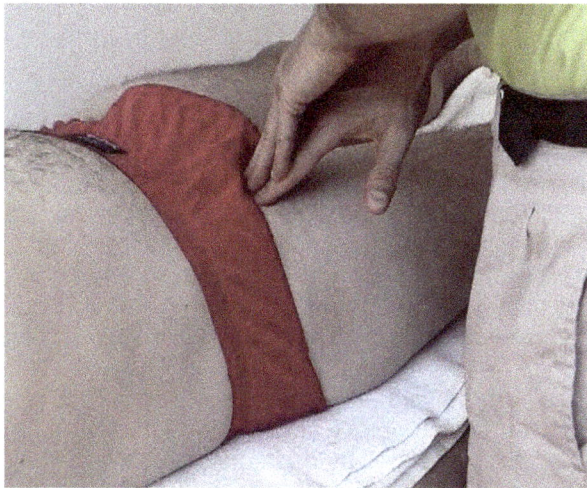

Picture 37.1

38. Piriformis, obturator internus and externus, the gamelli and quadratus femoris

Anatomy

Piriformis arises on the anterior sacrum, but a few fibres arise from a small area on the gluteal surface of the ilium near the posterior inferior iliac spine and from the capsule of the sacroiliac joint. The muscle passes through the greater sciatic foramen and attaches by a rounded tendon on the superior greater trochanter. The tendon may merge with the common tendon of the obturator internus and gamelli. The piriformis muscle may be partly or completely absent and exhibit anatomical variations such as dividing or merging with gluteus medius.

Obturator internus arises from within the true pelvis on the inner surface of the inferior pubic ramus, ischial ramus, the obturator membrane and its aponeurosis. The muscle fibres converge onto four tendinous bands, which makes a 90 degree bend over the ischium between its spine and tuberosity and exits the pelvis through the lesser sciatic foramen. The bands merge into a single flat tendon which receives fibres from the gamelli and then attaches on medial surface of the greater trochanter.

The **gamellus superior** arises on the posterior surface of the ischial spine and attaches on the medial surface of the greater trochanter via the common tendon. It may be absent.

The **gamellus inferior** arises on the upper ischial tuberosity and attaches on the medial surface of the greater trochanter via the common tendon.

Actions: Lateral rotation of the extended thigh and abduction of the flexed thigh.
Nerve supply: Piriformis L5, S1 and 2. Obturator internus and gamelli L5 and S1.

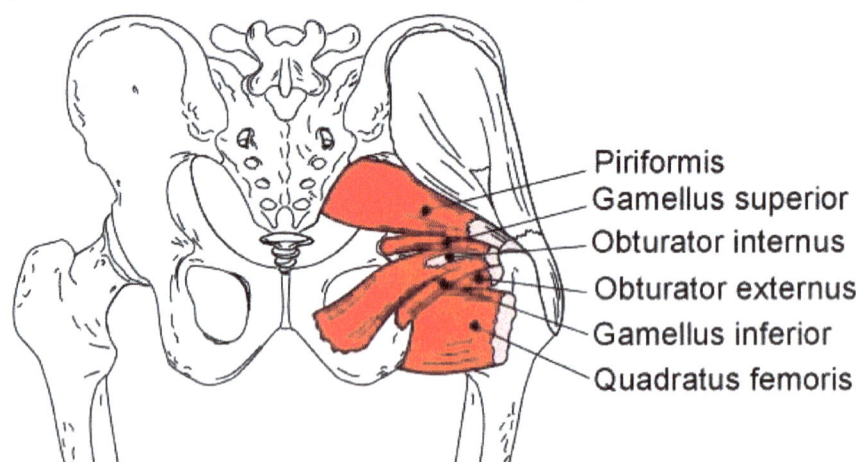

Piriformis
Gamellus superior
Obturator internus
Obturator externus
Gamellus inferior
Quadratus femoris

The **quadratus femoris** arises from the upper lateral ischial tuberosity and attaches on the upper trochanteric crest of the femur. It may be absent.
Actions: Lateral rotation of the thigh.
Nerve supply: L5 and S1.

Obturator externus arises from the pubic ramus, ischial ramus and the outer surface of the obturator membrane. The muscle fibres converge onto a tendon which passes over the neck of the femur and then attaches on the trochanteric fossa of the femur.
Actions: Lateral rotation of the thigh.
Nerve supply: L3 and 4.

Piriformis, Obturator internus and externus, the Gamelli and Quadratus femoris are deep and not easily palpable.
Actions generally: These are important postural muscles and help to stabilise the hip joint.

Sciatic nerve - derived from lumbarsacral plexus L4, 5, S1, 2 & 3. The sciatic nerve passes out of the pelvis through the greater sciatic foramen and normally passes under the piriformis. However, it may pass over the piriformis, pierce the piriformis or divide early and the division, usually the common peroneal nerve, pass over or through the muscle. If hypertonic the piriformis may result in sciatica.

A hypertonic piriformis also has the ability to displace the sacrum anteriorly and laterally, and thus distort the sacroiliac joint and stretch the ligaments over the joint. The piriformis should be checked in all back pain syndromes because displacement of the sacrum creates the possibility of nerve impingement of the sacral plexus.

A hypertonic obturator externus can irritate the **obturator nerve** as it passes through the obturator foramen and the obturator externus muscle. There may be symptoms of pain, burning and tingling in the anterior and medial thigh and groin.

Technique 38.1 Kneading and inhibition of the hip lateral rotator and gluteal muscles

Patient

- Prone with the head straight in a face hole or rotated towards the side you are standing.

Therapist

- Stand by the side of the table level with the patient's hips.
- Grasp the patient's ankle that is furthest from you with your caudad hand and flex their knee to 90 degrees.
- Reach over the patient's pelvis with your cephalad hand and make contact on the muscle to be treated with your applicator.

Applicator

- Olecranon process, knuckles of clenched fist, the tip of the thumb or pisiform bone.

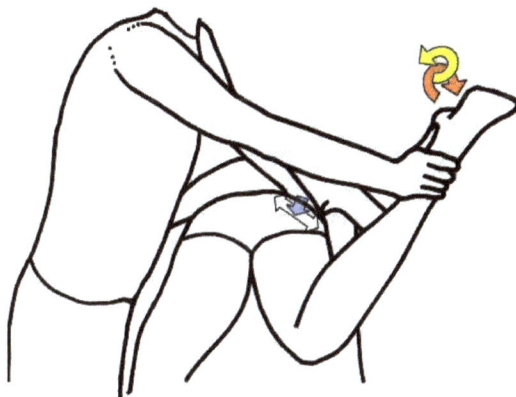
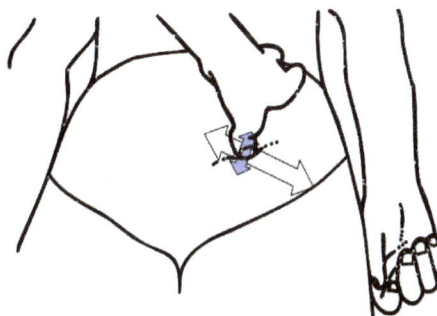

Figure 38.1   Figure 38.2

Muscle Fibres	⇕	Primary Force	⬇	Secondary Force	↻	Stretch Force	⬇	Contraction Force	⬇

Tissue tension

- Take up the primary tissue tension with compression and a transverse pressure by applying a cross fibre force on the muscles with your applicator.
- Take up the longitudinal tension by pushing the patient's leg away from you thereby increasing medial rotation at the hip.

Kneading

- Rotate the ankle in a circular motion thereby moving the hip through a cycle of internal and external rotation.
- Apply a rhythmical cycle of compression and transverse force.
- When the muscle is at an optimal point in the rotation cycle increase the primary forces.
- The optimum point of tension depends on which of the muscles you are treating.

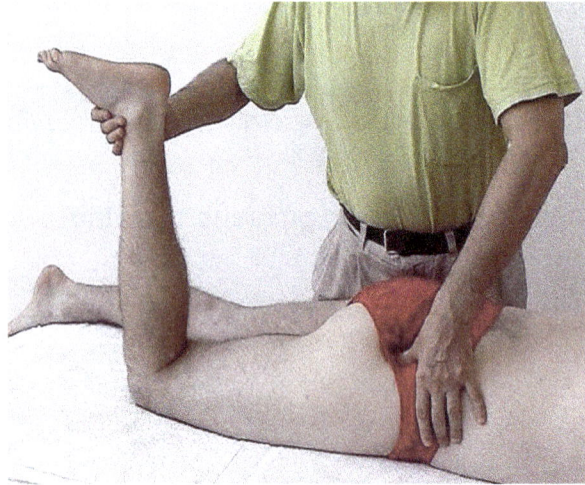

Picture 38.1

- For gluteus minimus the optimum place to emphasise the pressure of your contact is in external rotation. For piriformis and the other lateral rotators, it is in internal rotation.
- Your pressure should be just short of discomfort.
- To relax the muscle work with the patient's breathing cycle of 15 breaths per minute.
- To stimulate the muscle, increase your speed to about 40 cycles per minute.

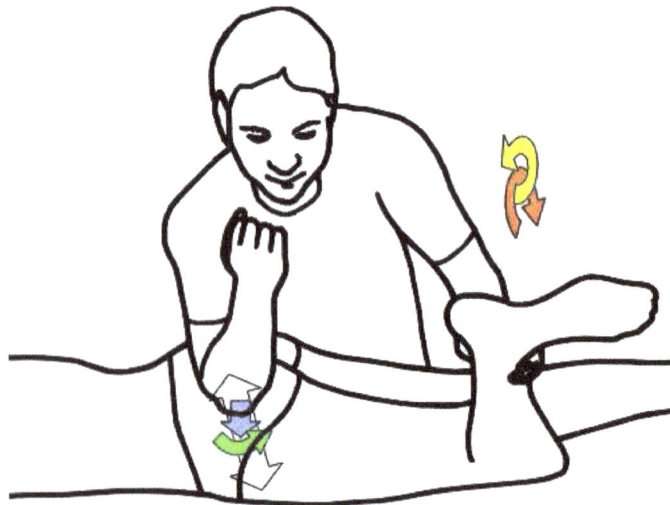

Figure 38.3 Shown for the lateral rotator muscles

Muscle Fibres	⇕	Primary Force	⬇	Secondary Force	↻	Stretch Force	⬇	Contraction Force	⬇

Active component

- Ask the patient to take a deep breath and hold it in.
- Ask the patient to attempt to contract their muscle for 3 to 5 seconds using a 10% effort.

- For gluteus maximus ask them to lift their thigh off the table.
- For gluteus medius and tensor fascia lata ask them to push their thigh to the side.
- For gluteus minimus ask them to rotate their hip inwards.
- For the lateral rotator muscles ask them to rotate their hip outwards.

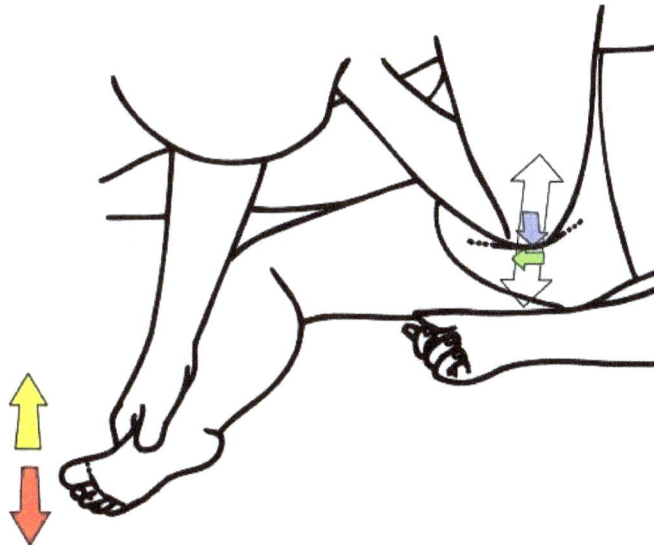

Figure 38.4

Muscle Fibres	⇕	Primary Force	⬇	Secondary Force	↻	Stretch Force	⬇	Contraction Force	⬇

- Resist their effort and maintain tissue lockup throughout inhalation.
- Ask the patient to exhale and to relax their muscle contraction.
- As soon as you feel that the patient has relaxed their gluteus maximus completely (about 3 seconds) take up the tissue slack by increasing the primary and secondary tension.
- Take up the slack after each contraction and during exhalation.
- Repeat 2 or 3 times or as required.

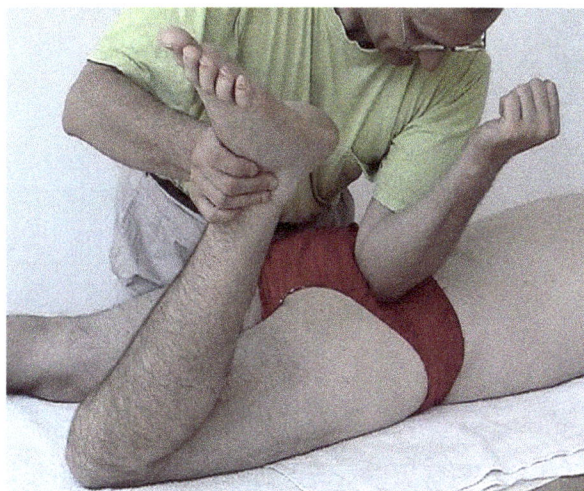

Picture 38.2

<u>Technique 38.2</u> Kneading and inhibition of the deep hip muscles and hip joint capsule

Patient

- Prone with head rotated towards you.

Therapist

- Stand by the side of the table opposite the patient's hips.
- Grasp the patient's ankle nearest you with your caudad hand and flex their knee to 90 degrees.
- Internally rotate the thigh for easier access to the deep hip rotators.
- Your cephalad applicator makes contact on the muscle to be treated.
- Find the deep hip rotators on the posterior aspect of the hip on the medial and superior edge of the greater trochanter.
- Press through the gluteal maximus.

Applicator

- Olecranon process.
- Alternatives: knuckles of index and middle finger, the tip of the thumb or the tips of both thumbs pointed toward each other.

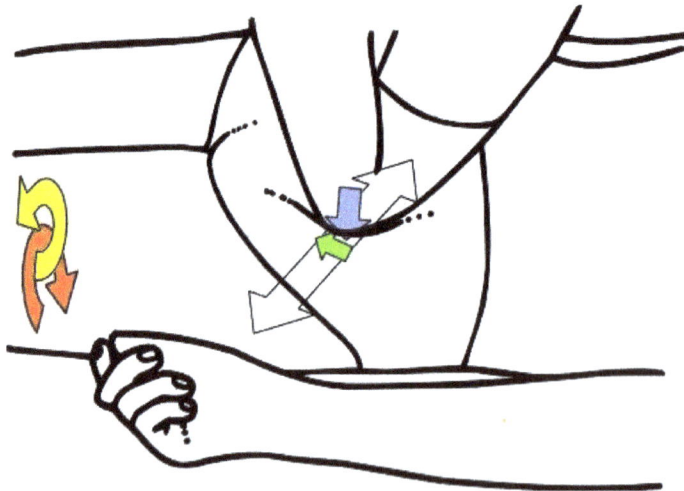

<u>Figure 38.5</u>

Muscle Fibres	⇕	Primary Force	⬇	Secondary Force	↻	Stretch Force	⬇	Contraction Force	⬇

Tissue tension

- Take up the primary tissue tension with compression by pushing into the muscle with your applicator and a transverse pressure by applying a cross fibre force on the muscles with your applicator.
- Take up the longitudinal tension by pulling the patient's leg towards you thus increasing medial rotation at the hip.

Kneading and inhibition

- Move the hip through a cycle of internal and external rotation by rotating the ankle in a circular motion. Alternatively use a fixed internal rotation position.
- Apply a rhythmical cycle of compression and transverse force.
- This is a generally in a superior-inferior direction.

- When the muscle is at an optimal point of longitudinal tension increase the primary forces. For the lateral hip rotator muscles, this is towards the end of internal rotation.

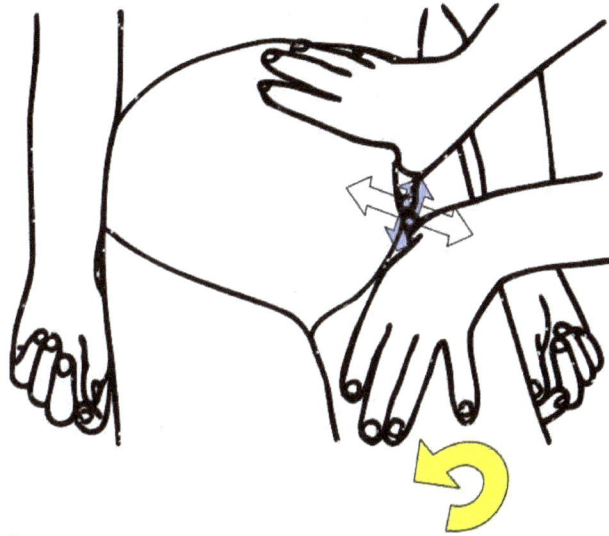

Figure 38.6

Muscle Fibres	⇕	Primary Force	⬇	Secondary Force	↻	Stretch Force	⬇	Contraction Force	⬇

- Your pressure should be just short of discomfort.
- Start at the head of the femur and work medially.
- Apply inhibition or cross fibre kneading with your applicator.
- Cover the entire area of the deep hip rotators.
- Work in a transverse direction across the piriformis, and then work on the other five deep hip rotators, which lie just inferior to it. These are superior and inferior gemellus, obturator internus and externus and quadratus femoris.
- To relax the muscle work with the patient's breathing cycle of 15 breaths per minute.
- To stimulate the muscle increase your speed to about 40 cycles per minute.

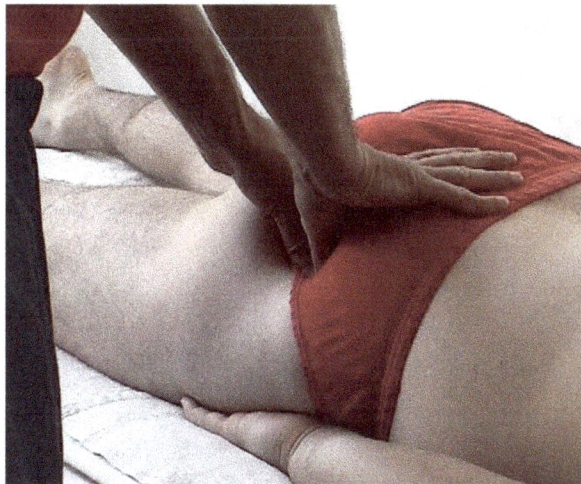

Picture 38.3

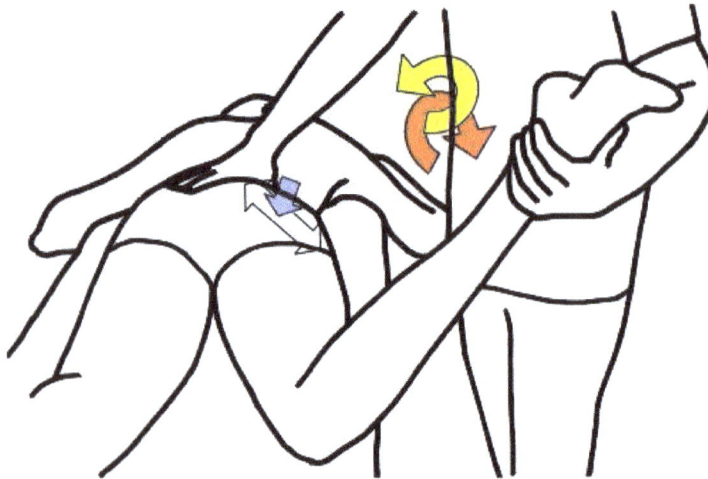

Figure 38.7

Muscle Fibres	⇕	Primary Force	⬇	Secondary Force	↻	Stretch Force	⬇	Contraction Force	⬇

Active component

- Ask the patient to take a deep breath and hold it in.
- Ask the patient to attempt to rotate their hip outwards contract the muscle for 3 to 5 seconds using 10% of full contraction. The lateral rotator muscles will contract.
- Resist their effort and maintain tissue lockup throughout inhalation.
- Ask the patient to exhale and to relax their muscle contraction.
- As soon as you feel that the patient has relaxed their deep hip muscles completely
- (about 3 seconds) take up the tissue slack by increasing the primary tension.
- Take up the slack after each contraction and during exhalation.
- Repeat 2 or 3 times or as required.

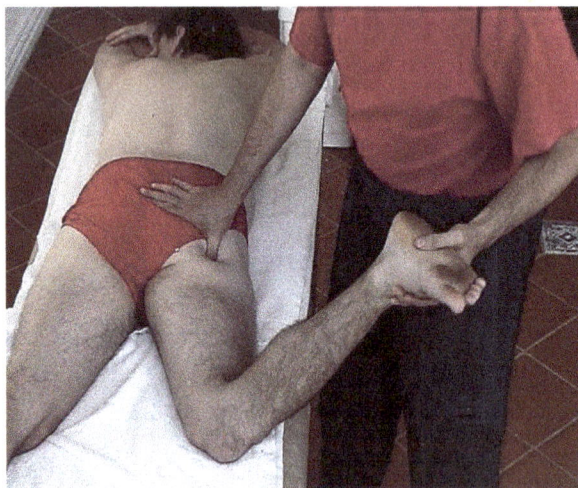

Picture 38.4

39. The anterior group of thigh muscles

Anatomy

Sartorius forms the lateral border of the femoral triangle. It is palpable. It arises on the anterior superior iliac spine of the ilium and attaches on the superior medial tibia.
Action: Flexes, abducts and laterally rotates the thigh and flexes and medially rotates the leg.
Nerve supply: Femoral nerve L2, 3 and 4.

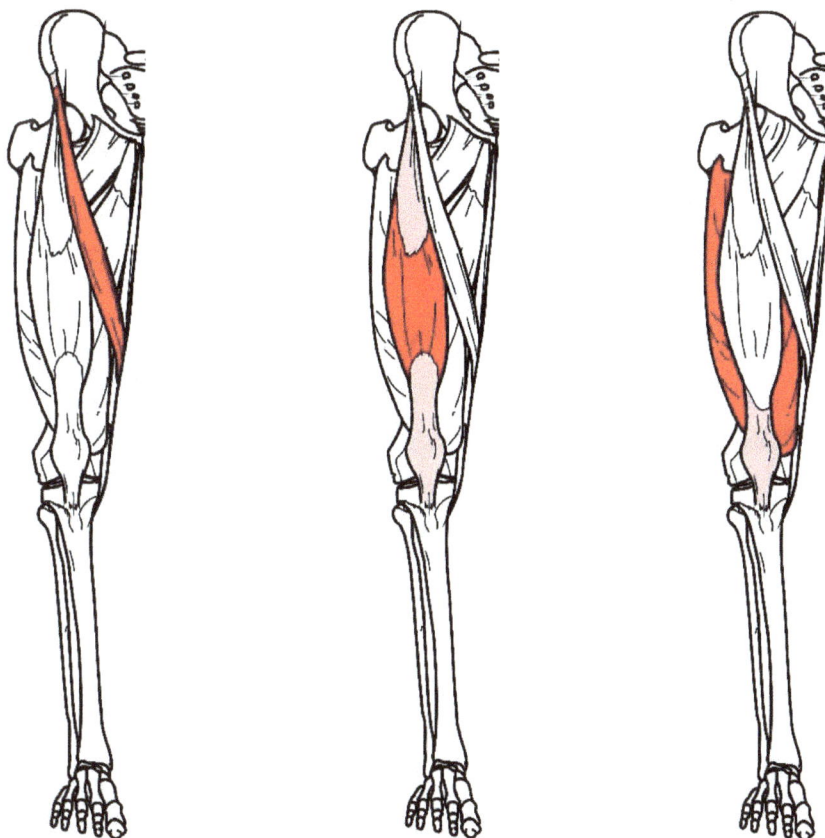

Quadriceps
Rectus femoris arises by two heads. The straight head arises from the anterior inferior iliac spine of the ilium and the reflected head arises from just above the acetabulum. The muscle attaches on the patella. This is the most superficial quadriceps muscle running down anterior thigh and is easily palpable.
Action: A knee extensor, a weak hip flexor and important for stability.

Vastus lateralis arises on the intertrochanteric line, the greater trochanter, the gluteal tuberosity and the lateral linea aspera. The muscle attaches on the lateral patella.

Vastus medialis arises on the intertrochanteric line, medial linea aspera and attaches on the medial patella. The muscle is prominent just above medial aspect of knee. It is important for knee stability.

Vastus intermedius is deep to rectus femoris. It arises on the upper anterior shaft of the femur and attaches on the base of the patella.
Action: Knee extensors
Nerve supply: Femoral nerve L2, 3 and 4.

The quadriceps tendon runs from the quadriceps muscles to the patella. The patella ligament runs from the patella to the tibial tuberosity. Fibrous expansions of the quadriceps tendon extend into the capsule, fascia and onto tibial condyles.

Technique 39.1 Kneading of vastus medialis

Patient

- Sidelying close to the side you are standing and facing away from you.
- The leg to be treated is closest to the table. Flex the knee to 90 degrees.
- The uppermost leg is flexed 90 degrees at the hip and 90 degrees at the knee and rests on a pillow.

Therapist

- Stand by the side of the table behind the patient and level with their hips.
- Grasp the patients ankle in your caudad hand.
- Grasp the patient's vastus medialis in your cephalad hand.

Applicator

- The fingers and thumb of your cephalad hand.
- Alternatively, the heel or pisiform bone of your cephalad hand.

Tissue tension

- Take up the primary tissue tension with compression and a transverse force by pushing away with your thumb or the heel of your hand.
- Take up the secondary (torsion) tissue tension by either flexing the fingers and pulling with your fingertips or twisting the wrist and pushing away with your pisiform. Take care not to pinch the skin.
- Take up the longitudinal tissue tension by flexing the patient's leg.

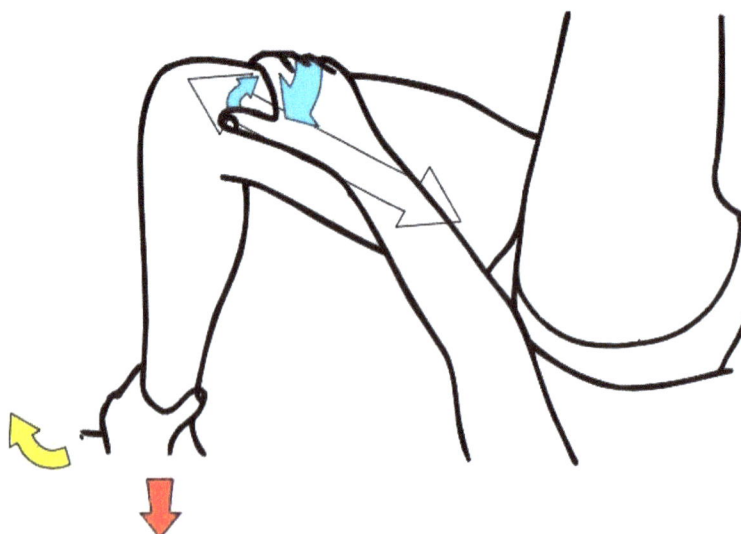

Figure 39.1

Muscle Fibres	⇕	Primary Force	⬇	Secondary Force	↻	Stretch Force	⬇	Contraction Force	⬇

Kneading

- Apply a rhythmical cycle of primary, secondary and longitudinal forces.
- When the muscle is at an optimal longitudinal tension increase the primary and secondary forces.
- Your pressure should be just short of discomfort.

254

- To relax the muscle work with the patients breathing cycle of 15 breaths per minute.
- To stimulate the muscle, increase your speed to about 40 cycles per minute.

Active component

- Ask the patient to take a deep breath and hold it in.
- Ask the patient to attempt to straighten their leg for 3 to 5 seconds using 10% of full contraction of their quadriceps.
- Resist their effort and maintain tissue lockup throughout inhalation.
- Ask the patient to exhale and to relax their muscle contraction.
- As soon as you feel that the patient has relaxed their muscles completely (about 1-3 seconds) take up the tissue slack by increasing the primary, secondary and longitudinal tension.
- Take up the slack after each contraction and during exhalation.
- Repeat 2 or 3 times or as required.

Clinical note: Measure circumference of thigh 8 cm above the knee for atrophy of vastus medialis.

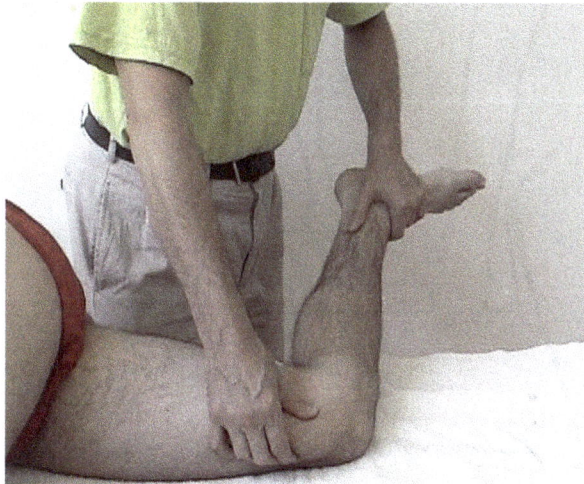

Picture 39.1

Technique 39.2 Kneading of rectus femoris

Patient

- Sidelying close to the side you are standing and facing away from you.
- The leg to be treated is closest to the table. Flex the knee to 90 degrees.
- The uppermost leg is flexed 90 degrees at the hip and 90 degrees at the knee and rests on a pillow.

Therapist

- Stand by the side of the table behind the patient and level with their hips.
- Grasp the patients ankle in your caudad hand.
- Grasp the patient's rectus femoris in your cephalad hand.

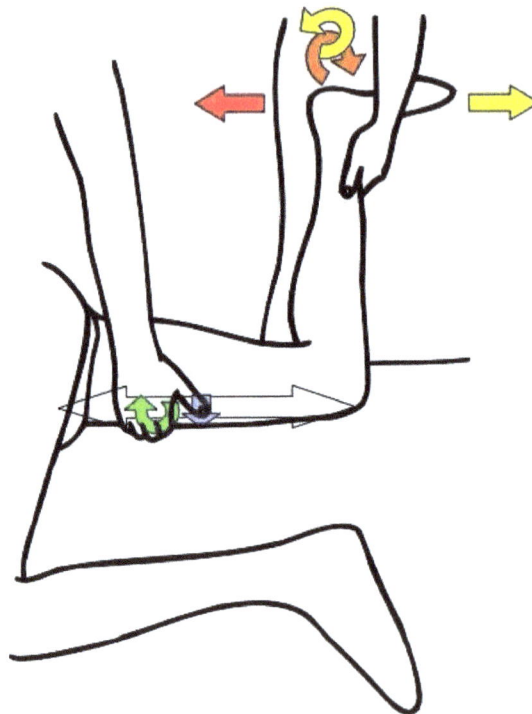

Figure 39.2

Muscle Fibres	⇕	Primary Force	⬇	Secondary Force	↻	Stretch Force	⬇	Contraction Force	⬇

Applicator

- The fingers and thumb of your cephalad hand.
- Alternatively, the heel or pisiform bone of your cephalad hand.

Tissue tension

- Take up the primary tissue tension with compression and a transverse force by pushing away with your thumb or the heel of your hand.
- Take up the secondary (torsion) tissue tension by either flexing the fingers and pulling with your fingertips or twisting the wrist and pushing away with your pisiform. Take care not to pinch the skin.
- Take up the longitudinal tissue tension by flexing the patient's leg.

256

Kneading

- Apply a rhythmical cycle of primary, secondary and longitudinal forces.
- When the muscle is at an optimal longitudinal tension increase the primary and secondary forces.
- Your pressure should be just short of discomfort.
- To relax the muscle work with the patients breathing cycle of 15 breaths per minute.
- To stimulate the muscle, increase your speed to about 40 cycles per minute.

Active component

- Ask the patient to take a deep breath and hold it in.
- Ask the patient to attempt to straighten their leg for 3 to 5 seconds using 10% of full contraction of their quadriceps.
- Resist their effort and maintain tissue lockup throughout inhalation.
- Ask the patient to exhale and to relax their muscle contraction.
- As soon as you feel that the patient has relaxed their muscles completely (about 1-3 seconds) take up the tissue slack by increasing the primary, secondary and longitudinal tension.
- Take up the slack after each contraction and during exhalation.
- Repeat 2 or 3 times or as required.

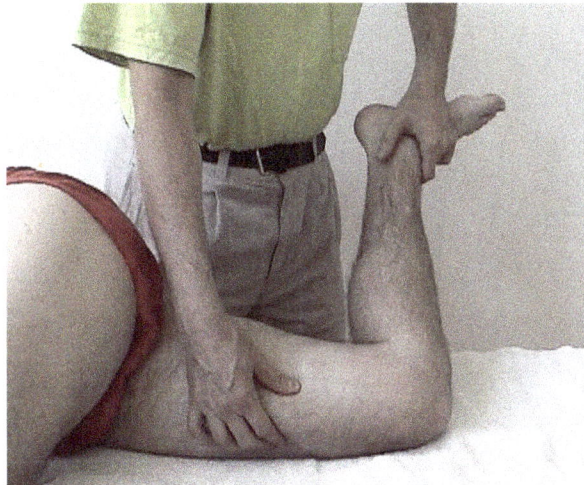

Picture 39.2

Technique 39.3 Kneading of sartorius

Patient

- Sidelying close to the side you are standing and facing away from you.
- The leg to be treated is closest to the table. Flex the knee to 90 degrees.
- The uppermost leg is flexed 90 degrees at the hip and 90 degrees at the knee and rests on a pillow.

Therapist

- Stand by the side of the table behind the patient and level with their hips.
- Grasp the patients ankle in your caudad hand.
- Grasp the patient's sartorius muscle in your cephalad hand.

Applicator

- The fingertips and thumb of your cephalad hand.
- Alternatively, the heel and pisiform bone of your cephalad hand.

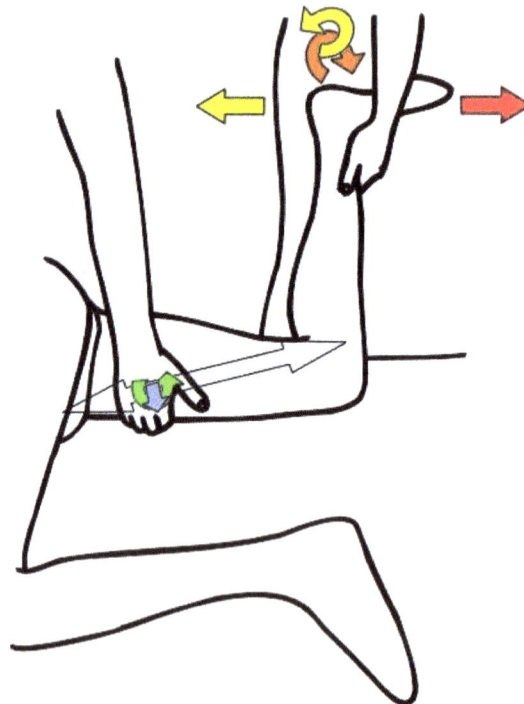

Figure 39.3

Muscle Fibres	⇕	Primary Force	⬇	Secondary Force	↻	Stretch Force	⬇	Contraction Force	⬇

Tissue tension

- Take up the transverse tissue tension by pushing away with the thumb or heel of your cephalad hand.
- Take up the secondary (torsion) tissue tension by either flexing the fingers and pulling with your fingertips or twisting the wrist and pushing away with your pisiform. Take care not to pinch the skin.
- Take up the longitudinal tissue tension by extending the patient's leg.

Kneading

- Apply a rhythmical cycle of primary, secondary and longitudinal forces.
- When the muscle is at an optimal longitudinal tension increase the primary and secondary forces.
- Your pressure should be just short of discomfort.
- To relax the muscle work with the patients breathing cycle of 15 breaths per minute.
- To stimulate the muscle, increase your speed to about 40 cycles per minute.

Active component

- Ask the patient to take a deep breath and hold it in.
- Ask the patient to attempt to flex their leg for 3 to 5 seconds using 10% of full contraction of their quadriceps.
- Resist their effort and maintain tissue lockup throughout inhalation.
- Ask the patient to exhale and to relax their muscle contraction.
- As soon as you feel that the patient has relaxed their muscles completely (about 1-3 seconds) take up the tissue slack by increasing the primary, secondary and longitudinal tension.
- Take up the slack after each contraction and during exhalation.
- Repeat 2 or 3 times or as required.

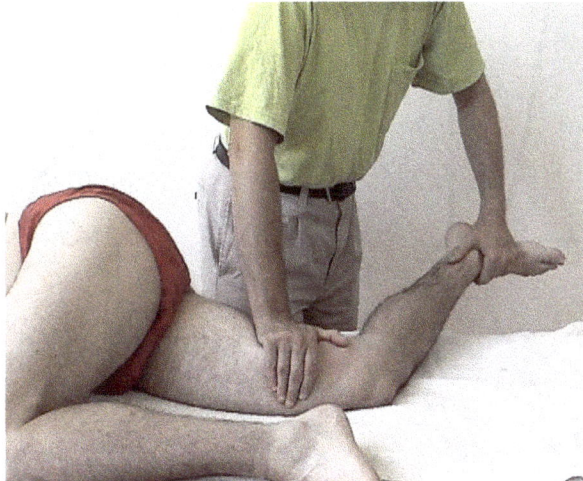

Picture 39.3

Technique 39.4 Kneading of rectus femoris

Patient

- Supine with the head on a pillow or folded towel.

Therapist

- Stand at the side of the table level with the patient's thighs.
- Flex the patient's hip and knee that is nearest you.
- Allow the patient's flexed knee to rest against your abdomen.
- The hip will abduct and externally rotate.
- Grasp the patients ankle in your caudad hand.
- Grasp the patient's rectus femoris in your cephalad hand.

Applicator

- The side of the thumb and fingertips of your cephalad hand.
- Alternatively, the heel and pisiform bone of your cephalad hand.

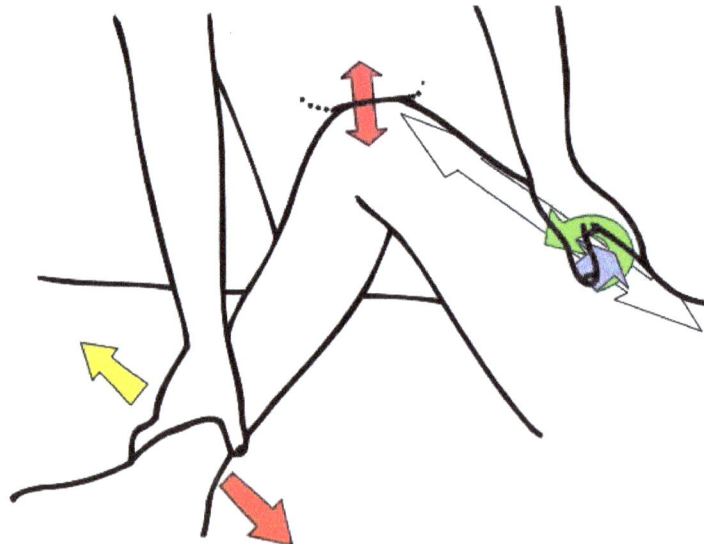

Figure 39.4

Muscle Fibres	↕	Primary Force	⬇	Secondary Force	↻	Stretch Force	⬇	Contraction Force	⬇

Tissue tension

- Take up the primary tissue tension with compression and a transverse force by pushing away with your thumb or the heel of your hand.
- Take up the secondary (torsion) tissue tension by either flexing the fingers and pulling with your fingertips or twisting the wrist and pushing away with your pisiform. Take care not to pinch the skin.
- Take up the longitudinal tissue tension by flexing the patient's leg.

Kneading

- Apply a rhythmical cycle of primary, secondary and longitudinal forces.
- When the muscle is at an optimal longitudinal tension increase the primary and secondary forces.

- Your pressure should be just short of discomfort.
- To relax the muscle work with the patients breathing cycle of 15 breaths per minute.
- To stimulate the muscle, increase your speed to about 40 cycles per minute.

Active component

- Ask the patient to take a deep breath and hold it in.
- Ask the patient to attempt to straighten their leg for 3 to 5 seconds using 10% of full contraction of their quadriceps.
- Resist their effort and maintain tissue lockup throughout inhalation.
- Ask the patient to exhale and to relax their muscle contraction.
- As soon as you feel that the patient has relaxed their muscles completely (about 1-3 seconds) take up the tissue slack by increasing the primary, secondary and longitudinal tension.
- Take up the slack after each contraction and during exhalation.
  Repeat 2 or 3 times or as required.

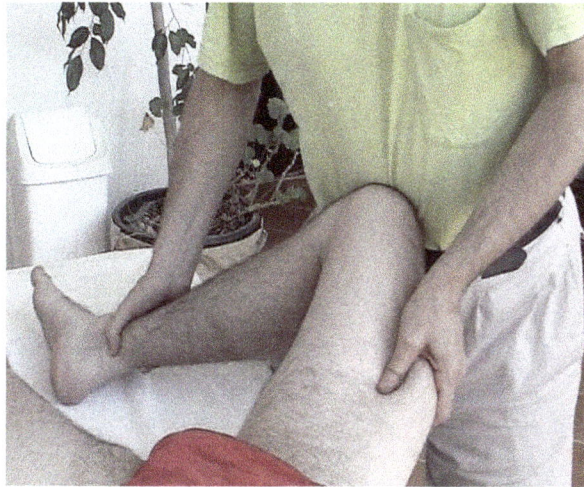

Picture 39.4

Technique 39.5 Kneading of sartorius

Patient

- Supine.
- The leg to be treated is flexed at the knee and hip and abducted at the hip.
- The patient's knee rests on your abdomen.

Therapist

- Stand by the side of the couch level with the patient's hips.
- Grasp the patients ankle in your caudad hand.
- Grasp the patient's sartorius in your cephalad hand.

Applicator

- The side of the thumb and fingertips of your cephalad hand.
- Alternatively, the heel and pisiform bone of your cephalad hand.

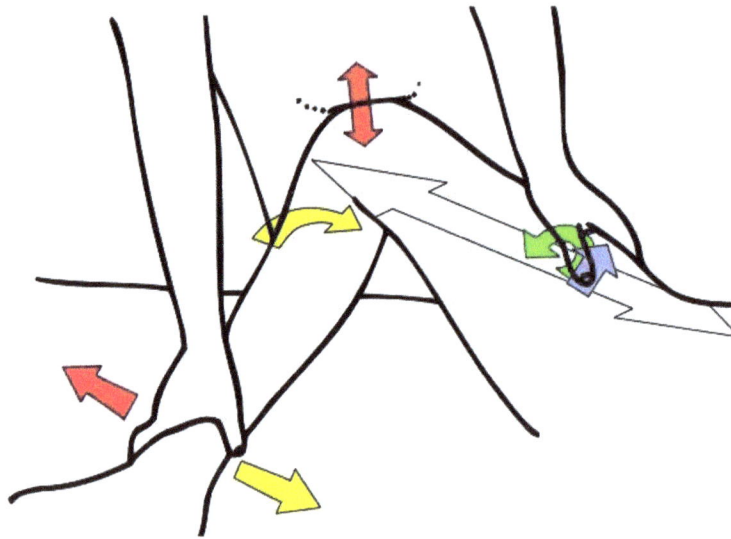

Figure 39.5

Muscle Fibres	↕	Primary Force	⬇	Secondary Force	↻	Stretch Force	⬇	Contraction Force	⬇

Tissue tension

- Take up the transverse tissue tension by pushing laterally with the side of your thumb.
- Take up the secondary (torsion) tissue tension by pulling with your fingertips or twisting your wrist. Take care not to pinch the skin.
- Take up the longitudinal tissue tension by extending the patient's leg.

Kneading

- Apply a rhythmical cycle of primary, secondary and longitudinal forces.
- When the muscle is at an optimal longitudinal tension increase the primary and secondary forces.
- Your pressure should be just short of discomfort.
- To relax the muscle work with the patients breathing cycle of 15 breaths per minute.
- To stimulate the muscle, increase your speed to about 40 cycles per minute.

Active component

- Ask the patient to take a deep breath and hold it in.
- Ask the patient to attempt to flex their leg and flex their hip for 3 to 5 seconds using 10% of full contraction of their sartorius.
- Resist their effort and maintain tissue lockup throughout inhalation.
- Ask the patient to exhale and to relax their muscle contraction.
- As soon as you feel that the patient has relaxed their muscles completely (about 1-3 seconds) take up the tissue slack by increasing the primary, secondary and longitudinal tension.
- Take up the slack after each contraction and during exhalation.
  Repeat 2 or 3 times or as required.

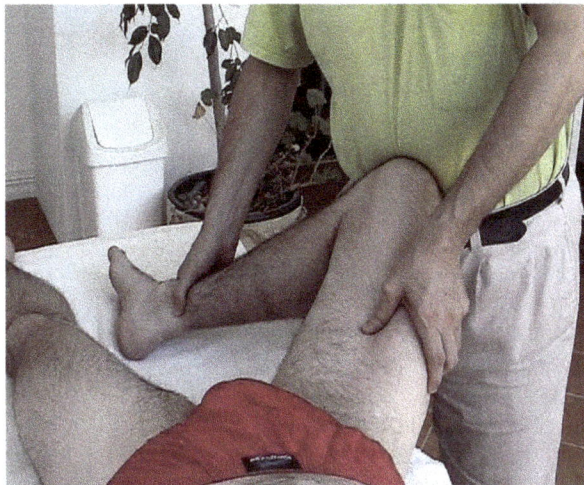

Picture 39.5

40. The hamstrings

Anatomy

Semimembranosus The tendon arises on the upper ischial tuberosity. It also receives fibres inferiorly and medially from the semitendinosus and biceps femoris tendon and from the adductor magnus tendon. The muscle and its upper tendon are deep to semitendinosus. It remains a muscle to its insertion on the tubercle on the posterior aspect of the medial tibial condyle. Fibres also attach on the medial tibia just posterior to the lateral collateral ligament, onto fascia overlying popliteus, and merge with the oblique popliteal ligament, which attaches on the lateral femoral condyle.
Variation: Fibres may attach on the sacrotuberous ligament or femur. The muscle varies in size and may be absent.

Semitendinosus The muscle arises on the medial ischial tuberosity by a short tendon, which it shares with the long head of biceps femoris. The fusiform muscle end about halfway down the thigh as a long round tendon. The tendon passes over and is separated from the medial collateral ligament by a pes anserine bursa. It attaches on the anteromedial tibia posterior and inferior to the tendons of gracilis and sartorius. The fibres of all three tendons merge and extend into the deep fascia of the leg.

Biceps femoris The long head arises on the medial ischial tuberosity by a tendon, which it shares with semitendinosus and from an inferior area of the sacrotuberous ligament. The short head arises on lateral linea aspera running along the posterior shaft of the femur and the lateral intermuscular septum. The tendon attaches on the head of the fibula, the lateral condyle of the tibia and part of it merges with fibres of the lateral collateral ligament.
Variations. The short head may be absent.

Actions: Extension of the thigh. Mainly the short head of biceps produces flexion of the leg. Semimembranosus and semitendinosus produce internal rotation of the leg. External rotation of the leg is produced by biceps femoris. The hamstrings give collateral support to the knee joint. The trochanteric bursa and several bursa in the knee may be palpable when inflamed.
Clinical indications: Strain and shortness
Nerve supply: Sciatic nerve. **L5, S1** and S2. The common peroneal nerve supplies the short head of biceps femoris. The tibial nerve supplies the long head of biceps femoris, semimembranosus and semitendinosus.

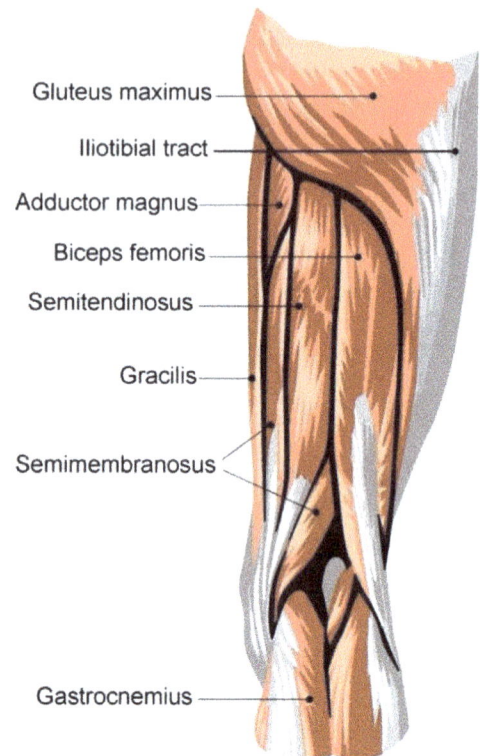

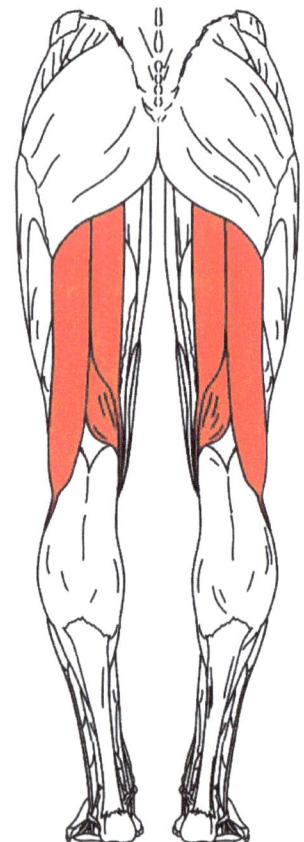

Gluteus maximus

Iliotibial tract

Adductor magnus

Biceps femoris

Semitendinosus

Gracilis

Semimembranosus

Gastrocnemius

Technique 40.1 Kneading the hamstrings

Patient

- Prone with head straight in a face-hole or rotated to one side.

Therapist

- Stand by the side of the table level with the patient's thighs.
- Grasp the ankle nearest you with your caudad hand and flex the knee to 90 degrees.
- Your cephalad hand makes contact on the muscle to be treated.

Applicator

- The heel of your hand and pisiform bone.
- Alternatively, the knuckles of your clenched fist or the side of the thumb.

Tissue tension

- Take up the primary tissue tension with compression and a transverse force by pushing across the muscle with your applicator.
- Take up the secondary (torsion) tissue tension by rotating your applicator. If this is the heel of your hand the axis of rotation passes through your hamate and is radial deviation.

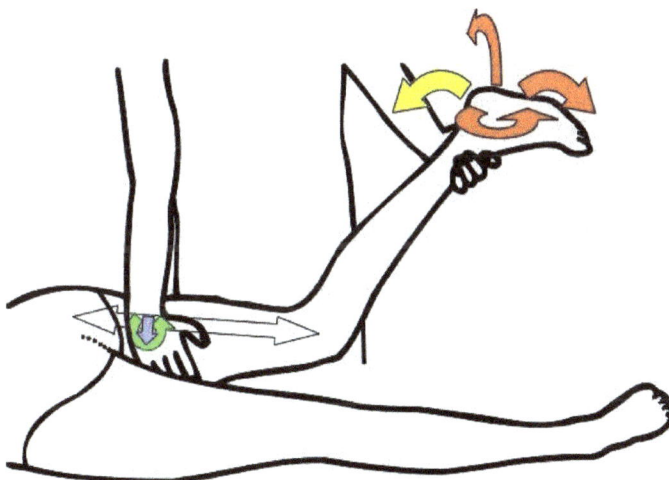

Figure 40.1

Muscle Fibres	⇕	Primary Force	⬇	Secondary Force	↻	Stretch Force	⬇	Contraction Force	⬇

Kneading

- Rotate the ankle in a circular motion thereby moving the hip through a cycle of internal and external rotation.
- Apply a rhythmical cycle of primary and secondary forces.
- When the muscle is at an optimal point in the rotation cycle increase the primary and secondary forces.
- Your pressure should be just short of discomfort.
- To relax the muscle work with the patient's breathing cycle of 15 breaths per minute.
- To stimulate the muscle, increase your speed to about 40 cycles per minute.

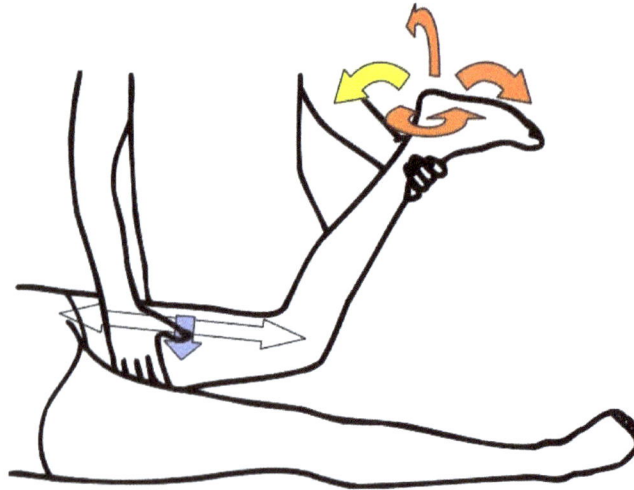

Figure 40.2

Muscle Fibres	↕	Primary Force	⬇	Secondary Force	↻	Stretch Force	⬇	Contraction Force	⬇

Active component

- Ask the patient to take a deep breath and hold it in.
- Ask the patient to attempt bend (flex) their knee for 3 to 5 seconds using 10% of full contraction. The hamstring muscles will contract.
- Resist their effort and maintain tissue lockup throughout inhalation.
- Ask the patient to exhale and to relax their muscle contraction.
- As soon as you feel that the patient has relaxed their hamstrings completely (about 3 seconds) take up the tissue slack by increasing the primary and secondary tension.
- Take up the slack after each contraction and during exhalation. Repeat as required.

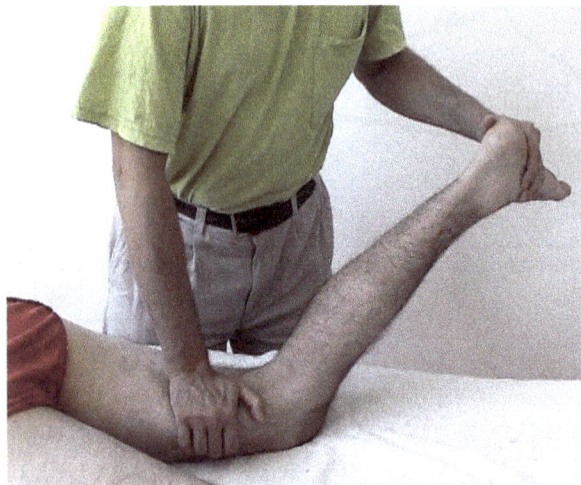

Picture 40.1

41. The hip adductors

Anatomy

Adductor longus is easily palpable in abduction especially at its tendon origin. It forms the medial border of the femoral triangle. It arises as a flat narrow tendon on the anterior pubis. The muscle runs inferiorly, posteriorly and laterally to attach along the middle third of the medial linea aspera of femur by an aponeurosis. Fibres of the muscle usually merge with those of adductor magnus. The muscle may be doubled.
Action: Adduction, flexion and rotation of the thigh depending on the position of the limb.
Nerve supply: Obturator nerve L2, **3** and 4.

Adductor brevis is not directly palpable deep to adductor longus and pectineus. It arises on the external aspect of the inferior pubic ramus and body. The muscle runs inferiorly, posteriorly and laterally to attach by an aponeurosis to a line which runs from lesser trochanter to the proximal linea aspera of the femur. The muscle may be split into separate parts or merge with adductor magnus.
Nerve supply: Obturator nerve L2, **3** and 4.

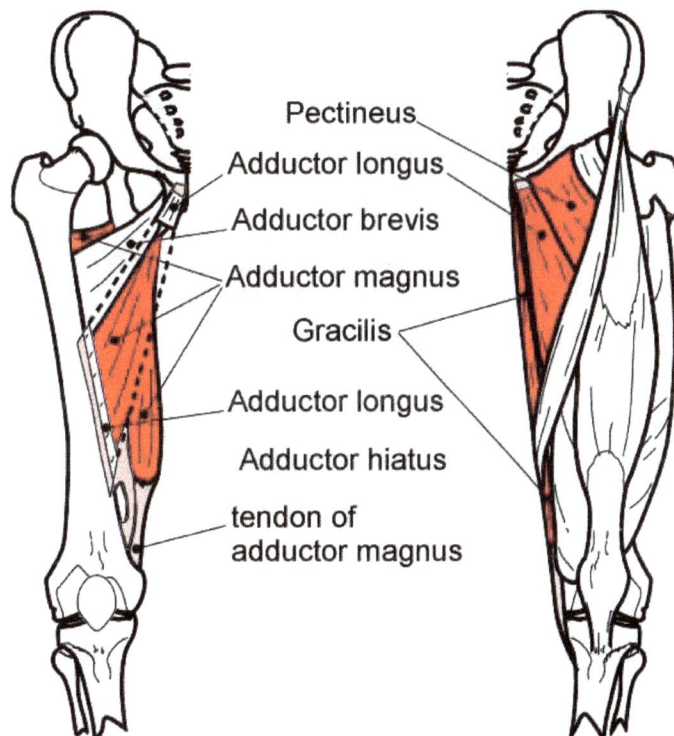

Pectineus
Adductor longus
Adductor brevis
Adductor magnus
Gracilis
Adductor longus
Adductor hiatus
tendon of adductor magnus

Adductor magnus is a large triangular sheet of muscle covered anteriorly by adductor longus and adductor brevis and posteriorly by the hamstrings. Although its tendons are palpable, the muscle is only directly palpable along its thicker medial border between the hamstrings and gracilis. It arises on the anterior surface of inferior ramus of pubis and ischium and ischial tuberosity. Its fibres fan out from their origin, with short fibres running horizontally to the medial edge of the gluteal tuberosity, intermediate fibres running diagonally to attach almost along the whole length of the linea aspera and proximal supra medial supracondylar line by an aponeurosis, and long fibres running almost vertically to a round tendon attaching on the adductor tubercle on the medial condyle of the femur. The aponeurotic attachment is broken at several places by tendinous arches, the most significant of which is the large adductor hiatus which allows the femoral vessels to pass between the anterior thigh and the popliteal fossa.

Actions: Its fibres adduct, flex, extend and may rotate the thigh depending on the position of the limb. Because of its posterior placement and attachment on the ischial tuberosity adductor magnus functionally acts like a hamstring.
Nerve supply: Obturator nerve and tibial division of the sciatic nerve L2, **3** and **4**.

Gracilis is a palpable thin flat muscle running down the medial thigh. It arises on the body and ramus of the pubis (pubic arch) and a small part of the ramus of the ischium. Its tendon merges with the tendon of sartorius and attaches on the medial surface of tibia distal to the condyle and just proximal to the semitendinosus tendon. Some of its fibre merge with the deep fascia of the leg.

Actions: The gracilis flexes and medially rotates the leg. It may be weak adductor of the thigh.

Nerve supply: Obturator nerve L2, 3 and 4 supplies above adductors & skin of upper medial thigh. Nerve descends through obturator foramen and is not palpable.

Pectineus is a flat rectangular muscle forming part of the floor of the femoral triangle. It arises on the pectineal line of pubis and its fibres run inferiorly, posteriorly and laterally to attach on the pectineal line between lesser trochanter & linea aspera. The muscle may be two layered and it may attach on the capsule of the hip joint.

Actions: Adduction and flexion of the thigh.

Nerve supply: Femoral nerve L2 and 3 and sometimes the accessory obturator nerve L3.

Actions: Although the adductors adduct the thigh, during normal standing they have minimal activity. Their major role is as synergists in controlling posture particularly during gait.

Technique 41.1 Kneading the hip adductors

Patient

- Supine with their head on a pillow or folded towel.

Therapist

- Stand by the side of the table level with and next to the thigh you are treating.
- Grasp the patients ankle in your caudad hand and abduct their thigh.
- Grasp the patients adductor muscles in your cephalad hand.

Applicator

- Heel of hand and the pisiform bone or the pads of the fingers of your cephalad hand.

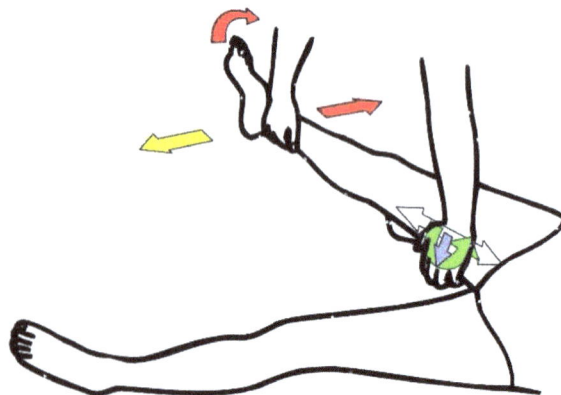

Figure 41.1

Muscle Fibres	⇕	Primary Force	⬇	Secondary Force	↻	Stretch Force	⬇	Contraction Force	⬇

Tissue tension

- Take up the primary tissue tension with compression and a transverse force by pushing away with the heel of your cephalad hand.
- Take up the secondary tissue tension by externally rotating the patient's leg.
- Add further tissue tension by abducting your wrist (radial deviation). Your pisiform rotates about an axis passing through the hook of the hamate. Take care not to pinch the skin.

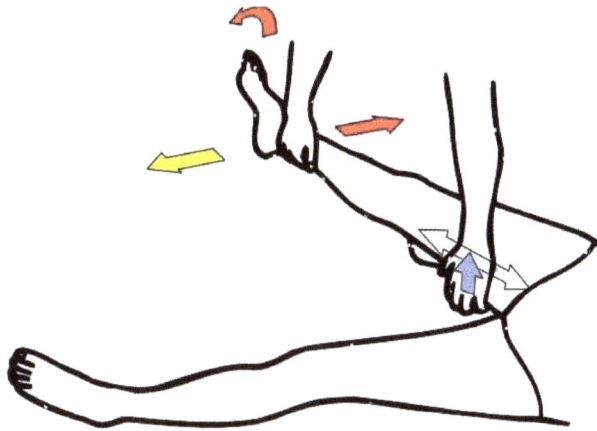

Figure 41.2

Muscle Fibres	⇕	Primary Force	⬇	Secondary Force	↻	Stretch Force	⬇	Contraction Force	⬇

- Take up the longitudinal tissue tension by abducting the patient's leg.
- Alternatively pull up with your fingertips while internally rotating the patient's leg.

Kneading

- Apply a rhythmical cycle of primary, secondary and longitudinal forces.
- When the muscle is at an optimal longitudinal tension increase the other forces.
- Your pressure should be just short of discomfort.
- To relax the muscles work with the patients breathing cycle of about 15 breaths a minute.
- To stimulate the adductors, increase your speed to about 40 cycles per minute.

Active component

- Ask the patient to take a deep breath and hold it in.
- Ask the patient to adduct and internally rotate their leg for 3 to 5 seconds using 10% of full contraction of their muscles.
- Resist their effort and maintain tissue lockup throughout inhalation.
- Ask the patient to exhale and to relax their muscle contraction.
- As soon as you feel that the patient has relaxed completely (about 1-3 seconds) take up the tissue slack by increasing the primary, secondary and longitudinal tension.
- Take up the slack after each contraction and during exhalation.
- Repeat 2 or 3 times or as required.

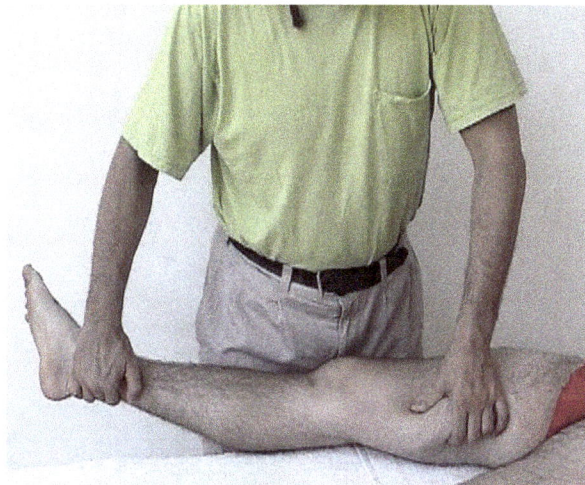

Picture 41.1

Technique 41.2 Kneading the hip adductors

Patient

- Sidelying near to the side of the table that you are standing.
- The leg to be treated is closest to the table.
- The uppermost leg is flexed 90 degrees at the hip and flexed 90 degrees at the knee and rests on a pillow.

Therapist

- Stand by the side of the table behind the patient and level with their hips.

Applicator

- A row of interdigitating fingers of both hands.
- The heels of your hands.
- Your knuckles.

Tissue tension

- Take up the primary tissue tension with compression and a posterior to anterior transverse force on the muscles with your applicator.
- There is no secondary or longitudinal force.

Kneading

- Start at the junction of adductor magnus and the hamstrings.
- Apply cross fibre kneading to the adductors as a rhythmical cycle of compression and a posterior to anterior transverse force.
- Your pressure should be just short of discomfort.
- To relax the muscle work with the patients breathing cycle, about 15 breaths per minute.
- To stimulate increase your speed to about 40 cycles per minute

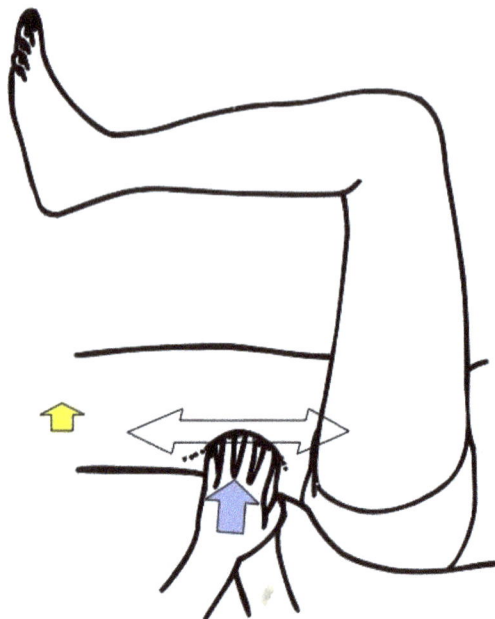

Figure 41.3

Muscle Fibres	⇕	Primary Force	⬇	Secondary Force	↻	Stretch Force	⬇	Contraction Force	⬇

Active component

- Ask the patient to take a deep breath and hold it in.
- Ask the patient to attempt to lift their leg off the table for 3 to 5 seconds using 10% of full contraction of their adductors.
- Resist their effort and maintain tissue lockup throughout inhalation.
- Ask the patient to exhale and to relax their muscle contraction.
- As soon as you feel that the patient has relaxed their muscles completely (about 1-3 seconds) take up the tissue slack by increasing the compression and transverse tension.
- Take up the slack after each contraction and during exhalation.
- Repeat 2 or 3 times or as required.

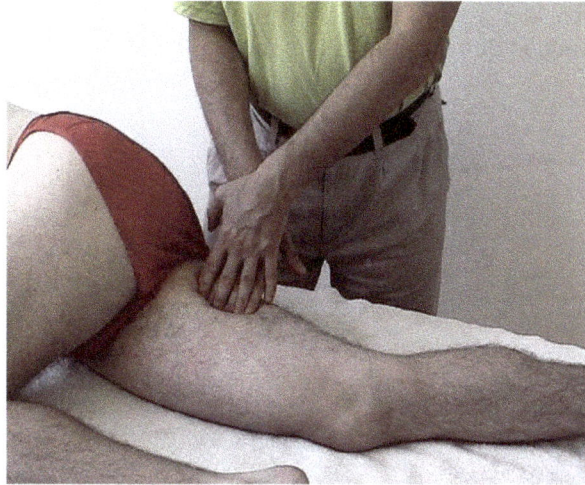

Picture 41.2

Technique 41.3 Kneading the hip adductors

Patient

- Sidelying near to the side of the table that you are standing.
- The leg to be treated is closest to the table. Flex the knee to 90 degrees.
- The uppermost leg is flexed 90 degrees at the hip and flexed 90 degrees at the knee and rests on a pillow.

Therapist

- Stand by the side of the table behind the patient and level with their hips.
- Grasp the patients ankle in your caudad hand.
- Grasp the patient's adductor muscle in your cephalad hand.

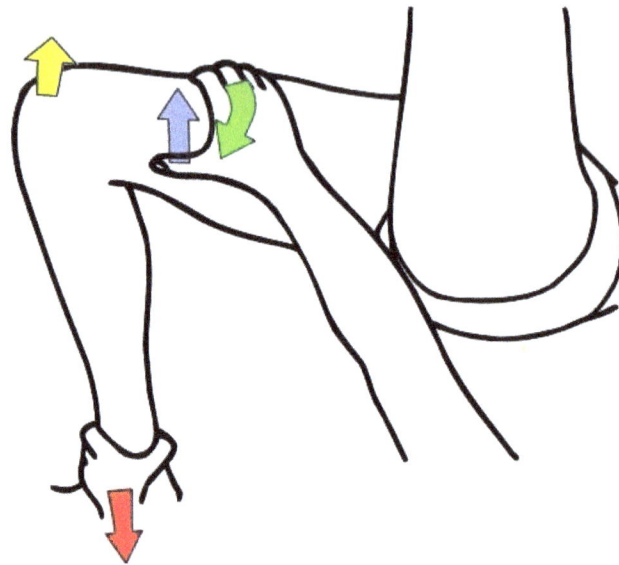

Figure 41.4

Muscle Fibres	⇕	Primary Force	⬇	Secondary Force	↻	Stretch Force	⬇	Contraction Force	⬇

Applicator

- The fingers and thumb of your cephalad hand.
- Alternatively, the heel and pisiform bone of your cephalad hand.

Tissue tension

- Take up the primary tissue tension with compression and a transverse force by pushing away with your thumb or the heel of your cephalad hand.
- Take up the secondary (torsion) tissue tension by pulling with your fingertips or twisting (radial deviation) the wrist. Take care not to pinch the skin.
- Take up further tension by taking the patient's foot towards the floor (internal rotation).

Kneading

- Apply a rhythmical cycle of primary and secondary forces.
- Your pressure should be just short of discomfort.
- To relax the muscle work with the patients breathing cycle of 15 breaths per minute.
- To stimulate the muscle, increase your speed to about 40 cycles per minute.

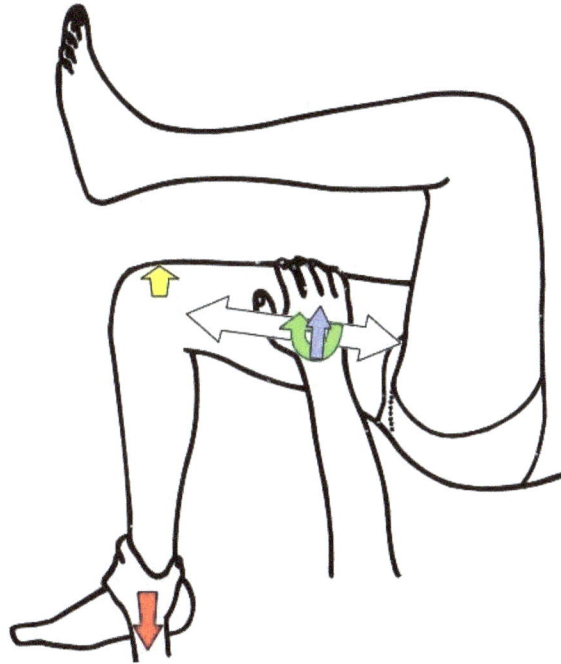

Figure 41.5

Muscle Fibres	⇕	Primary Force	⬇	Secondary Force	↺	Stretch Force	⬇	Contraction Force	⬇

Active component

- Ask the patient to take a deep breath and hold it in.
- Ask the patient to attempt to lift their knee off the table for 3 to 5 seconds using 10% of full contraction of their adductors.
- Resist their effort and maintain tissue lockup throughout inhalation.
- Ask the patient to exhale and to relax their muscle contraction.
- As soon as you feel that the patient has relaxed their muscles completely (about 1-3 seconds) take up the tissue slack by increasing the primary and secondary tension.
- Take up the slack after each contraction and during exhalation.
- Repeat 2 or 3 times or as required.

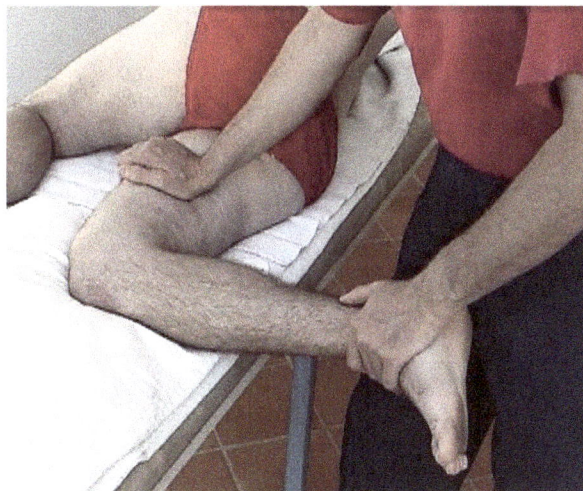

Picture 41.3

42. Popliteus

Anatomy

Popliteus arises on the lateral surface of the lateral condyle of the femur by a strong tendon and on the popliteal ligament and attaches on the posterior surface of the tibia, just above the soleal line. The tendon pierces the capsule laterally and its fibres merge with the joint capsule and the lateral meniscus. A layer of fascia derived from the semimembranosus tendon covers its superficial surface.

The Popliteal fossa is a fat filled cavity defined by the hamstring tendons and, medial and lateral heads of the gastrocnemius. Popliteal fascia forms the roof. The popliteus muscle and posterior femur form the floor. The presence of a cyst in the fossa may indicate pathology.

Actions: It is a knee flexor and is important in unlocking the extended knee at the beginning of flexion. It medially rotates the tibia on the femur or laterally rotates the femur on the tibia when the tibia is fixed. It is a meniscus stabiliser and it pull the lateral meniscus backwards and prevents it getting crushed between the tibia and femur during flexion and lateral rotation of the femur.
Nerve supply: Tibial nerve L4, 5 and S1.

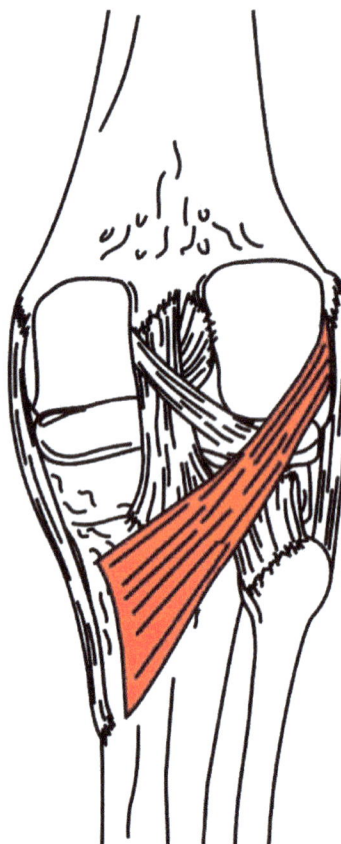

Technique 42.1 Inhibition of popliteus

Patient

- Prone with head straight in a face-hole or rotated to one side.

Therapist

- Stand by the side of the table level with the patient's thighs.
- Grasp the ankle nearest you with your caudad hand and flex the knee to 90 degrees.
- The applicator of your cephalad hand makes contact on the muscle to be treated.

Applicator

- The tip of your thumb.

Tissue tension

- Position the patient's leg where the popliteal fascia is at its most relaxed state and also so you can access the popliteus muscle (about 90 degrees flexion is fine).
- Take up the primary tissue tension with compression.
- Your force is in an anterior direction

Inhibition

- Take up the tissue tension by gradually increasing your thumb pressure on the muscle.
- Your pressure should be just short of discomfort.
- To relax the muscle work with the patients breathing cycle, about 15 breaths per minute.
- Maintain some compression throughout the technique but increase it during exhalation.

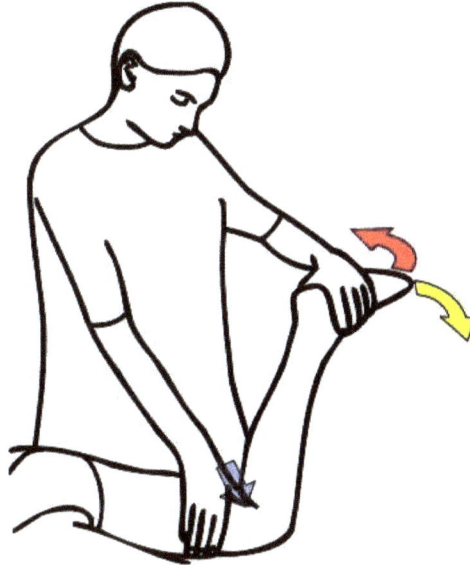

Figure 42.1

Muscle Fibres	↕	Primary Force	⬇	Secondary Force	↻	Stretch Force	⬇	Contraction Force	⬇

Active component

- Ask the patient to take a deep breath and hold it in.
- Ask the patient to attempt to turn their foot inward for 3 to 5 seconds using a 10% effort. The popliteus muscle will contract.
- Maintain tissue compression.
- Ask the patient to exhale and to relax their muscle contraction.
- As soon as you feel that the patient has relaxed their muscle completely (about 1-3 seconds) take up the tissue slack by increasing the compression.
- Take up the slack after each contraction and during exhalation.
- Repeat 2 or 3 times or as required.

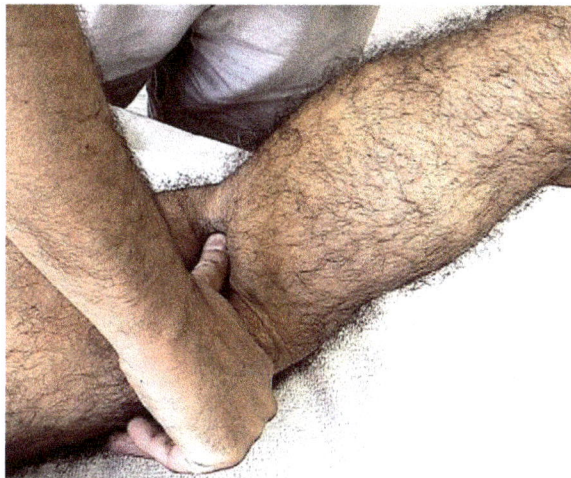

Picture 42.1

43. Knee medial and lateral collateral ligaments

Anatomy

The **medial or tibial collateral ligament** arises on the medial epicondyle of the femur just below the adductor tubercle. It descends and runs slightly anteriorly to attach on the medial condyle and medial shaft of the tibia. It is a wide, flat and strong ligament and overlies the joint capsule and medial meniscus. Although it is separated from the capsule by a bursa some of its fibre merge with it. The medial meniscus may be palpated anteromedially along the joint line when the tibia is internally rotated.

The **lateral or fibular collateral ligament** arises on the lateral epicondyle of the femur and attaches just in front of the apex of the head of the fibula. It is palpable as a round band when the knee is flexed and the hip abducted and externally rotated - such as when the ankle is resting above the knee. It is set apart from the joint capsule and lateral meniscus. The meniscus may be palpable along tibial margin when the knee is flexed.

The **tibiofibular ligament** arises on the fibular head and attaches on the tibial condyle.

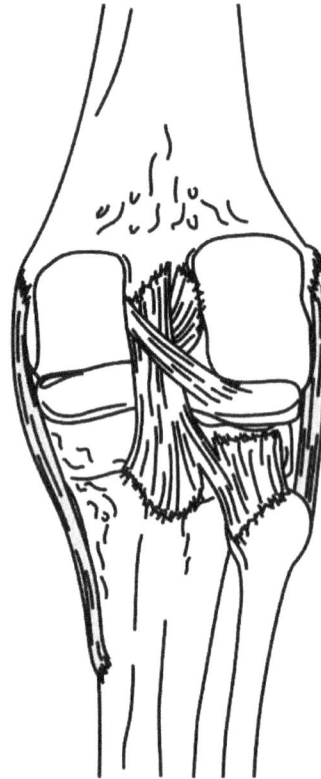

Clinical indications: Strain and rupture and bursitis. The menisci will be tender if torn.

Technique 43.1 Friction over the collateral ligaments (shown for the lateral collateral ligament)

Patient

- Sidelying near to the side of the table that you are standing.
- The head is resting on a pillow.

Therapist

- Stand at the side of the table level with the patient's knee.

Applicator

- The tip of the thumb of your cephalad hand.

Tissue tension

- Find the joint line. You may need to flex the knee.
- The plateau of the tibia is easily palpable anteriorly.
- Follow the joint line posteriorly until you are on the most lateral (or medial) side of the knee.
- Place your thumb on the ligament.
- The ligament runs inferior to superior
- Take up the tissue tension by gradually increasing your thumb pressure on the ligament.

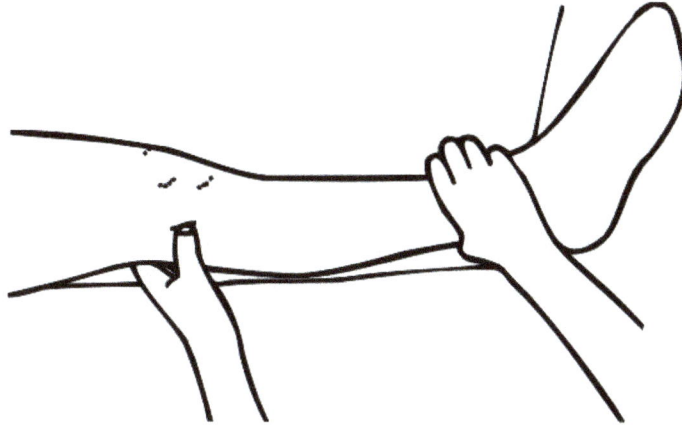

Figure 43.1 Lateral collateral ligament

Transverse Friction

- Work across the ligament with transverse friction.
- Apply firm pressure over a small area.

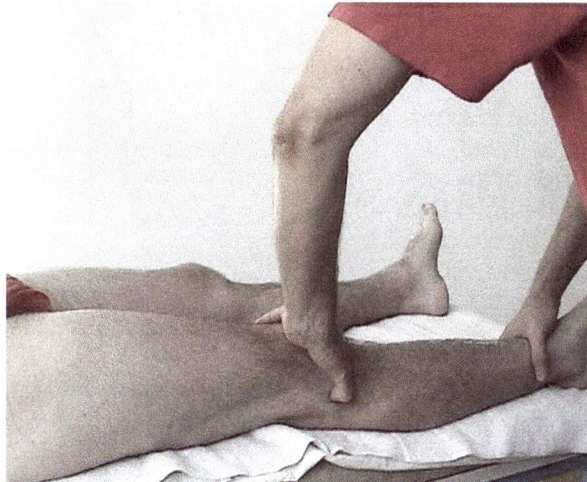

Picture 43.1

44. Knee tendons

Anatomy

Medial tendons

The **sartorius, gracilis** and **semitendinosus tendons** all attach close to each other on an area of the superior, anterior and medial tibia. Fibrous expansions extend from their attachment into the deep fascia covering the anterior compartment of the leg. Sartorius has the most anterior tendon insertion and is muscular to its insertion, the gracilis tendon is anterior and medial and the semitendinosus tendon is the most posterior and inferior and is easily palpable as a thick round tendon with the knee flexed 90 degrees. **Semimembranosus** is muscular to its insertion on the posterior tibia and lies deep to all the other muscles.

Lateral tendons

The **biceps femoris tendon** is easily palpable when the knee is flexed, inserting on the lateral side of the knee on the fibular head. The **iliotibial tract** is palpable anteriorly and inserts on the lateral tibial tubercle. The iliotibial tract helps stabilises the knee.

Anterior tendons

The **quadriceps tendon** runs from the quadriceps muscles to the patella. The **patellar ligament** runs from the patella to the tibial tuberosity. Fibrous expansions of the quadriceps tendon extend into the capsule, fascia and onto tibial condyles.

Alar folds consisting of a fat pad and synovium lie deep to the patella ligament.

Clinical indications: The superficial infrapatellar bursa, prepatellar bursa and several other bursae lie adjacent to the knee tendons and may become swollen, tender and palpable if irritated.

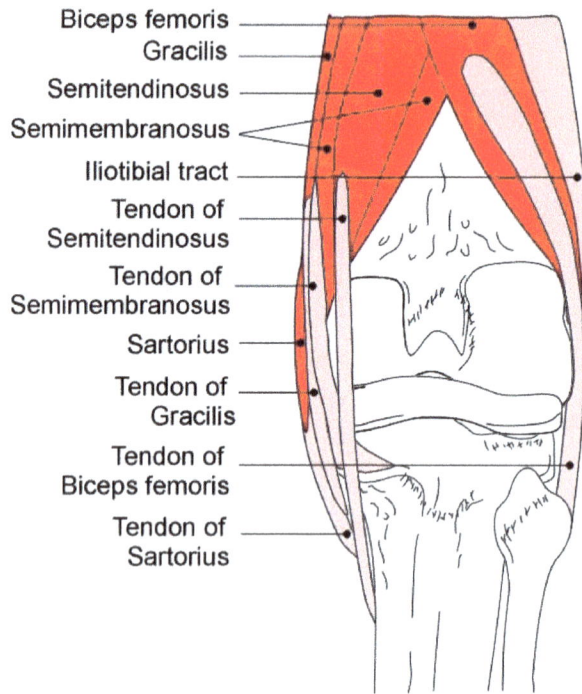

Biceps femoris
Gracilis
Semitendinosus
Semimembranosus
Iliotibial tract
Tendon of Semitendinosus
Tendon of Semimembranosus
Sartorius
Tendon of Gracilis
Tendon of Biceps femoris
Tendon of Sartorius

Posterior view

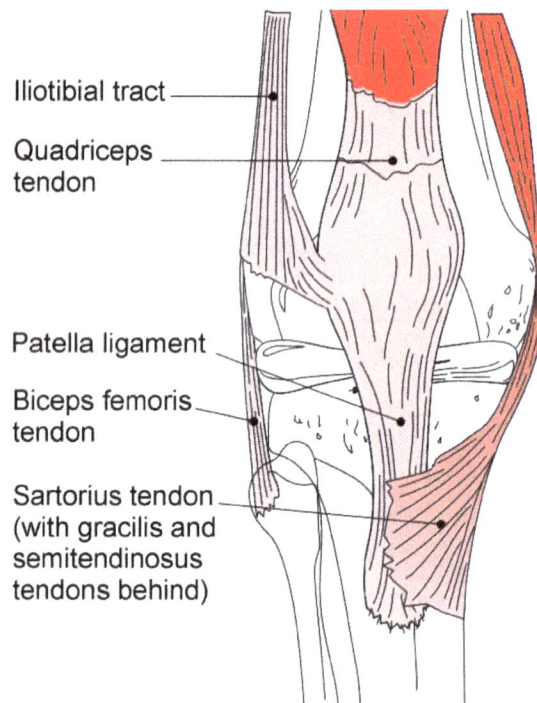

Iliotibial tract
Quadriceps tendon
Patella ligament
Biceps femoris tendon
Sartorius tendon (with gracilis and semitendinosus tendons behind)

Anterior view

Technique 44.1 Friction over the medial and lateral knee tendons

Patient

- Prone with head straight in a face-hole or rotated to one side.
- Treatment of some of the medial tendons may be best done supine.

Therapist

- Stand by the side of the table level with the patient's knee.
- Grasp the ankle nearest you with your caudad hand and flex the knee to 90 degrees.
- The applicator of your cephalad hand makes contact on the tendon to be treated.

Applicator

- The tip of your thumb or a T-bar.

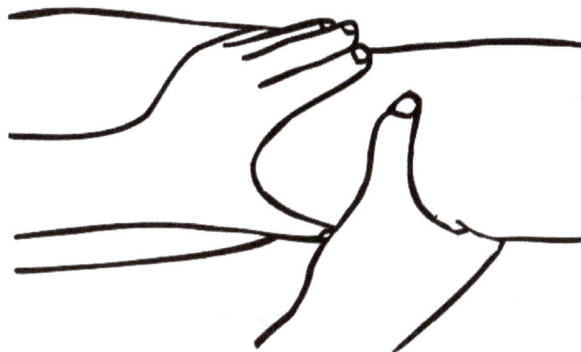

Figure 44.1 Friction over medial tendons.

Tissue tension

- Position the patient's leg so you can access the appropriate tendon.
- Place the tip of your thumb on the tendon and take up the tissue tension by gradually increasing your thumb pressure on the tendon.

Transverse Friction

- Work across the tendon with transverse friction.
- Apply firm pressure over a small area.
- Move along the tendon towards its attachment on the bone.
- Cover the entire surface area of the bone-tendon junction.

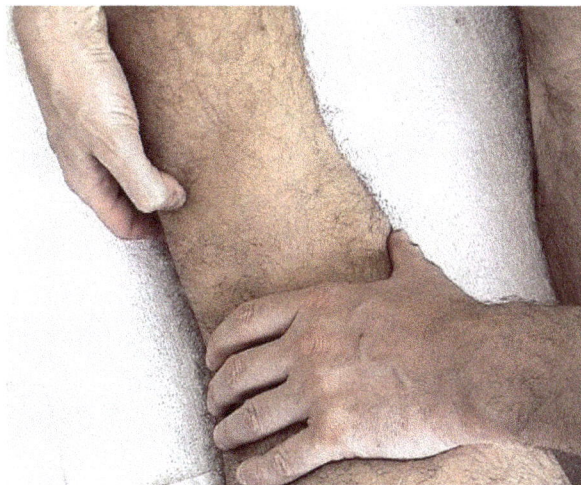

Picture 44.1

Technique 44.2 Friction over the quadriceps tendon or the patellar ligament

Patient

- Supine with the head on a pillow or folded towel.

Therapist

- Stand at the side of the table level with the patient's knee.
- Grasp the patella between the fingers and thumb of your hand.
- Place your applicator on the quadriceps tendon or patellar ligament.

Applicator

- The tip of your thumb or a T-bar.

Tissue tension

- Fix the patella against the femur.
- Take up the tissue tension by gradually increasing your thumb pressure on the quadriceps tendon or patellar ligament.

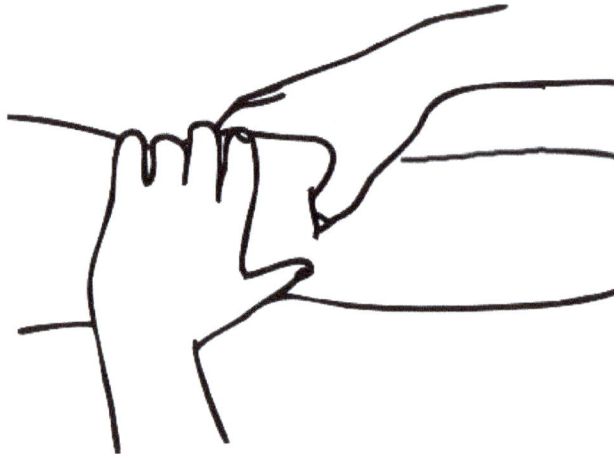

Figure 44.2 Patellar ligament

Transverse Friction

- Work across the quadriceps tendon or patella ligament with transverse friction.
- Apply firm pressure over a small area.

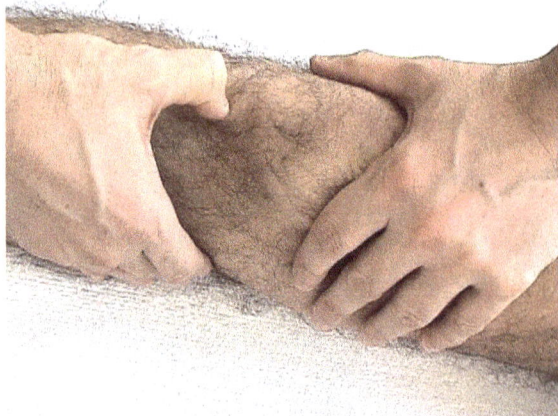

Picture 44.2

45. Gastrocnemius and soleus

Anatomy

Gastrocnemius Two heads arise on the upper posterior medial and lateral femoral condyles and femur above this and from the knee joint capsule. Both heads attach on the anterior surface of a tendinous expansion that forms the tendo calcaneus. The heads are separated by an aponeurosis and attached to its posterior surface. The muscle forms the bulk of the calf.

Actions: Plantar flexion, knee flexion, stability and balance.
Nerve supply: Tibial nerve S**1** and 2.

Soleus arises on the head and upper fibula, soleal line, the upper medial tibia via the posterior surface of an aponeurosis, which spans between the tibia and fibula. The muscle fibres insert on the anterior surface of the tendo calcaneus. The tendo calcaneus inserts onto the middle of the posterior calcaneus. Soleus is deep to gastrocnemius and only directly palpable at the distal aspect of the medial and lateral sides of the leg.

Actions: Plantar flexion and balance. During standing, soleus is continuously active whereas gastrocnemius exhibits only intermittent contraction.
Nerve supply: Tibial nerve S1 and **2**.

The **tendo calcaneus** or **Achilles tendon** extends about half the length of the leg. It is broad and flat superiorly and becomes thicker and rounded as it descends. Its fibres spiral and give the tendon elastic properties which facilitate gait. The tendon is strong but may be ruptured. A minor strain can be treated with transverse friction but anything greater may require immobilisation and surgery.

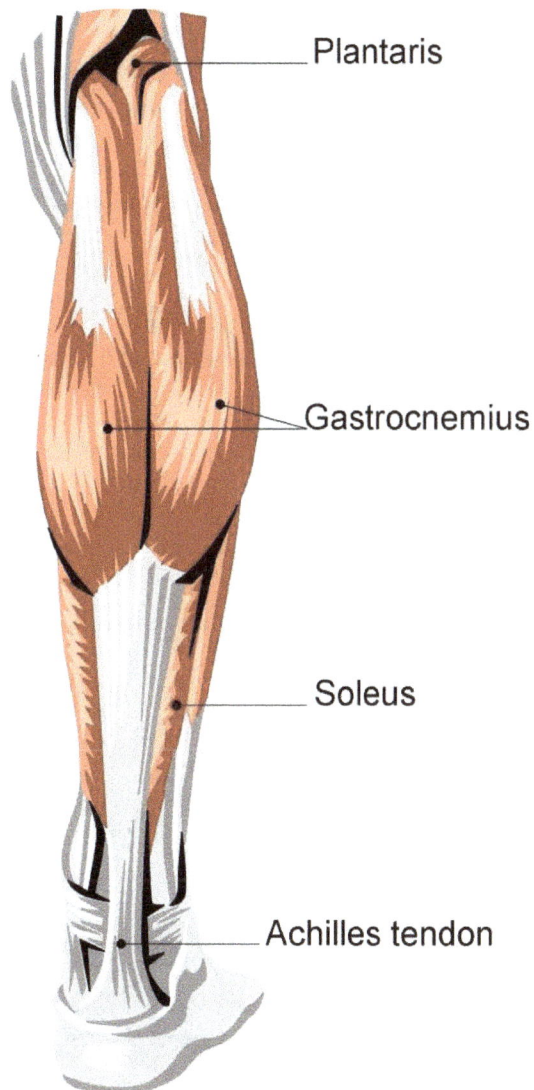

Plantaris

Gastrocnemius

Soleus

Achilles tendon

Technique 45.1 Kneading of gastrocnemius and soleus

Patient

- Supine and near to the side of the table that you are standing.
- Treat the lower limb nearest to the side that you are standing.
- The patient's hip is flexed to about 45 degrees and the knee flexed to about 90 degrees.

Therapist

- Sit on the side of the table and on the patient's foot to fix it to the table.
- Grasp the patient's knee with your cephalad hand.
- Reach around the lateral side of the patient's leg and grasp the lateral head of gastrocnemius between your fingertips and thumb.
- Alternatively, you can extend your reach and grasp the medial head with your fingertips.
- The same principle applies if you reach around the medial side of the patient's leg.

Tissue tension

- Take up the primary tissue tension with compression and a transverse force achieved by flexing your fingertips.
- Your force is perpendicular to the muscle and in a medial to lateral or lateral to medial direction depending on which side of the leg you are working.
- Take up the secondary tissue tension with a torsion force achieved by flexing your thumb. (optional)

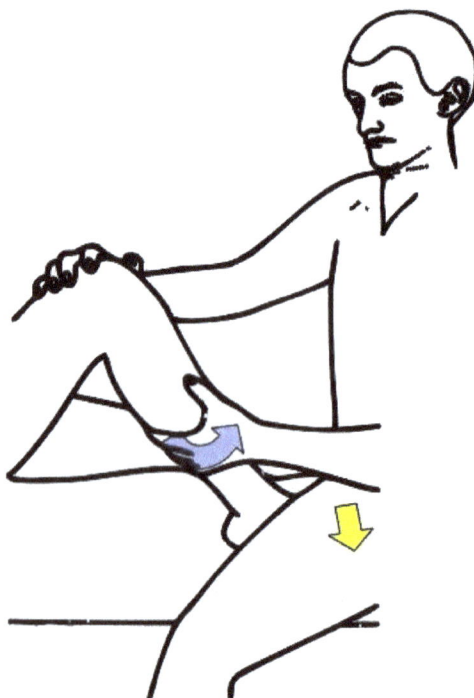

Figure 45.1

Muscle Fibres	⇕	Primary Force	⬇	Secondary Force	↻	Stretch Force	⬇	Contraction Force	⬇

Kneading

- With the fingertips of one hand apply a rhythmical cycle of primary and secondary forces.
- Your hooked fingertips pull back on the muscle as your thumb pushes away.
- If you have grasped the medial head with your fingertips, then as you pull back on the medial head you can simultaneously pull back on the lateral head with the heel of your hand. In other word you can treat the medial head and the lateral head together.
- Your pressure should be just short of discomfort.
- Start at the proximal attachment of the muscle and work your way down the leg.
- To relax the muscle, work with the patients breathing cycle, about 15 breaths per minute.
- To stimulate increase your speed to about 40 cycles per minute.

Active component

- Ask the patient to plantarflex their foot by pushing the toe end of their foot into the table for 3 to 5 seconds using a 10% effort. The gastrocnemius and soleus will contract.
- Resist the patient's effort and maintain tissue lockup throughout the technique.
- Ask the patient to exhale and to relax their muscle contraction.
- When you feel that the patient has relaxed their muscles completely (about 1-3 seconds) take up the tissue slack by increasing the primary and secondary tension.
- Take up the slack after each contraction and during exhalation.
- Repeat 2 or 3 times or as required.

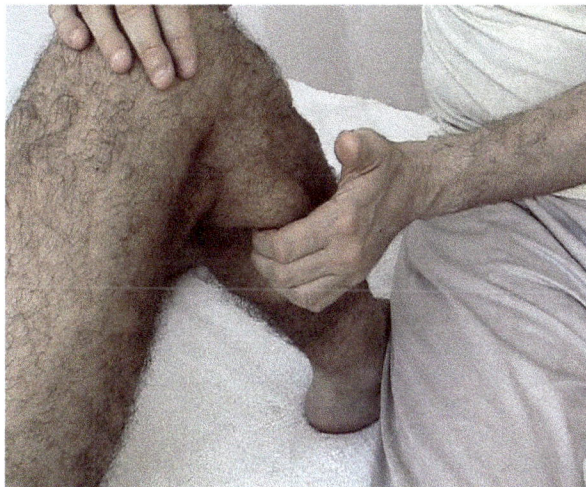

Picture 45.1

Technique 45.2 Kneading of gastrocnemius and soleus

Patient

* Prone with head straight in a face-hole or rotated to one side.

Therapist

* Stand at the side of the table level with the patient's leg.
* Grasp the patient's ankle on the side nearest you with your caudad hand and flex their leg to 90 degrees.
* Grasp around the calcaneus with your caudad hand.
* Your fingers extend along the Achilles tendon and your forearm extends along the plantar surface of the foot.
* Dorsiflex the patient's foot.
* Reach around the back of the patient's leg with your cephalad hand and hook your fingertips around the medial side of the medial head of the gastrocnemius muscle.
* Move to the other side of the table to treat the lateral head of gastrocnemius.
* Grasp the leg furthest from you. Hook your fingertips around the lateral side of the lateral head of the gastrocnemius muscle.

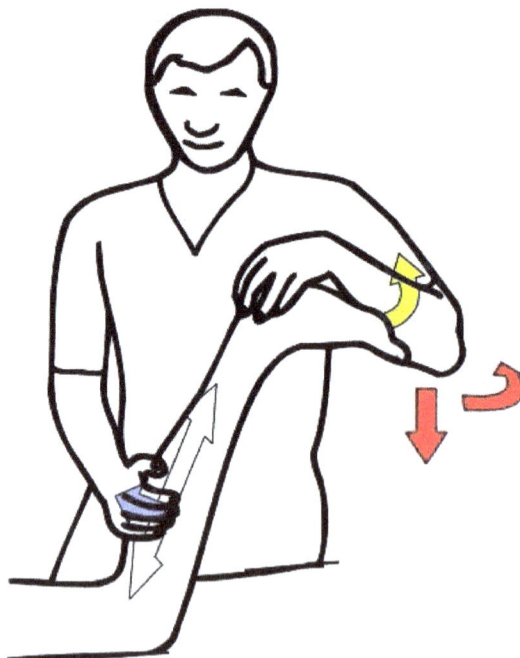

Figure 45.2

Muscle Fibres	⇕	Primary Force	⬇	Secondary Force	↻	Stretch Force	⬇	Contraction Force	⬇

Applicator

* The fingertips of your cephalad hand. You fingertips should be together.
* You may use your thumb, pisiform bone or thenar eminence as a secondary applicator.

Tissue tension

* Take up the primary tissue tension with compression and a transverse force achieved by pulling across the muscle with your fingertips.
* The force is generated by adducting and externally rotating your shoulder.

- Your force is perpendicular to the muscle and in a medial to lateral direction if you are working on the medial head and a lateral to medial direction if you are working on the lateral head.
- Longitudinal tension is taken up by dorsiflexing the patient's foot.
- Secondary tension is taken up by externally rotating the patient's leg when you are working on the medial head and internally rotating the patient's leg when you are working on the lateral head. This is always in the opposite direction to your primary force.

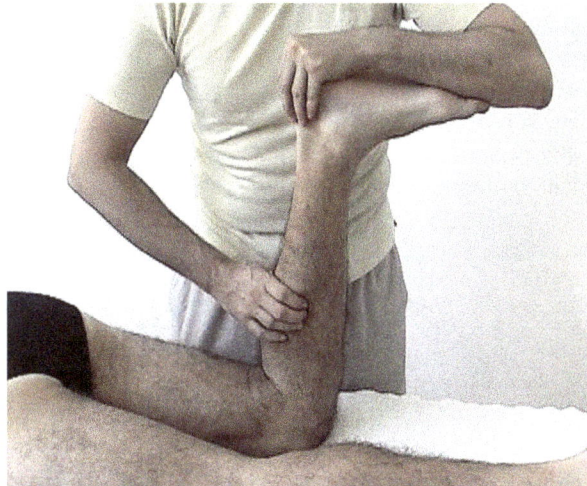

Picture 45.2

Kneading

- With the fingertips of one hand apply a rhythmical cycle of primary, secondary and longitudinal forces.

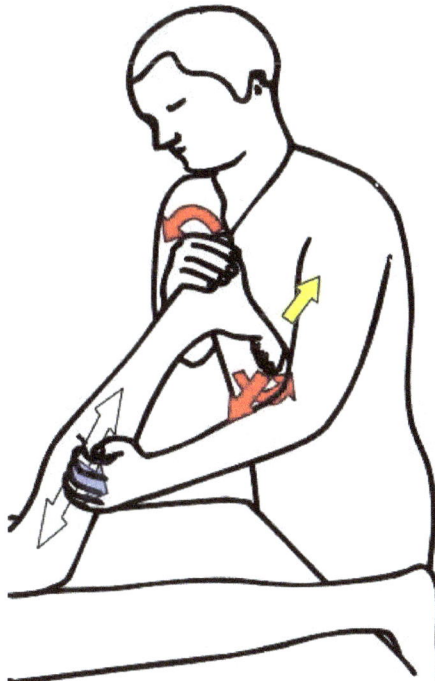

Figure 45.3 Alternative position. Place the ball of the patient's foot on your sternum and use your body weight to dorsiflex their foot.

Muscle Fibres	⇕	Primary Force	⬇	Secondary Force	↻	Stretch Force	⬇	Contraction Force	⬇

- Your hooked fingertips pull back on the muscle as you dorsiflex the foot and rotate the leg.
- Your pressure should be just short of discomfort.
- Start at the proximal attachment of the muscle and work your way down the leg.
- To relax the muscle, work with the patients breathing cycle, about 15 breaths per minute.
- To stimulate increase your speed to about 40 cycles per minute.

Active component

- Ask the patient to plantarflex their foot.
- Contract the muscles for 3 to 5 seconds using a 5% effort.
- Resist the patient's effort and maintain tissue lockup throughout the technique.
- Ask the patient to exhale and to relax their muscle contraction.
- When you feel that the patient has relaxed their muscles completely (about 1-3 seconds) take up the tissue slack by increasing the primary, secondary and longitudinal tension.
- Take up the slack after each contraction and during exhalation.
- Repeat 2 or 3 times or as required.

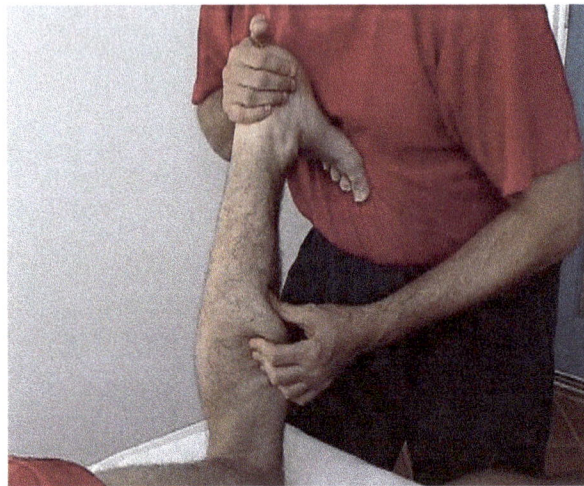

Picture 45.3

46. The posterior compartment

Anatomy

Tibialis posterior is the deepest of the flexor muscles. It arises on the lateral side of the proximal half of the posterior shaft of the tibia, along the medial side of the proximal two thirds of the posterior shaft of the fibula and the posterior interosseous membrane. It also arises from the deep transverse fascia and intermuscular septa. The tendon passes over a groove behind the medial malleolus with the flexor digitorum longus tendon just posterior to it and separated from it by a fibrous septum and its own synovial sheath. In the foot the tendon encloses a sesamoid fibrocartilage. After passing over the plantar calcaneonavicular ligament the tendon splits into a larger direct branch which runs more superficially to attach on the navicular tuberosity, the first cuneiform and the sustentaculum tali of the calcaneus. The deeper branch sends fibrous expansions laterally to the second cuneiform and the bases of metatarsals 2, 3, and 4. The cuboid, and third cuneiform may also receive slips. The tendon is prominent below the malleolus with resisted inversion and plantar flexion of the foot.

Action: Plantar flexion, adduction and inversion of the foot and supports the arch during gait.
Nerve supply: Tibial nerve L4 and 5.

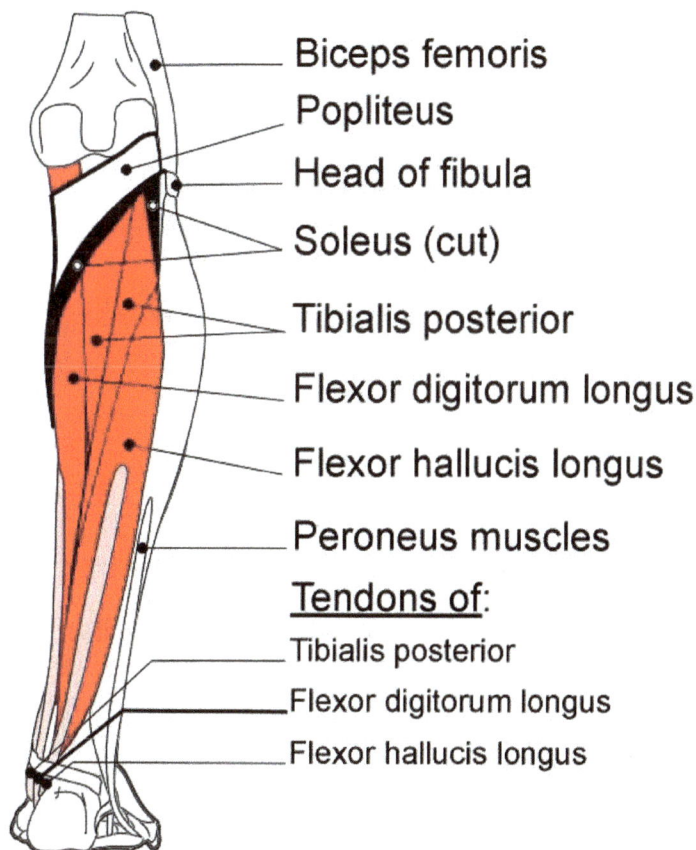

Biceps femoris
Popliteus
Head of fibula
Soleus (cut)
Tibialis posterior
Flexor digitorum longus
Flexor hallucis longus
Peroneus muscles
Tendons of:
Tibialis posterior
Flexor digitorum longus
Flexor hallucis longus

Flexor Digitorum longus arises along the medial side of the posterior shaft of the tibia, medial to tibialis posterior and just below the soleal line. The muscle also arises on the fascia covering tibialis posterior. The tendon passes over a groove behind the medial malleolus. It passes over the medial side of the sustentaculum tali. More distally it crosses the tendon of flexor hallucis longus and may send a slip to it. It also receives slips from flexor accessorius. It attaches on the bases of the distal phalanges of the lateral four toes. The tendon is palpable posterior and inferior to the medial malleolus. It is prominent on resisted toe flexion.

Action: It flexes toes and plantar flexes the foot.
Nerve supply: Tibial nerve S 2 and 3.

Flexor Hallucis longus arises along two thirds of the medial side of the posterior shaft of the fibula, the interosseous membrane and the fascia covering tibialis posterior. It lies deep to soleus and the Achilles tendon and is separated from it by the deep transverse fascia. The tendon runs the whole length of the muscle. As it descends it passes over a groove on the posterior tibia, a groove on the posterior talus and a groove on the inferior side of the sustentaculum tali of the calcaneus. More distally it crosses over the tendon of flexor digitorum longus and receives slips from it. It attaches on the base of the distal phalanx of the big toe.

Actions: It flexes the big toe.
Nerve supply: Tibial nerve S **2** and 3.

Posterior tibial Artery and *Tibial Nerve* (an) The posterior tibial artery carries the major blood supply to foot. A pulse is palpable when the tendons are relaxed. Palpate the tibial nerve deep against the calcaneus near the insertion of the Achilles tendon. In the foot it divides into the medial and lateral plantar nerves which supply the skin and small muscles of the foot.

From medial to lateral the structures passing behind the medial malleolus and into the foot are: Tibialis posterior tendon (Tom), Flexor Digitorum longus tendon (Dick), the Posterior tibial Artery and Tibial Nerve (an) and the Flexor Hallucis longus tendon (Harry).

The tendons of the deep posterior muscles pass behind the medial malleolus deep to the flexor retinaculum but superficial to the deltoid ligament. The deltoid ligament or medial collateral ligament is broad and strong. It runs from the medial malleolus to the talus and calcaneus. The deep transverse fascia divides the superficial and deep muscles of the posterior compartment of the leg and at the ankle forms a thickening, the flexor retinaculum, which supports the flexor tendons, blood vessels and nerves as they pass into the foot. The flexor retinaculum runs from the tip of the medial malleolus to the medial process of the calcaneal tuberosity. It also attaches on the sustentaculum tali above and below the flexor hallucis longus tendon and merges with the deep fascia of the dorsum of the foot and plantar aponeurosis.

Technique 46.1 Inhibition of posterior compartment muscles

Patient

- Supine with the hips and knees flexed.

Therapist

- Sit on the side of the table and on the patient's foot to fix it to the table.
- Grasp the patient's knee with one hand.
- With the other hand place your applicator on the muscle to be treated.

Applicator

- Pad or tip of thumb or fingertips.

Tissue tension

- Position the patient's leg where the superficial leg muscles are at their most relaxed state.
- Take up the primary tissue tension with compression.
- Your force is perpendicular to the muscle and in an anterior direction.
- Take up the tissue tension by gradually increasing your applicator pressure on the muscle.

Inhibition

- Apply pressure (compression) on the area of muscle covered by your applicator.
- Your pressure should be just short of discomfort.
- To relax the muscle work with the patients breathing cycle, about 15 breaths per minute.

- Maintain some compression throughout the technique but increase it during exhalation.
- Start at the proximal attachment of the muscle and work your way down the leg.

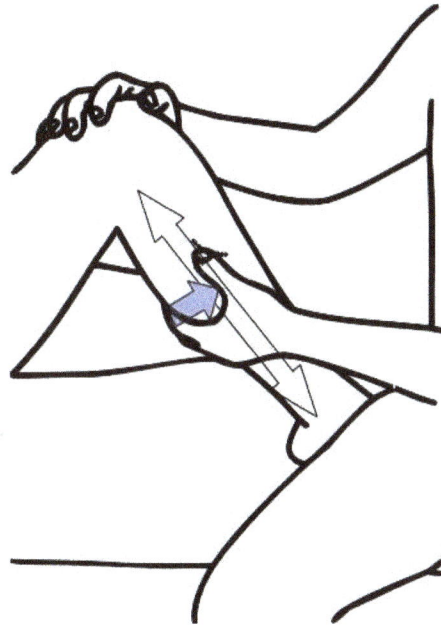

Figure 46.1

Muscle Fibres	↕	Primary Force	⬇	Secondary Force	↻	Stretch Force	⬇	Contraction Force	⬇

Active component

- Ask the patient to take a deep breath and hold it in.
- Ask the patient to attempt to flex their toes and curl their foot inwards into the table for 3 to 5 seconds using a 10% effort. The posterior compartment muscles will contract.
- Maintain tissue compression.
- Ask the patient to exhale and to relax their muscle contraction. As soon as you feel that the patient has relaxed their muscles completely (about 1-3 seconds) take up the tissue slack by increasing the compression.
- Take up the slack after each contraction and during exhalation.
- Repeat 2 or 3 times or as required.

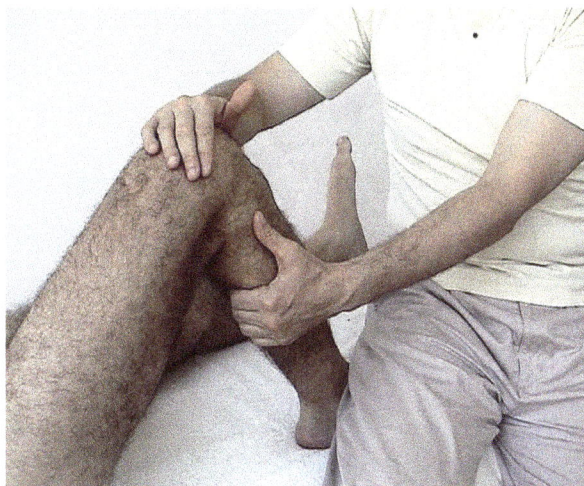

Picture 46.1

Technique 46.2 Inhibition of posterior compartment muscles and soleus

Patient

- Prone.

Therapist

- Stand at the side of the table opposite the patient's leg.
- Grasp the patient's ankle with your caudad hand and flex their leg to 90 degrees.
- Grasp around the calcaneus. Your fingers extend along the Achilles tendon and your forearm extends along the plantar surface of the foot.
- Dorsiflex and plantarflex the patient's foot until you find the position where the superficial leg muscles are at their most relaxed state.
- Place your applicator on the muscle to be treated.

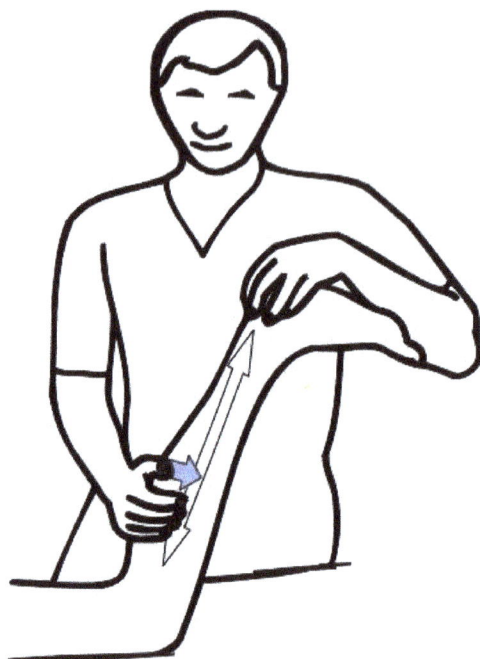

Figure 46.2

Muscle Fibres	⇕	Primary Force	⬇	Secondary Force	↻	Stretch Force	⬇	Contraction Force	⬇

Applicator

- The pad or tip of your thumb or fingertips or the knuckle of your index and middle finger.

Tissue tension

- Take up the primary tissue tension with compression.
- Your force is perpendicular to the muscle and in an anterior direction.

Inhibition

- Gradually increase your applicator pressure on the muscle.
- Your pressure should be just short of discomfort.
- To relax the muscle work with the patients breathing cycle, about 15 breaths per minute.
- Maintain some compression throughout the technique but increase it during exhalation.
- Start at the proximal attachment of the muscle and work your way down the leg.

Active component

- Ask the patient to take a deep breath and hold it in.
- Ask the patient to attempt to flex their toes and foot and curl their foot inwards for 3 to 5 seconds using a 10% effort. The posterior compartment muscles will contract.
- Maintain tissue compression.
- Ask the patient to exhale and to relax their muscle contraction. As soon as you feel that the patient has relaxed their muscles completely (about 1-3 seconds) take up the tissue slack by increasing the compression.
- Take up the slack after each contraction and during exhalation.
- Repeat 2 or 3 times or as required.

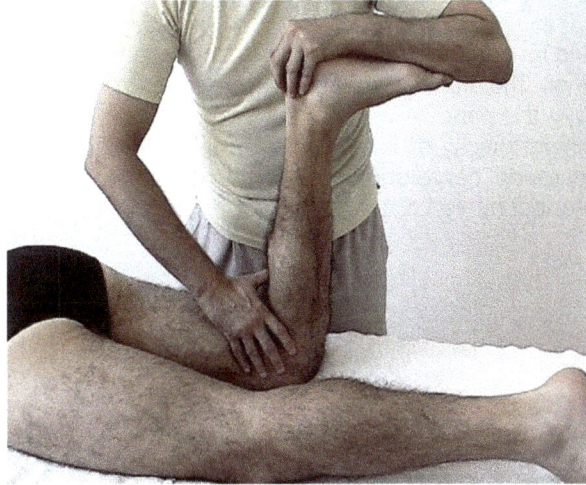

Picture 46.2

47. The anterior compartment

Anatomy

Tibialis anterior arises on the lateral tibial condyle and proximal two thirds of the anterolateral surface of the tibia, the interosseous membrane, the intermuscular septum between it and extensor digitorum longus, and on the deep surface of the deep fascia (fascia cruis) of the leg. The tendon attaches on the medial and inferior side of the first cuneiform and the base of the first metatarsal. Tibialis anterior is the most superficial muscle in the anterior compartment and lies lateral to the sharp subcutaneous border of the tibia. Its tendon is prominent with resisted dorsi flexion of the foot.
Variations: Attachments may occur on the talus, first metatarsal head or proximal phalanx.

Actions: It dorsiflexes and inverts the foot. It is active during gait.
Clinical indications: When the tibialis anterior becomes extremely hypertonic, its muscle attachment may pull away the periosteum from the tibia. This results in the conditions of shin splints and periostitis. Hypertonicity of the muscles of the anterior compartment can result in ischaemia of the deep peroneal nerve and cause toe drop.
Nerve supply: Deep Peroneal nerve L**4** and 5.

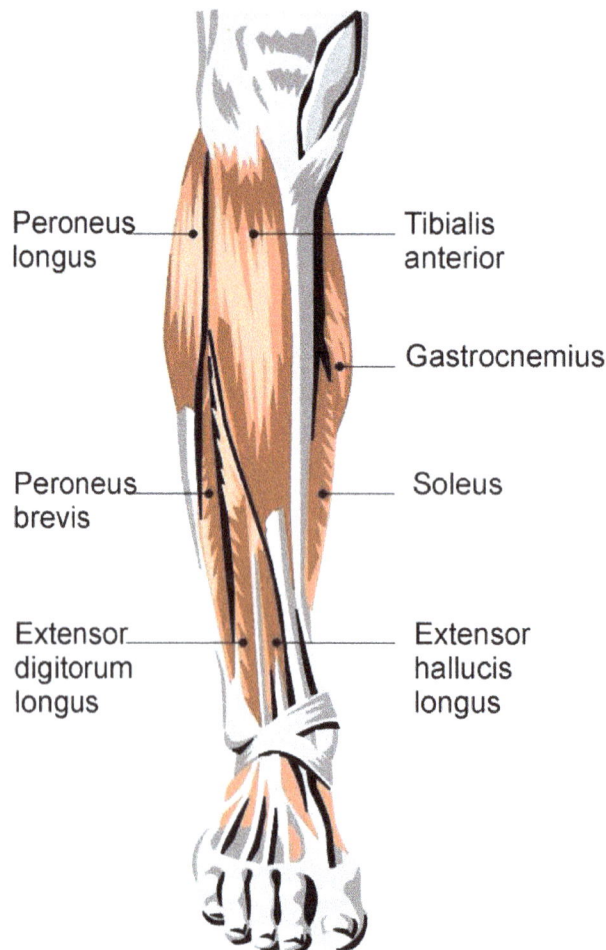

Extensor hallucis longus arises on the middle of the fibula shaft and interosseous membrane and attaches on the base of the distal phalanx of the big toe. A slip to the base of the proximal phalanx is usual. The muscle lies deep in the anterior compartment. The tendon is prominent with resisted extension of the big toe.

Actions: It extends the big toe, dorsiflexes the foot.
Nerve supply: Deep Peroneal nerve L5 and S1

Extensor digitorum longus arises on the lateral tibial condyle, upper 2/3 of the anterior fibula, interosseous membrane, the intermuscular septum between it and tibialis anterior and on the deep surface of the deep fascia (fascia cruis) of the leg. It may be palpated lateral to tibialis anterior but part of it lies deep to tibialis anterior. The tendon passes under the extensor retinaculum lateral to extensor hallucis longus and on the dorsum of the foot splits into four tendons, which attach on the bases of the middle and distal phalanges of the lateral four toes. The tendon is prominent with resisted extension of the toes. Variations include attachment on the metatarsals or big toe.

Action: It extends the toes, dorsiflexes the foot. Nerve supply: Deep Peroneal nerve L5 and S1

Peroneus tertius is part of extensor digitorum longus. It arises on a lower part of the fibula, interosseous membrane and anterior crural intermuscular septum. The tendon passes under the extensor retinaculum with extensor digitorum longus and attaches on the base of the fifth metatarsal. It may be absent.

Action: It dorsiflexes the foot. It may aid eversion of the foot.
Nerve supply: Deep Peroneal nerve L5 and S1

Technique 47.1 Inhibition of anterior compartment muscles

Patient

- Supine with the hips and knees flexed.

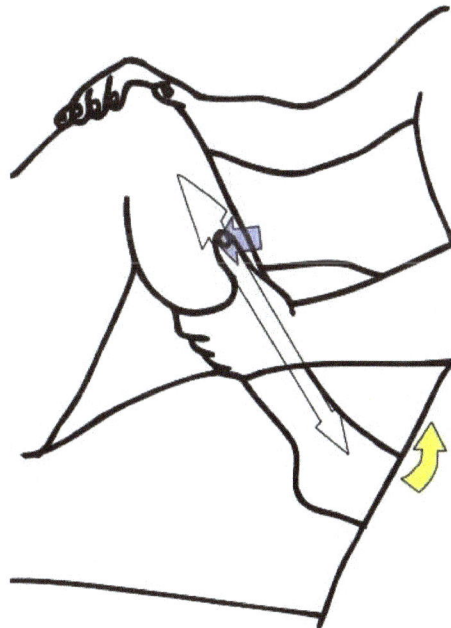

Figure 47.1

Muscle Fibres	⇕	Primary Force	⬇	Secondary Force	↻	Stretch Force	⬇	Contraction Force	⬇

Therapist

- Sit on the side of the table and on the patient's foot to fix it to the table.
- Grasp the patient's knee with your cephalad hand.
- Place the applicator of your caudad hand on the muscle to be treated.

Applicator

- Pad of thumb or knuckle of clenched fist.

Tissue tension

- Take up the primary tissue tension with compression.
- Your force is perpendicular to the muscle and in a posterior direction.

Inhibition

- Apply pressure (compression) on the area of muscle covered by your thumb.
- Take up the tissue tension by gradually increasing your thumb pressure on the muscle.
- Your pressure should be just short of discomfort.
- To relax the muscle work with the patients breathing cycle, about 15 breaths per minute.
- Maintain some compression throughout the technique but increase it during exhalation.
- Start at the proximal attachment of the muscle and work your way down the leg.

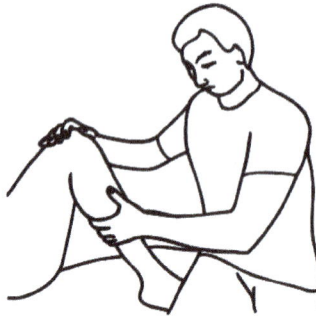

Figure 47.2

Active component

- Ask the patient to take a deep breath and hold it in.
- Ask the patient to attempt to lift their foot upward off the table but leave their heel fixed on the table for 3 to 5 seconds using a 10% effort. The anterior compartment muscles will contract.
- Maintain tissue compression.
- Ask the patient to exhale and to relax their muscle contraction. As soon as you feel that the patient has relaxed their muscles completely (about 1-3 seconds) take up the tissue slack by increasing the compression.
- Take up the slack after each contraction and during exhalation.
- Repeat 2 or 3 times or as required.

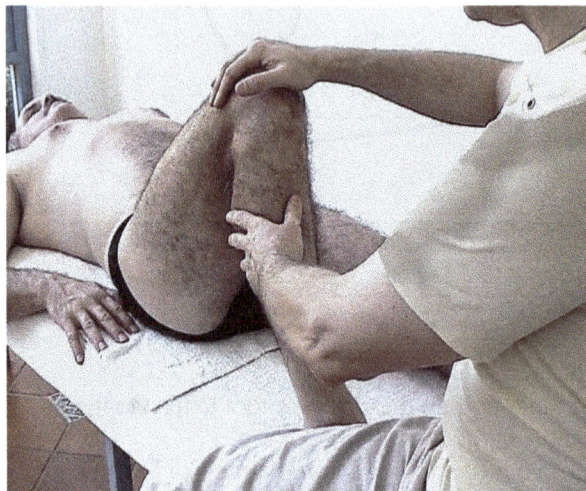

Picture 47.1

48. Peroneus longus and peroneus brevis

Anatomy

Peroneus longus arises on the head of the fibula and upper two-thirds of the lateral shaft of the fibula, the deep fascia of the leg (the fascia cruris) and from the anterior and posterior intermuscular septum. A few fibres may arise on the lateral tibial condyle.
The tendon is long and passes over a groove on the posterior aspect of lateral malleolus, which it shares with the peroneus brevis tendon. It runs over the lateral calcaneus going anteriorly and inferiorly and passing below the peroneal tubercle/ trochlea. A sesamoid fibrocartilage or bone is present in a thickening of the tendon as it changes direction at the cuboid. It goes deep, passing over a groove in the cuboid, and is covered by the long plantar ligament. It stays hard up against the tarsals running diagonally under the plantar surface of the foot, over the third cuneiform and second metatarsal bone.
It attaches on the lateral side of the base of the first metatarsal and on the anterolateral corner of the first cuneiform and sometimes the second metatarsal.
Variations include attachments on the third, fourth or fifth metatarsals or the adductor hallucis and fusion with peroneus brevis.

Action: Plantar flexion and eversion of the foot. It helps supports the arch.
Nerve supply: Superficial peroneal nerve L **5**, S**1** and 2.

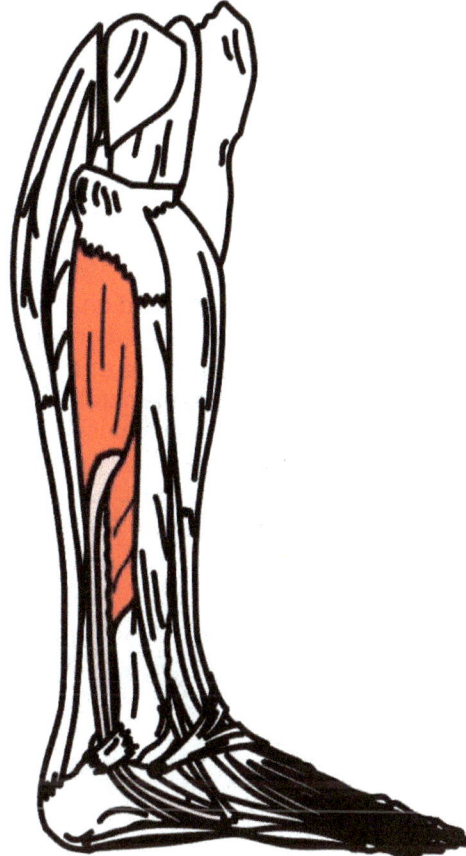

Peroneus brevis arises on the middle third of the lateral shaft of the fibula and on the anterior and posterior crural intermuscular septum. It lies deep to peroneus longus.
Behind the lateral malleolus the peroneus brevis tendon lies anterior to the peroneus longus tendon. Both tendons run close together under the superior peroneal retinaculum and share a common synovial sheath. On the lateral side of the calcaneus the tendons diverge, the peroneus brevis above the peroneal tubercle/ trochlea and peroneus longus runs anteriorly. It attaches on the dorsal lateral side of tuberosity of the fifth metatarsal (the styloid process).

Action: Eversion and plantar flexion of the foot. It may give support to the lateral ligaments and steady the leg on the foot.
Nerve supply: Superficial peroneal nerve L **5**, S**1** and 2.

Peroneus longus and brevis tendons are held in place by fibrous bands, the superior and inferior peroneal retinaculum. The superior retinaculum attaches on the lateral calcaneus, the posterior lateral malleolus and merges with the deep transverse fascia of the leg. It forms a canal for peroneus longus and brevis tendons as it covers the groove behind the lateral malleolus. The inferior retinaculum attaches on the lateral calcaneus and merges with the inferior extensor retinaculum. Some fibres attach on the periosteum of the peroneal trochlea/ tubercle thus forming a septum, which separates the peroneus longus and brevis tendons.
Synovial sheaths encloses the tendons for a distance of about 4 cm proximal and 4 cm distal to the tip of the lateral malleolus.

Following a severe lateral ankle sprain, it is not uncommon for a person to complain of tenderness in the ankle years after the actual sprain has taken place. The sprain itself usually leaves the peroneus longus and peroneus brevis in a hypertonic state. This chronic hypertonicity usually causes the person to complain of pain in the ankle, particularly under the lateral malleolus. The hypertonicity of the brevis and longus causes the tendons to be pulled against the lateral malleolus, thus chronically irritating them. Releasing the peroneus brevis and longus and treating the tendons usually produces immediate relief.

Technique 48.1 Kneading of peroneus longus and brevis

Patient

- Supine with the hips and knees flexed.

Therapist

- Sit on the side of the table and on the patient's foot to fix it to the table.
- Grasp the patient's knee with your cephalad hand.
- Reach around the lateral side of the patient's leg with your caudad hand and place your fingertips just posterior to the peroneus muscle and your thumb just anterior to the peroneus muscle. Grasp the peroneus muscle between your fingertips and thumb.
- Alternatively reach around the medial side of the patient's leg and place your fingertips anterior to the peroneus muscle and pull with your fingertips. Flex your fingertips or slide your flexed fingertips over the skin.

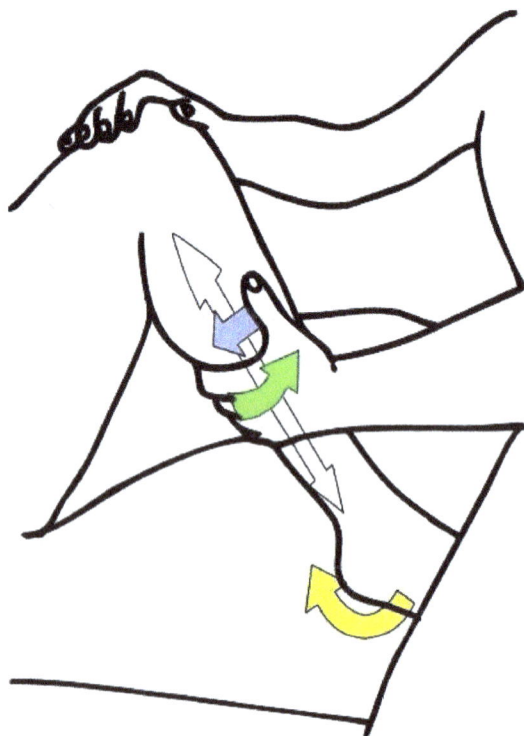

Figure 48.1

Muscle Fibres	↕	Primary Force	⬇	Secondary Force	↻	Stretch Force	⬇	Contraction Force	⬇

Tissue tension

- Take up the primary tissue tension with compression and a transverse force achieved by flexing your fingertips.
- Your force is perpendicular to the muscle and in an anterior direction.
- Take up the secondary tissue tension with a torsion force achieved by flexing your thumb.

Kneading

- With the fingertips of one hand apply a rhythmical cycle of primary and secondary forces.
- Your hooked fingertips pull back on the muscle as your thumb pushes away.
- Your pressure should be just short of discomfort.
- Start at the proximal attachment of the muscle and work your way down the leg.
- To relax the muscle, work with the patients breathing cycle, about 15 breaths per minute.
- To stimulate increase your speed to about 40 cycles per minute.

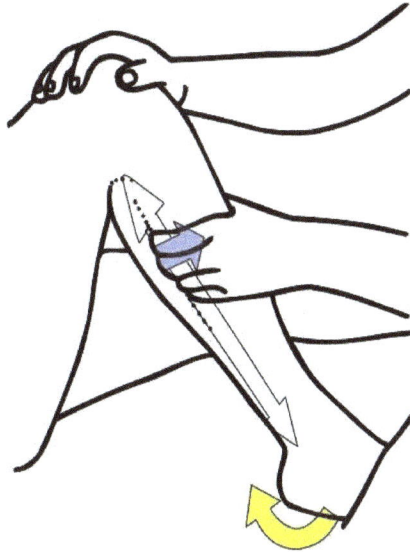

Figure 48.2

Muscle Fibres	↕	Primary Force	↓	Secondary Force	↻	Stretch Force	↓	Contraction Force	↓

Active component

- Ask the patient to rotate their foot outwards (eversion) and contract the peroneus muscles for 3 to 5 seconds using a 10% effort.
- Resist the patient's effort and maintain tissue lockup throughout the technique.
- Ask the patient to exhale and to relax their muscle contraction.
- When you feel that the patient has relaxed their muscles completely (about 1-3 seconds) take up the tissue slack by increasing the primary and secondary tension.
- Take up the slack after each contraction and during exhalation.
- Repeat 2 or 3 times or as required.

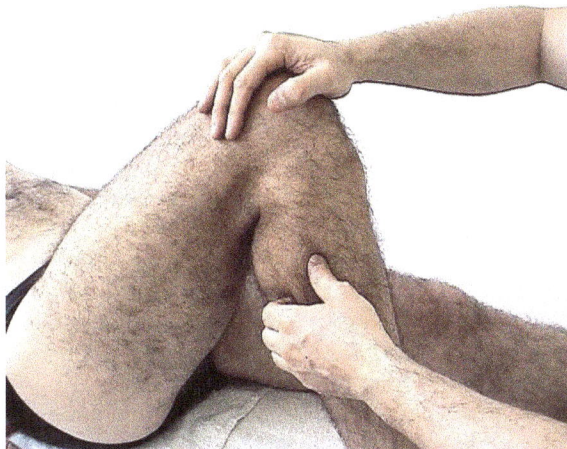

Picture 48.1

49. The peroneus tendons

Anatomy

The **peroneus longus tendon** passes behind the lateral malleolus in a groove, which it shares with the peroneus brevis tendon. The peroneal tendons also share a common synovial sheath. At the malleolus it runs behind the peroneus brevis tendon, but the tendons diverge at the peroneal trochlea of the calcaneus with the peroneus longus tendon passing below and the peroneus brevis tendon passing above the peroneal trochlea of the calcaneus. The peroneus longus passes over the lateral surface of the cuboid and then in a groove running under the cuboid. It passes through a second synovial sheath as it runs obliquely under the sole of the foot. It attaches on the base of the first metatarsal and first cuneiform. Slips may also attach on the bases of the other metatarsals. Rarely the peroneus longus and brevis are fused. Action - plantar flexes and everts foot and supports arch.

The **peroneus brevis tendon** passes behind the lateral malleolus anterior to the peroneus longus tendon and then runs above the trochlea to insert on the lateral surface of the tubercle on the base of the fifth metatarsal. Action - everts and plantar flexes foot.

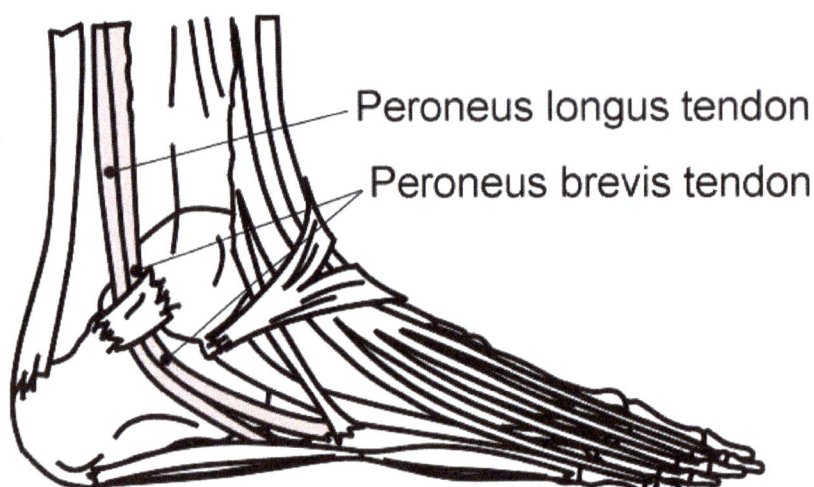

A superior and an inferior peroneal retinaculum hold down the peroneal tendons against the lateral side of the ankle. The superior peroneal retinaculum arise from the lateral surface of the calcaneus and from deep transverse fascia of the leg and inserts on the posterior of the lateral malleolus. The inferior peroneal retinaculum also arises from the lateral surface of the calcaneus but is continuous with the inferior extensor retinaculum anteriorly. Some fibres attach on the peroneal trochlea of the calcaneus thereby forming a septa which separates the two tendons.

Clinical considerations
When the peroneal retinaculum is ruptured the peroneal tendon dislocates from the malleolus. Pain over the lateral malleolus is more often due to a sprained anterior talofibular ligament and less frequently is due to tenosynovitis of the peroneal tendons. A subluxated tendon will be palpable and a history of twisting over on the ankle will suggest a ligament injury.
A dislocated peroneal tendon requires surgery. Myofascial manipulation should be used after surgery to remove scar tissue and restore structural integrity to the damaged tissues. Tenosynovitis is characterised by pain and swelling behind the lateral malleolus and is usually as a result of a previous fracture or injury and/or overuse. Transverse friction over the tendon and sheath for 3-5 minutes twice a week is required until the condition improves. Rest and strapping are indicated initially. Ice packs may be applied to the tendon for 15 minutes three times a day. Use kneading and MET if the peroneus longus or brevis muscles are hypertonic and short, perhaps as a result of a chronic ankle sprain. In this case also treat the ligament. Appropriate joint manipulation and an orthotic may be required to correct joint dysfunction in the foot, ankle or superior tibiofibular joint.

Technique 49.1 Friction over the peroneus tendons

Patient

- Supine with their head on a pillow or folded towel.

Therapist

- Stand at the side of the table opposite the patient's foot.

Applicator

- The tip of your thumb.

Tissue tension

- Find the tendon.
- Place your thumb on the tendon and take up the tissue tension by gradually increasing your thumb pressure on the tendon.

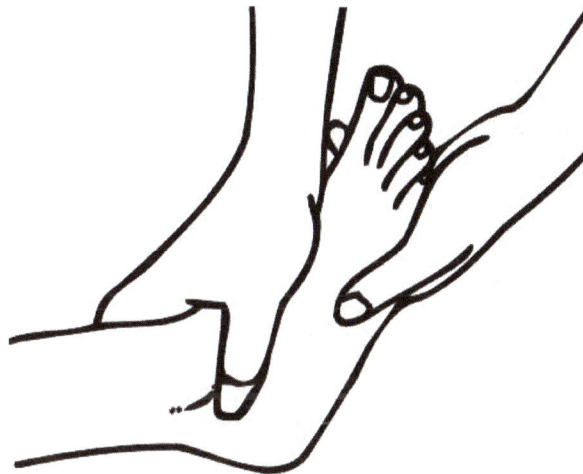

Figure 49.1 Peroneus tendons

Transverse Friction

- Work across the tendon with transverse friction.
- Apply firm pressure over a small area.

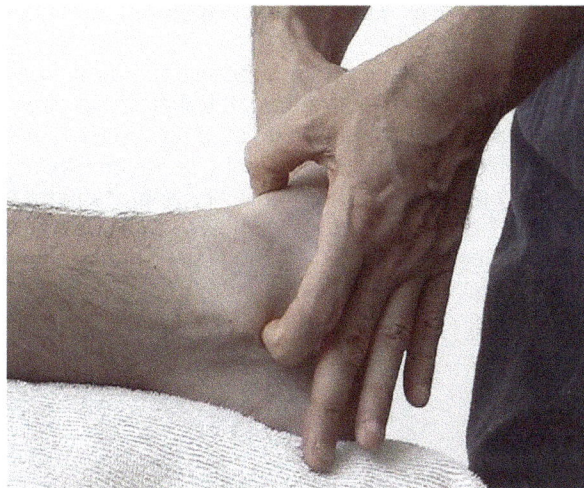

Picture 49.1

50. The ankle and toe extensor tendons

Anatomy

From medial to lateral the structures passing over the dorsum of the foot include tendons of: tibialis anterior, extensor hallucis longus, and extensor digitorum longus. The dorsalis pedis artery, the secondary blood supply to the foot passes between the extensor hallucis longus, and extensor digitorum longus tendons. It may be absent in 15% population.

The tendons of the muscles in the anterior compartment pass over the dorsum of the foot and ankle deep to the superior and inferior extensor retinaculum above and below the ankle joint. The retinacula are a thickening of the deep fascia of the leg, which support the tendons, blood vessels and nerves. The superior extensor retinaculum is attached laterally to the lower anterior fibula and medially to the anterior tibia. The inferior extensor retinaculum is Y shaped. The stem is attached laterally on the superior aspect of the calcaneus. The upper diverging band has a superficial and deep layer and attaches on the medial malleolus. The lower band attaches on the plantar aponeurosis medially. Synovial sheaths enclose and lubricate the tendons as they pass under the retinaculum and for short distance above and below the retinaculum.

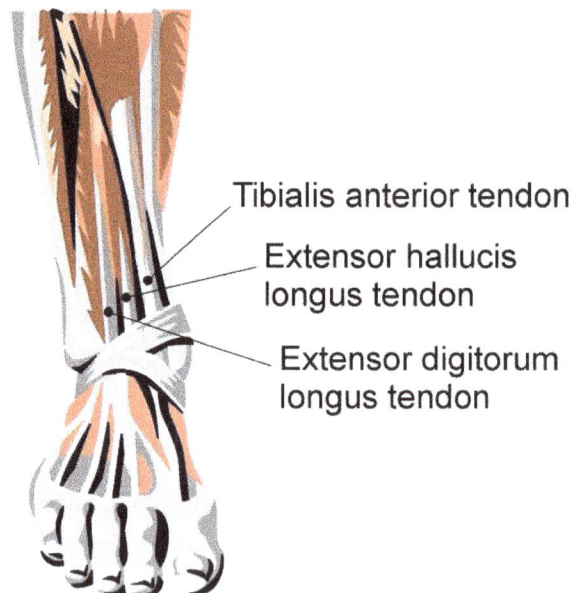

Tibialis anterior tendon

Extensor hallucis longus tendon

Extensor digitorum longus tendon

<u>Technique 50.1</u> Friction over the extensor tendons

Pain over the tendon is frequently due to a strain (tendonitis) but may be due to tenosynovitis. Myofascial manipulation should be used to treat both. It will increase circulation to the area and help remove scar tissue and with appropriate exercise it will restore structural integrity to the damaged tendon. These conditions are characterised by pain and swelling in front of the ankle and is usually as a result of a previous fracture or injury and/or overuse. Transverse friction over the tendon and sheath for 3-5 minutes twice a week is required until the condition improves. Rest and strapping may be indicated for the first 48 hours after injury. Ice packs may be applied to the tendon for 15 minutes three times a day.

Patient

- Supine.

Therapist

- Stand at the side of the table opposite the patient's foot.

Applicator

- Tip of thumb.

Tissue tension

- Find the tendon.
- Place your thumb on the tendon and take up the tissue tension by gradually increasing your thumb pressure on the tendon.

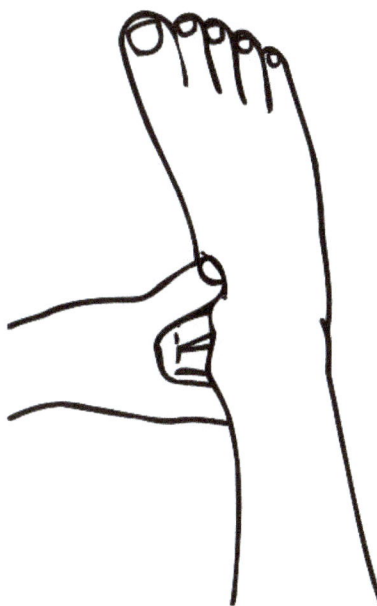

Figure 50.1 Extensor tendons

Transverse Friction

- Work across the tendon with transverse friction.
- Apply firm pressure over a small area.

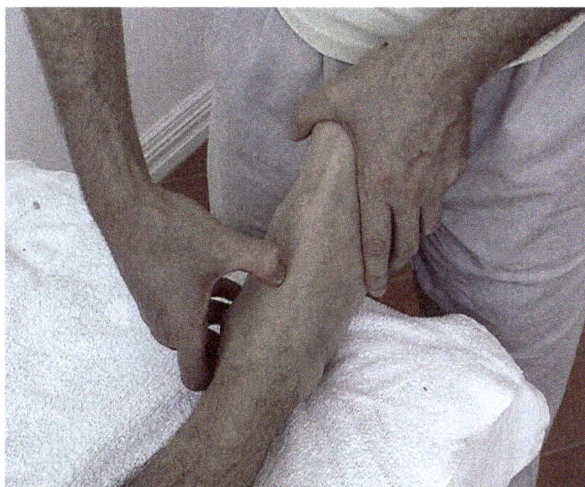

Picture 50.1

51. Short muscles of foot

Anatomy

Dorsal aspect
Extensor digitorum brevis arises on the distal, lateral and superior surface of the calcaneus and the inferior extensor retinaculum. The medial tendon attaches to the dorsal aspect of the base of the proximal phalanx of the big toe. It is sometimes referred to as **extensor hallucis brevis**. The other three tendons attach to the lateral side of the long extensor tendons of the second, third and fourth toes. Variations include additional slips arising from the talus, navicular and dorsal interosseous muscles, missing tendons or additional tendons.

Actions: Extension of the medial four toes. Nerve supply: Deep peroneal nerve S1 and 2.

The **dorsal interossei** lie between the metatarsal bones. They arise by two heads on adjacent sides of two metatarsal bones and attach to the base of the proximal phalanx of the toes. Actions: Abducts toes, flexes proximal phalanx and extends distal phalanges of the toes. Nerve supply: Deep branch of the lateral plantar nerve S2 and **3**.

The deep fascia is thin. Proximally it arises on the inferior extensor retinaculum. On each side of the foot it merges with the plantar aponeurosis. Distally if ensheathes the extensor tendons.

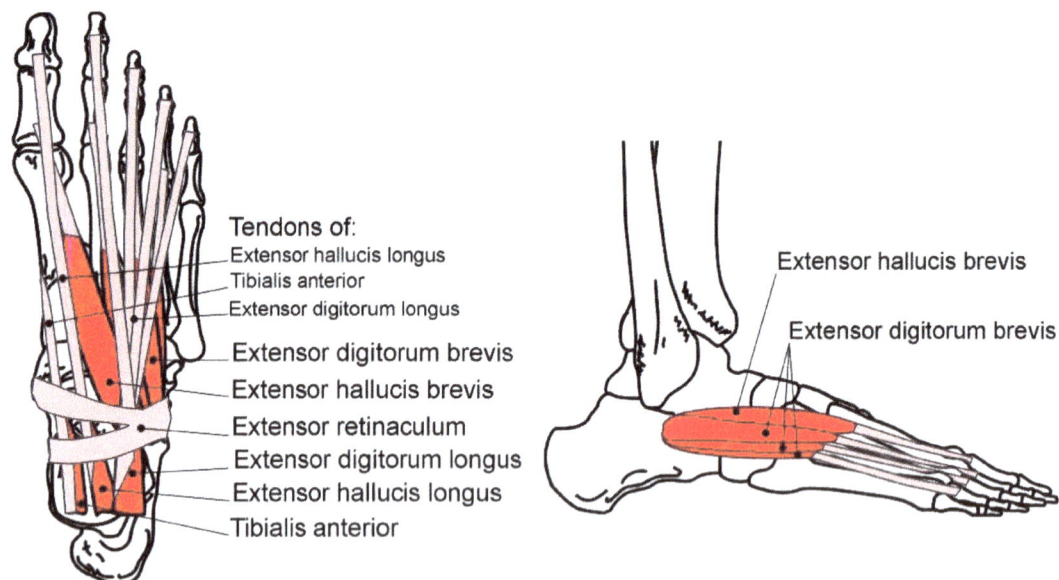

Tendons of:
Extensor hallucis longus
Tibialis anterior
Extensor digitorum longus

Extensor digitorum brevis
Extensor hallucis brevis
Extensor retinaculum
Extensor digitorum longus
Extensor hallucis longus
Tibialis anterior

Extensor hallucis brevis
Extensor digitorum brevis

Plantar aspect
Flexor digitorum brevis arises as a tendon on the medial process of the calcanean tuberosity, plantar aponeurosis and fascia attached to adjacent muscles. It splits into four tendons which attach on the middle phalanx of the lateral four toes. The tendon to the fifth toe is frequently absent.
Actions: Flexes toes. Nerve supply: The medial plantar nerve S2 and **3**.

Flexor hallucis brevis arises on the plantar surface of the cuboid and third cuneiform bone and on the tibialis posterior tendon and plantar fascia. It attaches to the base of the proximal phalanx and to the abductor tendon. A sesamoid bone is found within the tendon.
Actions: Flexes proximal phalanx of big toe. Nerve supply: The medial plantar nerve S2 and **3**.

Abductor hallucis arises on the flexor retinaculum, medial process of the calcanean tuberosity, plantar aponeurosis and fascia between it and flexor digitorum brevis. It attaches via a tendon to the medial side of the base of the proximal phalanx of the big toe. A slip may attach to the medial sesamoid bone. The muscle lies on the medial side of the foot.

Actions: Flexes and abducts the big toe. Nerve supply: The medial plantar nerve S2 and **3**.

Adductor hallucis arises by two heads. The oblique head arises from the base of the second, third and fourth metatarsals bones and the sheath of the peroneus longus tendon. The transverse head arises from capsules and overlying ligaments of the third, fourth and fifth metatarsophalangeal joints. It attaches to the lateral side of the base of the proximal phalanx of the big toe and merges with flexor hallucis brevis and lateral sesamoid bone. It is important for the internal strength of the foot. Variations include additional attachments on the first metatarsal and the proximal phalanx of the second toe.

Actions: Adducts and flexes the proximal phalanx of the big toe.

Nerve supply: The lateral plantar nerve S2 and **3**.

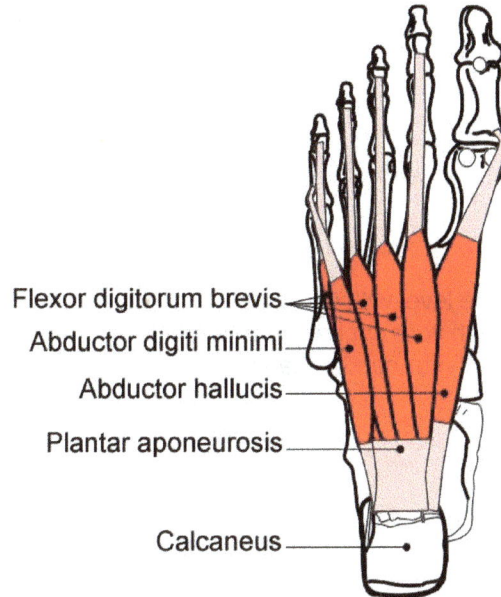

Flexor digitorum brevis
Abductor digiti minimi
Abductor hallucis
Plantar aponeurosis

Calcaneus

Flexor digiti minimi brevis arises on the medial side of the plantar surface of the base of the fifth metatarsal bone and the sheath of the peroneus longus tendon. It attaches on the lateral side of the base of the proximal phalanx of the fifth toe. Some of its fibres may attach on the lateral and distal area on the fifth metatarsal bone.

Actions: Flexes the proximal phalanx of the little toe.

Nerve supply: The lateral plantar nerve S2 and **3**

Abductor digiti minimi arises on the lateral and medial processes of the calcanean tuberosity and the area of bone between, plantar aponeurosis and fascia between it and flexor digitorum brevis. It attaches by a single tendon to the lateral side of the base of the proximal phalanx of the fifth toe. The muscle runs down the lateral side of the foot, frequently with intermediate attachments on the base of the fifth metatarsal bone.

Actions: It is more a flexor than an abductor of the little toe.

Nerve supply: The lateral plantar nerve S2 and **3**.

The **plantar interossei** lie below the metatarsal bones. They arise on the base and proximal shaft on the medial sides of the third, fourth and fifth metatarsal bones and attach to the base on the medial sides of the proximal phalanx of the toes.

Actions: Abducts toes, flexes proximal phalanx and extends distal phalanges of the toes.

Nerve supply: Deep branch of the lateral plantar nerve S2 and **3**.

The dome of calcaneus flares outward at it base. The medial tubercle is the weight bearing medial part. As well as serving as the attachment for muscle the medial tubercle serves as the attachment for the plantar aponeurosis. The plantar aponeurosis lies superficially and acts as a tie-beam to support the longitudinal arch of the foot. From the medial calcaneal tuberosity, it fans out to attach on the metatarsal heads. The skin is thickened and supported with subcutaneous fibro-fatty tissue.

Clinical indications: Pes planus and other structural variations, shortness, strains and spasms. Heel spurs and plantar fasciitis can develop at or near the medial tubercle and will be tender. The treatment is to correct the biomechanics, which caused the problem and remove any further weight being placed on the spur with an orthotic. A hole or depression is cut into the upper surface of a thick sole and the sole is inserted into a shoe. The spur sits in the depression. A sole of similar height should be inserted in the other shoe to maintain equal leg length. The patient should self-treat by soaking their foot in a bath of warm water for five or ten minutes and then perform transverse friction over the plantar fascia for five minutes daily.

Technique 51.1 Kneading the short toe flexor muscles and plantar aponeurosis

Patient

- Prone with their head rotated or straight and in a face hole.

Therapist

- Stand at the side of the table level with the patient's foot.
- Grasp the patient's ankle with your cephalad hand and flex their knee to 90 degrees.
- Grasp the patient's toes with your caudad hand and extend the patient's toes.

Applicator

- The tip of your thumb or a T bar.

Tissue tension

- Take up the primary tissue tension with compression and a transverse force achieved by moving across the muscle with your thumb in a fixed flexed position.
- Your force is perpendicular to the muscle and in a medial-lateral direction.
- Longitudinal tension is taken up by extending the patient's toes.

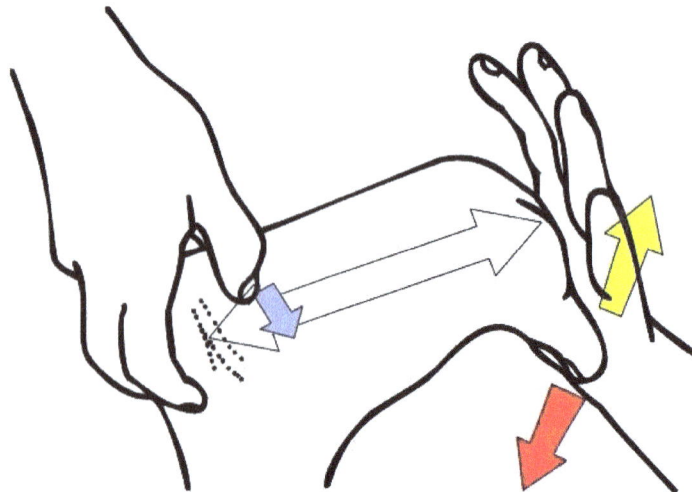

Figure 51.1

Muscle Fibres	⇕	Primary Force	⬇	Secondary Force	↻	Stretch Force	⬇	Contraction Force	⬇

Kneading

- Apply a rhythmical cycle of primary and longitudinal forces.
- Your pressure should be just short of discomfort.

- Start at the proximal attachment of the muscle and work down the sole of the foot.
- To relax the muscle work with the patients breathing cycle, about 15 breaths per minute.
- To stimulate increase your speed to about 40 cycles per minute.

Active component

- Ask the patient to flex their toes and contract the short toe muscles for 3 to 5 seconds using a 10% effort.
- Resist the patient's effort and maintain tissue lockup throughout the technique.
- Ask the patient to exhale and to relax their muscle contraction.
- When you feel that the patient has relaxed their muscles completely (about 1-3 seconds) take up the tissue slack by increasing the primary and longitudinal tension.
- Take up the slack after each contraction and during exhalation.
- Repeat 2 or 3 times or as required.

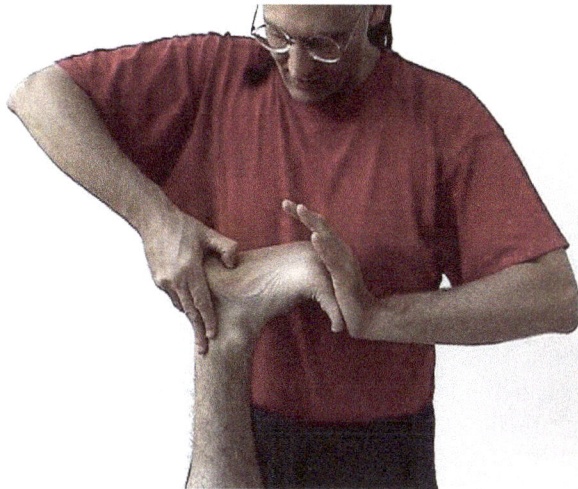

Picture 51.1

Technique 51.2 Kneading the short toe extensor muscles

Patient

- Supine with hips and knees flexed.
- The soles of the feet are flat on the table with the toes over the edge of the table.

Therapist

- Stand at the end of the table level with the patient's foot.
- Grasp the patient's ankle with one hand.
- Grasp the patient's toes with your other hand and flex the patient's toes. The toes should be made to curl over the edge of the table.

Applicator

- The tip of your fingers or thumb.

Tissue tension

- Take up the primary tissue tension with compression and a transverse force achieved by flexing your fingers.
- Your force is perpendicular to the muscle and in a medial-lateral direction.
- Longitudinal tension is taken up by flexing the patient's toes.

Kneading

- Apply a rhythmical cycle of primary and longitudinal forces.
- Your pressure should be just short of discomfort.
- Start at the proximal attachment of the muscle and work down the dorsum of the foot.
- To relax the muscle work with the patients breathing cycle, about 15 breaths per minute.
- To stimulate increase your speed to about 40 cycles per minute.

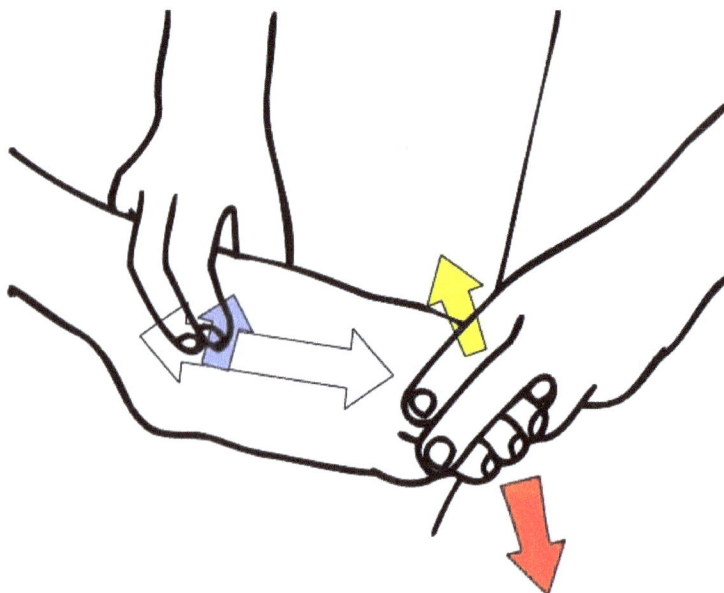

Figure 51.2

Muscle Fibres	⇕	Primary Force	⬇	Secondary Force	↻	Stretch Force	⬇	Contraction Force	⬇

Active component

- Ask the patient to attempt to pull up (extend) their toes.
- The toe extensor muscles contract for 3 to 5 seconds using a 10% effort.
- Resist the patient's effort and maintain tissue lockup throughout the technique.
- Ask the patient to exhale and to relax their muscle contraction.
- When you feel that the patient has relaxed their muscles completely (about 1-3 seconds) take up the tissue slack by increasing the primary and longitudinal tension.
- Take up the slack after each contraction and during exhalation.
- Repeat 2 or 3 times or as required.

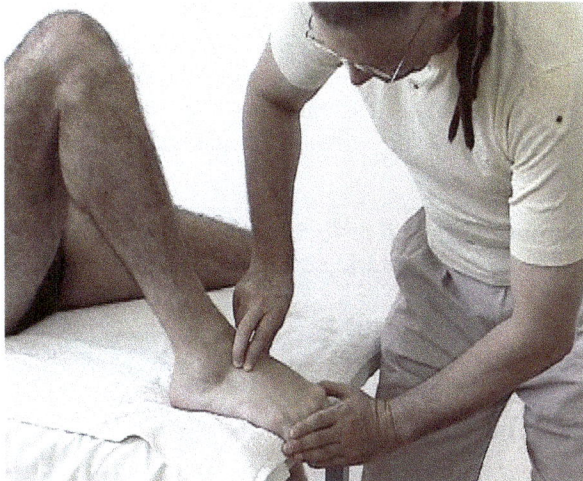

Picture 51.2

52. Ankle ligaments

Anatomy

Medial aspect
The **medial collateral ligament** also known as the deltoid ligament is broad and made up of two layers. It arises on the medial malleolus and fans out in a generally inferior direction to attach on the talus, calcaneus and navicular. Its great strength plus the fact the distal end of the fibula the lateral malleolus projects more distally than the medial malleolus means eversion sprains are much less common than inversion strains.

Lateral aspect
The **anterior talofibular ligament** arises on the anterior lateral malleolus and runs anteriorly and medially to the neck of the talus. It is the smallest, weakest and the most commonly sprained of the ankle ligaments. Swelling is usually localised in the sinus tarsi a depression just anterior to the lateral malleolus.

The **calcaneofibular ligament** arises on the inferior lateral malleolus and runs posteriorly and slightly inferiorly to a tubercle on the lateral surface of the calcaneus. Peroneus longus and brevis tendons pass over it.

The **posterior talofibular ligament** arises on the posterior lateral malleolus and runs posteriorly to lateral tubercle of the talus.

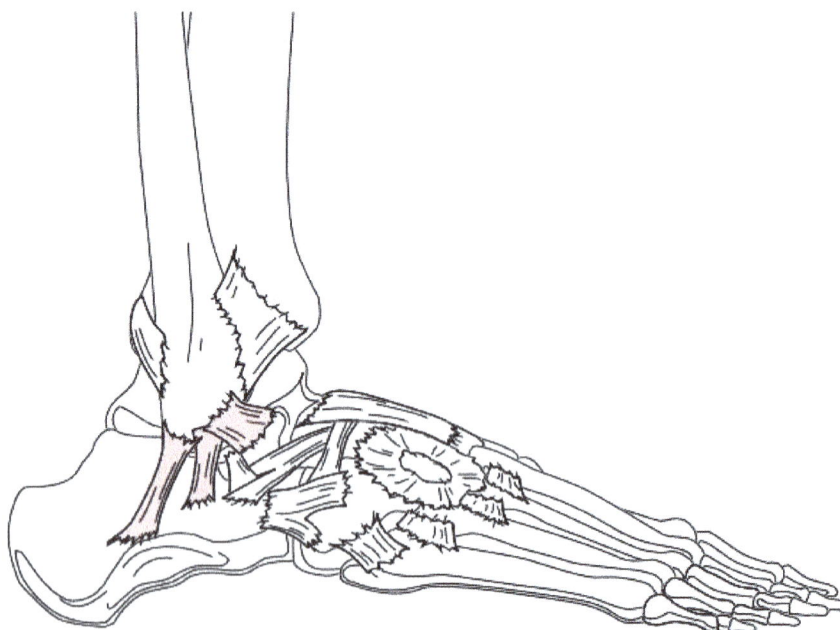

Treatment
During the initial acute phase which usually lasts about 24 hours the ankle should be **rested**, **elevated** above the body, **strapped** with a compression bandage, and an **ice pack** applied to the area for about 15 minutes every 3 hours.

The patient should attempt walking as soon as pain will permit but avoid prolonged standing as this may slow down the rate at which the swelling subsides. The rate also depends on the integrity of the lymphatic system and its efficiency at reabsorbing the oedema.

Apply **effleurage** over the entire lower limb to support lymphatic drainage. The elevated leg may be supported on the therapist's shoulder. Begin at the thigh. Use light but broad strokes towards the heart. Then cover the leg, foot and ankle. Use effleurage for about 10 minutes every couple of hours.

Lymphatic pumps and **passive joint movements** may be used on the lower limb. See the section on lymph pumps for a description of the techniques.

After a couple of days or when the swelling has subsided use **transverse friction** over the damaged ligament with your fingertip or a T bar as the applicator for about 1 minute. Apply strapping over the ankle and encourage the patient to engage in progressively greater levels of activity for a few days.

After a few days repeat the treatment. Increase the duration and pressure of your applicator depending on the patient's tolerance to pain. Transverse friction over a torn ligament will be painful and it should be explained to the patient that it is a technique, which is necessary to facilitate the removal of temporary scar tissue and its replacement by a stronger permanent ligament.

Strapping involves placing a layer of tubigrip elastic stocking over the leg, foot and ankle and covering this with 5 cm (2 inch) Zinc Oxide tape. The tape must be applied while the foot is held in eversion. Strapping is applied in the following order: anchor strapping, then stirrup strapping and finally figure of eight strapping. It must be firm enough to limit ankle movement yet not so tight as to inhibit circulation or cause discomfort.

After the strapping it is essential that the patient cooperates by performing vigorous ankle exercises. Stressing the ligament while it is protected against over-stretching or repeating the injury with the strapping is the key to restoring structural integrity to the ligament. In order of decreasing importance the following exercises or activities are recommended: soft sand running, tennis, dancing, balancing on the one foot while juggling balls, a wobble board. In all of these activities it is important that the movements are generally: quick and vigorous, change direction, from side to side and are not anticipated. Repeat the treatment, strapping and exercises.

Technique 52.1 Friction over the lateral ankle ligaments

Patient

- Supine with their head on a pillow or folded towel.

Therapist

- Stand at the side of the table level with the patient's foot.

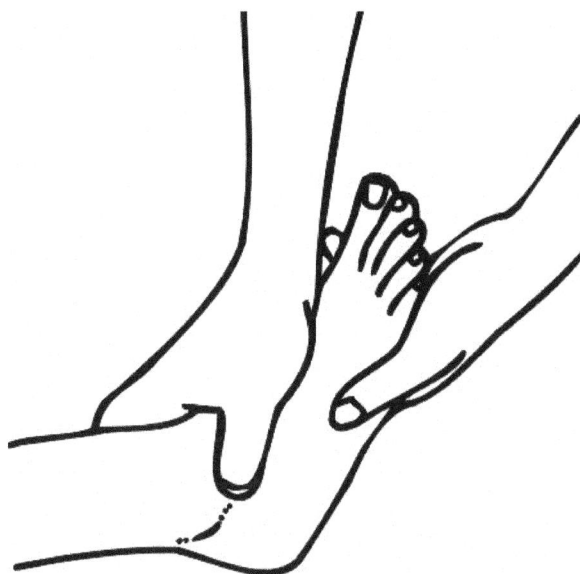

Figure 52.1 Lateral ankle ligament (shown for the anterior talofibular ligament)

Applicator

- The tip of your thumb.

Tissue tension

- Find the joint line.
- Place your thumb on the ligament. It will be tender to touch.
- The three lateral ligaments run obliquely inferiorly.
- Usually, it is only the anterior talofibular ligament that is damaged.
- Take up the tissue tension by gradually increasing your thumb pressure on the ligament.

Transverse Friction

- Work across the ligament with transverse friction.
- Apply firm pressure over a small area.
- Follow the joint line around the lateral malleolus.

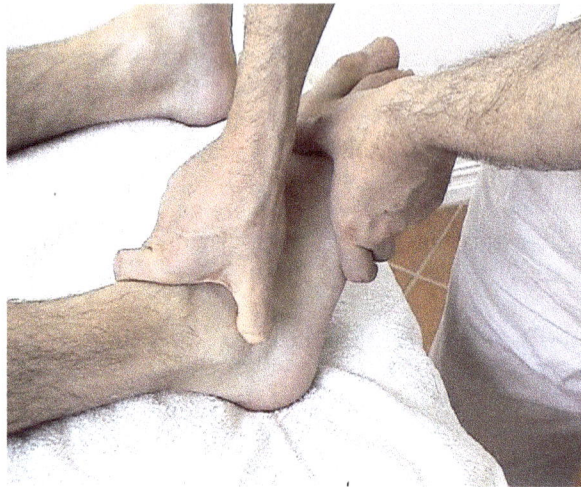

Picture 52.1

53. The lymphatic system and superficial veins

The lymphatic system drains away excess protein and fluid, mainly water, which escapes from the blood. Lymph vessels are found in most tissues. They begin small and gradually join together to form larger vessels. Lymph is drawn into the small vessels by the movement of muscles, which push against the thin walled vessels with assistance from the diaphragm.

The Diaphragm is a musculotendinous dome that arches into the thoracic and forms the roof of the abdomen. The muscle attaches to the xiphisternum, lower six costal cartilages and ribs, L1-3 vertebral bodies, via crura and inserts into a central tendon. The right dome may extend up to T8 or 9 and ribs 4 or 5 at the mid-clavicular line. In quiet respiration the dome move vertically 1 cm and in forced respiration it may move 3 to 10 cm. Its position depends on the respiration cycle, stomach size, posture (ie standing or supine) and the build of the person.
Its functions include respiration (especially in males), defecation, urination and parturition.

Valves inside the vessels prevent the backward flow of lymph. On its way through the lymphatic system the lymph is filtered by lymph nodes. These remove foreign bodies such as bacteria. The lymph eventually empties into the blood just below the lower cervical spine.

If the lymphatic system is not working efficiently there may be a build up of protein in the tissues and this will be followed by fluid entering the tissues. Swelling reduces the oxygenation of the tissues and interferes with their normal functioning. If sustained the inflammation may eventually lead to the formation of fibrous tissue in the area affected.

The causes of lymphatic dysfunction include trauma, inactivity and paralysis, infection, parasites, organ disease such as hepatitis, radiotherapy for cancer, surgery such as a mastectomy, long term venous insufficiency and sometimes very trivial things such as a bee-sting, sunburn, or a long aircraft flight.

Anatomy of the superficial venous system

Upper limb
The **Basilic vein** runs superficially up and around the ulnar border of the forearm, passes anteriorly to the medial epicondyle where it is joined by the median cubital vein from the cephalic vein. It continues up the medial arm into the axilla.

The **Cephalic vein** runs superficially over the anatomical snuffbox and up the radial side of forearm. From the lateral border of the cubital fossa it passes up the anterolateral arm over the lateral side of the biceps to the deltopectoral groove. It goes deep to the pectoral fascia to enter the axillary vein.

Lower limb
The **Long saphenous vein** arises from the venous arch and becomes superficial in the medial aspect of the dorsum of the foot. It may be visible anterior to the medial malleolus and running up the anteromedial aspect of the leg. The vein passes behind the medial condyle of tibia and femur and follows sartorius to the inguinal region where it becomes the femoral vein (deep).

The **Short saphenous vein** arises from the dorsum of the foot and runs behind the lateral malleolus and up the posterior leg to the middle of the popliteal fossa, where it becomes the popliteal vein (deep).

The deep veins follow the major arteries.

Lymphatic drainage techniques - lymph pumps
The classic techniques for assisting lymph drainage are described in this chapter. Any repeated active or passive movement of a limb would however, result in the movement of lymph and venous blood. Improvised techniques should also be utilised by the therapist.

Technique 53.1 Arm method

Patient

- Supine.

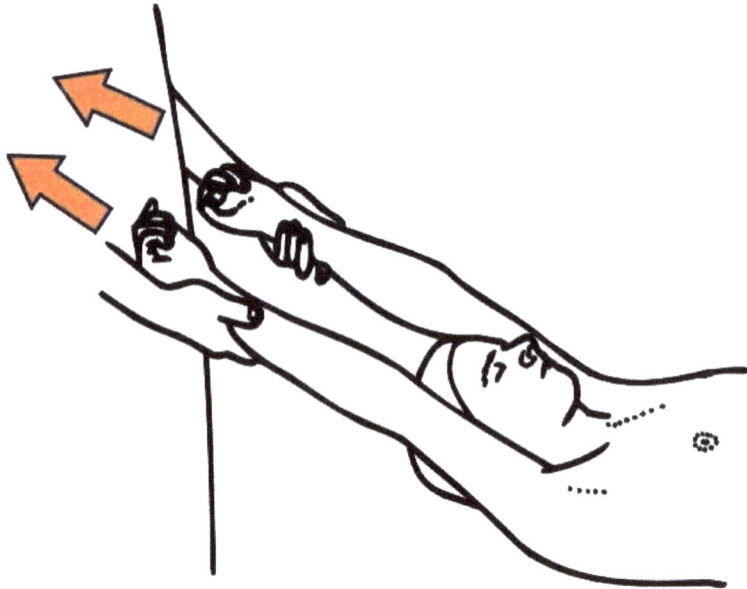

Therapist

- Stand at the head of the table.
- Grasp the patient's wrists and abduct arms fully overhead.
- Apply a rapid push-pull, oscillatory movement of the arms for about one minute.

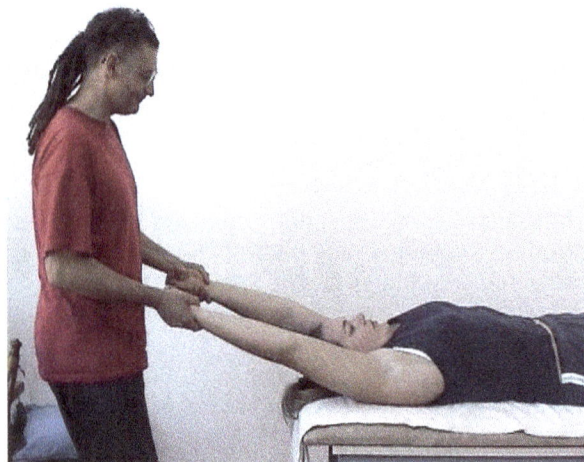

Picture 53.1

Technique 53.2 Foot method

Patient

- Supine.

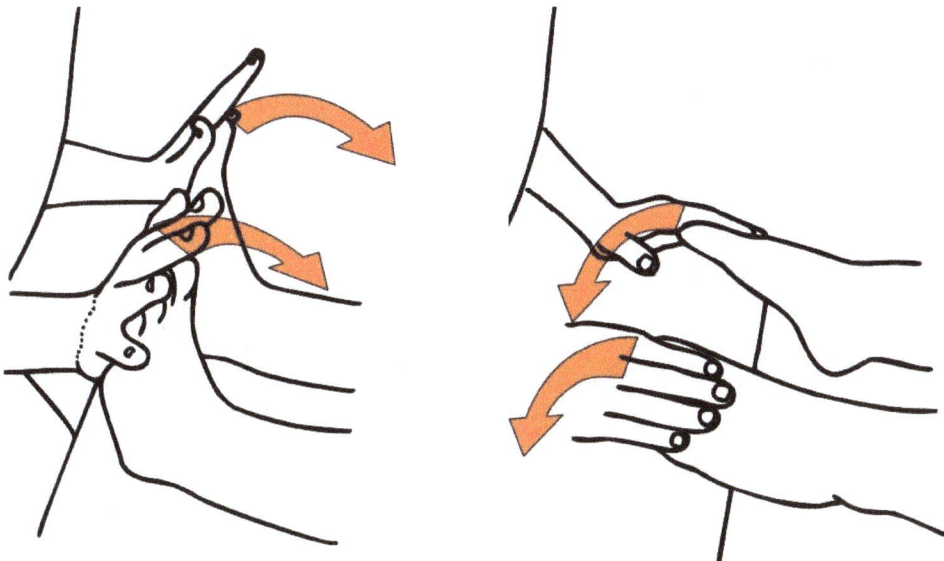

Therapist

- Stand at foot of table and grasp the patient's feet.
- Apply a rapid push-pull, oscillatory movement with your hands to plantarflex and dorsiflex the patient's feet.
- Continue for about one minute.

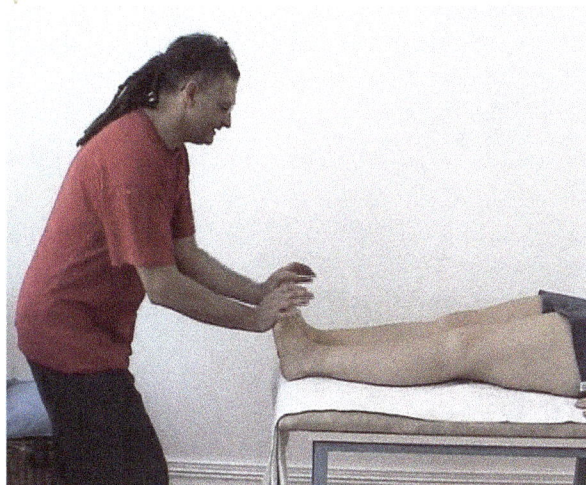

Picture 53.2

Technique 53.3 Respiratory method

Patient

- Supine.

Therapist

- Stand at the head of table.
- Place your palms on either side of the rib cage just lateral to the sternum.

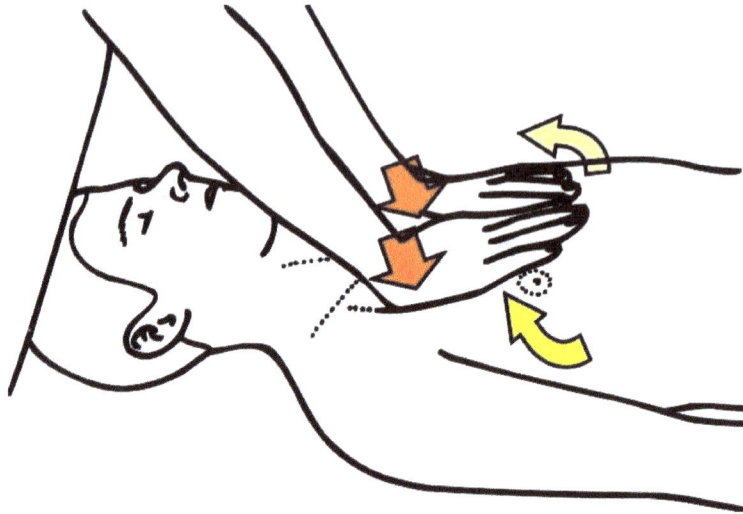

Action

- Ask the patient to inhale deeply.
- As patient exhales fully press down on ribs to assist exhalation.
- At the point of maximum exhalation ask the patient to inhale, then suddenly release the pressure of your hands.
- A suction sound may be heard.
- Continue for about one minute.

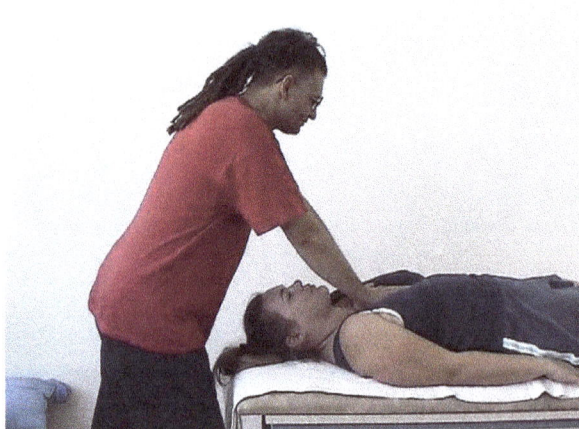

Picture 53.3

Technique 53.4 Spleen/Liver pump

Patient

- Sidelying with hips and knees flexed.

Therapist

- Stand at the side of the table.
- Place your palms on the side of the lower rib cage.

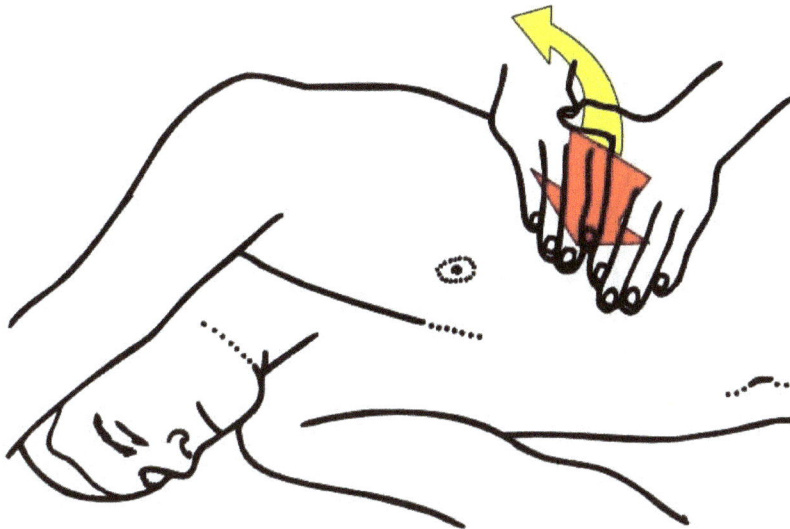

Action

- Ask the patient to inhale deeply.
- As patient exhales apply a downward pressure over the lower rib cage and then release in an oscillatory manner.
- Continue for about one minute.

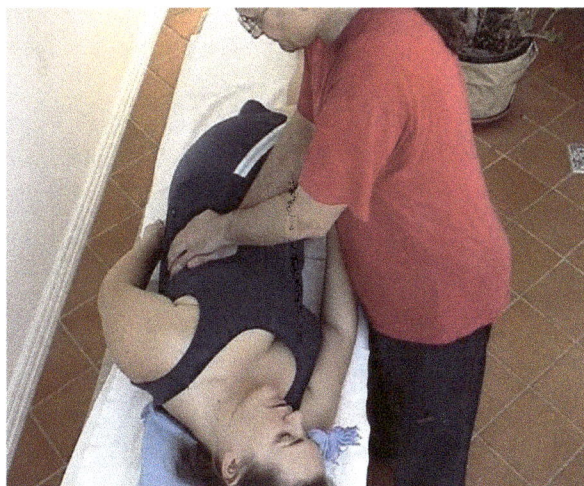

Picture 53.4

Technique 53.5 Sacral rocking method

Patient

- Prone.

Therapist

- Stand at the side of the table, adjacent to the patient's sacrum.
- Place both hands over the patient's sacrum, with the fingers of one hand pointing cephalad and the fingers of the other hand pointing caudad.

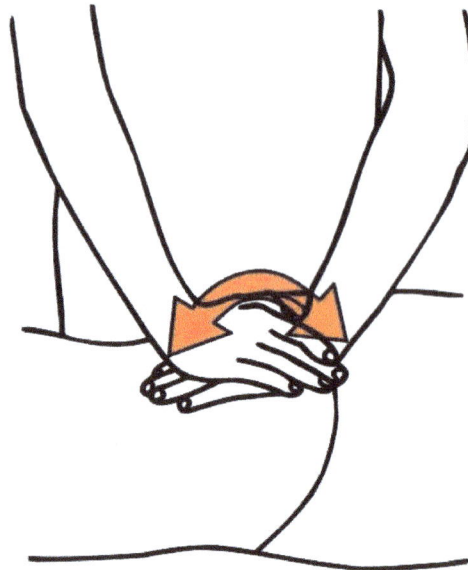

Action

- Keep your elbows extended.
- Apply rhythmic rocking to the sacrum in a direction of flexion and extension.
- Continue for about one minute.

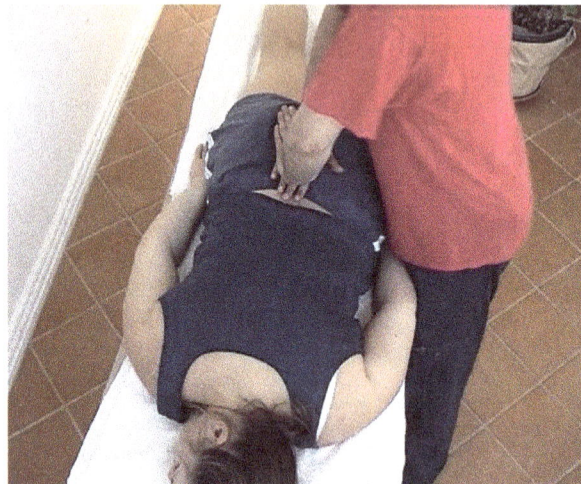

Picture 53.5

Technique 53.6 Effleurage

Apply gentle stroking over the skin in the direction of the heart.

54. Somafeedback

Somafeedback assesses the patient's ability to relax a single muscle or a group of muscles and corrects the muscle problems that are identified. The therapist gently supports and then lets go of the body part. The rate of oscillation varies from a slow movement of 10 -15 cycles per minute to a vibration of about 150 cycles per minute. The body part is usually the distal end of a long bone, but may be a group of vertebrae or ribs, or any point on the scull or pelvis.

The operator uses verbal and tactile systems to encourage maximum relaxation and correct the passive mechanism. Key words or verbal triggers are used. Overuse behaviour may be conscious or unconscious. Unconscious overuse behaviour may need to be exposed and brought to the patient's awareness. There are three types of statements:

a) provoking statements b) distracting statements c) relaxing statements.

Provoking statements are used to help identify overuse problems by provoking muscle contraction in a resting muscle. They are used to teach the patient to relax their muscle overuse during times of stress. It is during times of stress and mental concentration that muscle overuse is most likely to occur and if the problem is to be corrected it is essential that the patient learn to break this habit during these times. Provocative statements work by helping to stimulate the habitual muscle contractions in the patient. Use statements that are true or likely to be true and are likely to irritate the patient and trigger an overuse response in the muscle. Statements such as 'you are uptight', 'you are neurotic', 'you smoke/bite your nails' may be used. Warn the patient in advance that the technique will be provoking and stressful. Explain that this should not be regarded as a personal attack and that it is just part of the treatment.

Once the muscle tension is brought to the patient's awareness then the patient will have a better idea which muscle or group of muscles to relax. Another way to force the muscle to contract, thereby bringing the muscle tension to the patient's awareness is by lightly prodding the muscle, or in the spine by springing the vertebra. It is insufficient to learn to relax muscles in a stress-free environment. For lasting benefit, it must be learned in a stressful or challenging environment.

Relaxing statements are used to help the patient to let go of muscle tension. They are the first to be used once the problem has been identified. For example, say to the patient 'let go' or 'just relax'.

Distracting statements are used when you are confident that the patient is able to voluntarily relax their muscles when you prompt them with relaxing statements. These test whether or not the patient can relax in a more neutral situation. For example, say to the patient 'have you seen any good films lately?' or 'what day is good for your next appointment?'

Always finish with provoking statements to determine if the patient can relax their muscle or muscles in a stressful situation. Provoking statements test whether the patient is able to relax in a situation that is more realistic to life. Only when the patient can relax the muscle when under stress can they be cured of their overuse problem.

Move the joint or body part in a variety of randomly changing speeds and directions. Some positions are more convenient for controlling the patient's body part or more effective for revealing overuse patterns. The cervical spine, shoulder muscles, muscles of mastication, scapulo-thoracic muscles, the spinal muscles and the posterior hip muscles are the areas of the body most prone to muscle overuse and tension.

Testing the passive component of myofascia

Technique 54.1 Frontalis and occipitalis

- The patient is supine or seated.
- Cup the crown of the head in the palm of your hand and ensure a firm grip on the scalp or galea aponeurotica.
- Move the galea aponeurotica anteriorly, posteriorly, laterally and medially and rotate it.
- Feel for loss of free movement in any particular direction, especially after making distracting and provoking statements.
- Encourage the patient to relax their frontalis and occipitalis muscles and feel for better movement of the scalp.

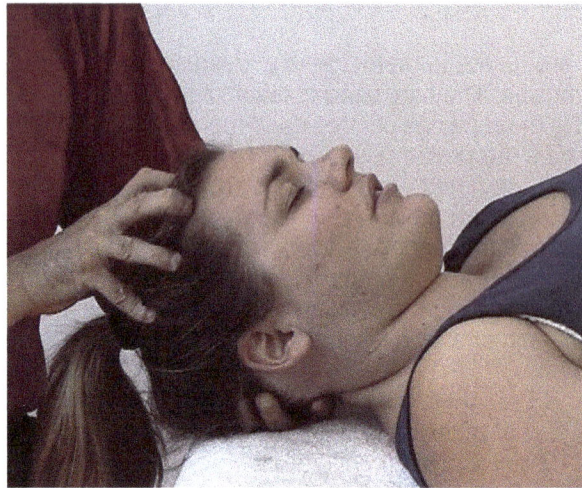

Picture 54.1

Technique 54.2 Muscles of mastication

- The patient is supine or seated.
- Open and close the patient's mouth.
- Move the patient's jaw from side to side.
- Assess the patient's ability to relax.

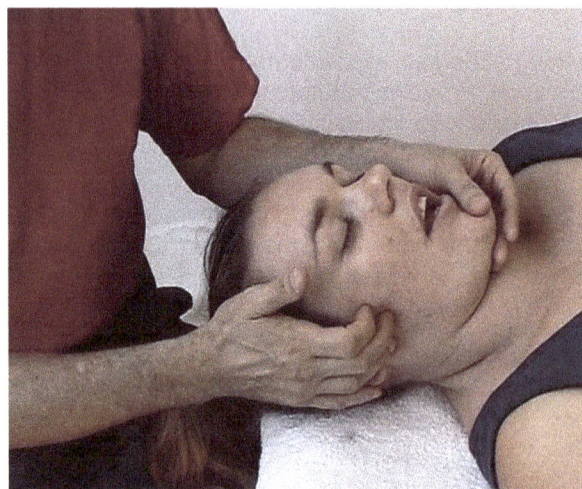

Picture 54.2

Technique 54.3 Cervical prevertebral muscles and sternocleidomastoid

- (a) The patient is supine.
- Lift up on the spines of the mid-cervical region.
- Expect the head to drop back into extension.
- (b) The patient is sitting or supine with their head over the end of the table.
- Support the patient's head in both hands.
- Take the patient's head and neck into extension and then bring it back to neutral.
- Assess the patient's ability to relax.

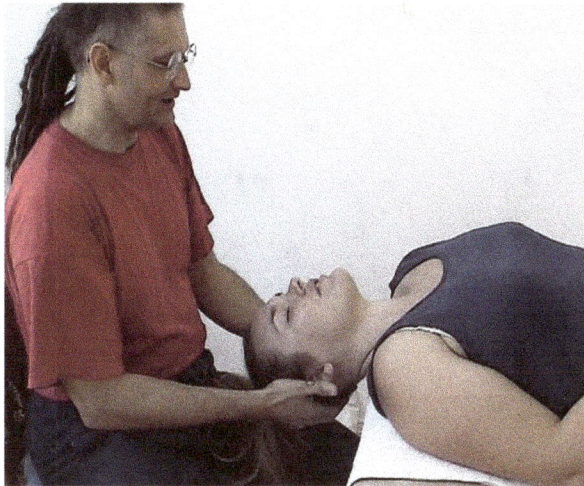

Picture 54.3

Technique 54.4 Superior and inferior hyoid muscles

- Grasp the hyoid bone between the index finger and thumb of your hand.
- Move it from side to side.
- Assess the patient's ability to relax.

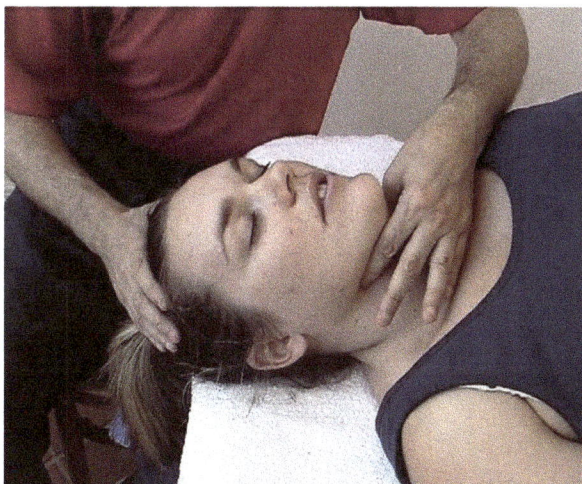

Picture 54.4

Technique 54.5 Suboccipital muscles

- The therapist slides the fingers of both hands under the patient's head until the patient's occiput rests on the operator's fingertips.
- The point of contact under the occiput must allow the patient's head to be perfectly balanced over the fingertips.
- Ask the patient to relax.
- Flex and extend your fingers so your fingertips rock the patient's head in flexion and extension.
- Also flex the fingers of one hand while extending the fingers of the other hand to rotate the patient's head.
- Assess the patient's ability to relax.

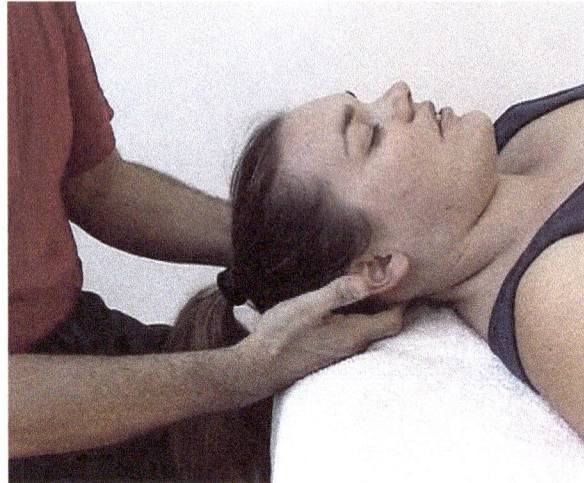

Picture 54.5

Technique 54.6 Cervical vertebral muscles

- The patient is supine.
- Slide the fingers of both hands under the patient's cervical spine with one hand either side of the spine.
- The articular pillars of the patient's cervical spine rest on the therapist's fingertips.
- Ask the patient to relax.
- Flex the fingers of one hand while extending the fingers of the other hand to rotate or sidebend the patient's neck.
- Alternatively, roll the patient's head from side to side by passing it between the fingertip of your hands.
- Assess the patient's ability to relax.

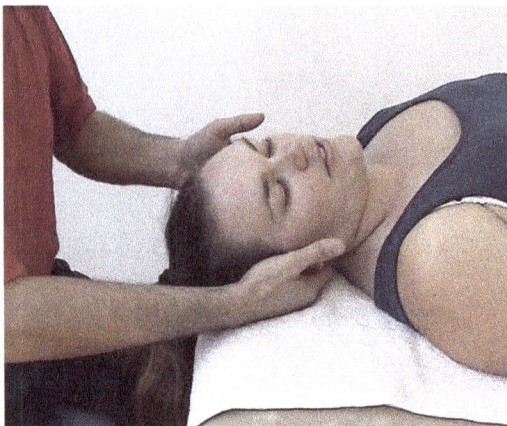

Picture 54.6

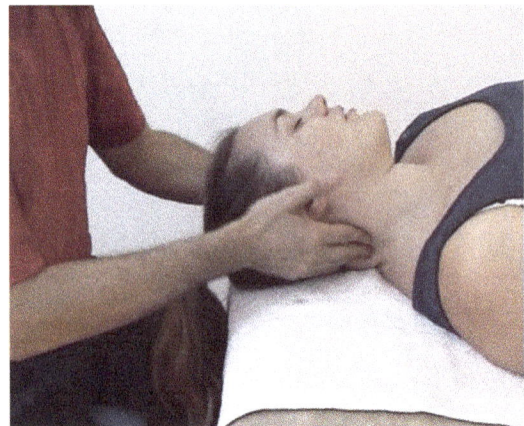

Picture 54.7

Technique 54.7 Cervical vertebral and prevertebral muscles, scalene, trapezius and levator scapulae

- Patient seated.
- Support the patient's head in both hands.
- Ask the patient to relax their head and neck completely.
- Push the patient's head from side to side and forwards and back.
- Pass it between your hands.
- Assess the patient's ability to relax.

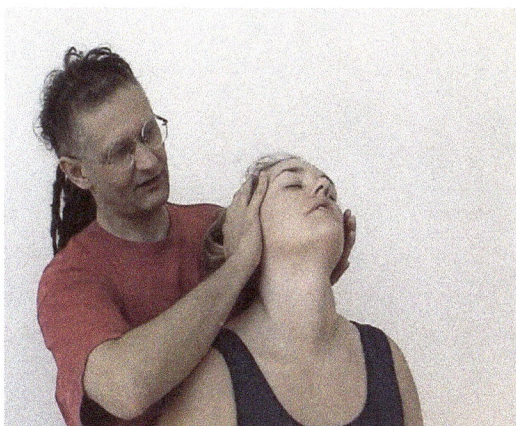

Picture 54.8

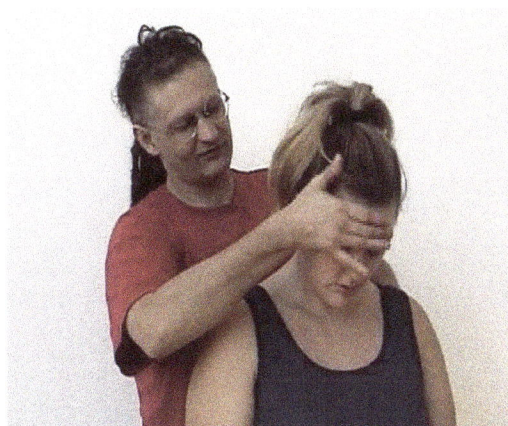

Picture 54.9

Technique 54.8 Erector spinae

- The patient is seated.
- Support the patient's forehead in one hand.
- Contact the erector spinae with the fingertips of the other hand.
- Ask the patient to relax their head, neck and upper thoracic spine completely.
- Support the weight of the patient's head and allow the spine to flex.
- To maintain the patient over their centre of gravity, take their thoracic backwards as their head drops forwards.
- Support the patient's head in varying degrees of flexion.
- Assess the patient's ability to relax

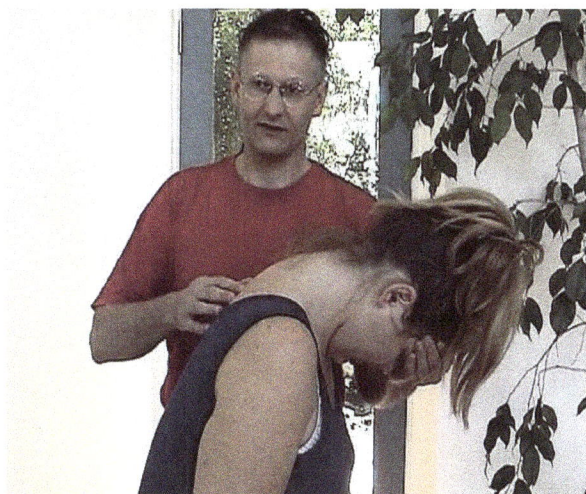

Picture 54.10

Technique 54.9 Trapezius and levator scapulae

- The patient is seated, the elbows are fully flexed and the arms are held close to the side of the rib cage.
- Grasp under both elbows and support the patient's shoulders through their arms.
- Elevate and depress the patient's shoulders.
- Ask the patient to relax their shoulders completely.
- Assess the patient's ability to relax.

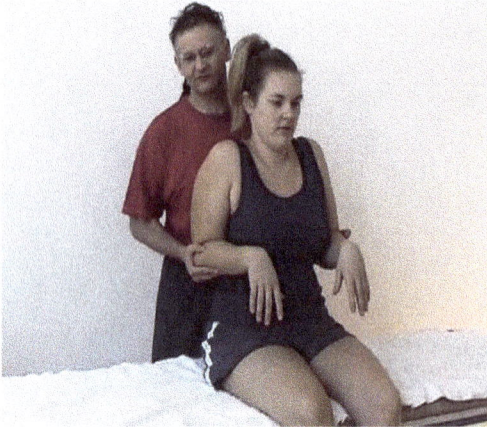

Picture 54.11

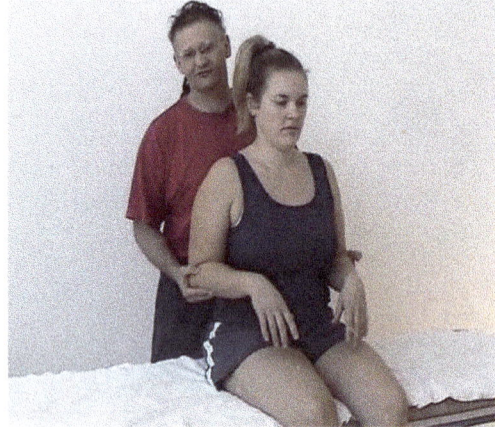

Picture 54.12

Technique 54.10 Pectoralis major and minor

- Patient supine.
- Ask the patient to relax their pectoralis muscles and allow their arm to fall outwards (abducted and externally rotated).
- Assess the patient's ability to relax in different positions.

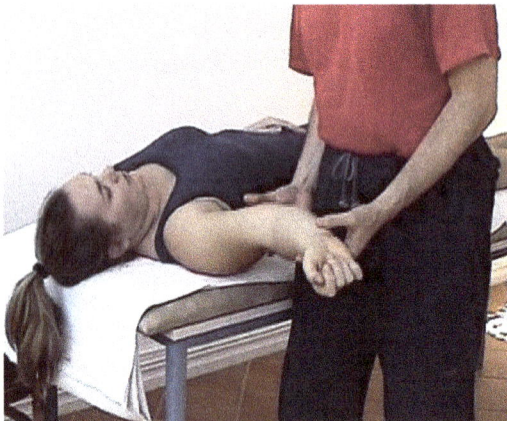

Picture 54.13

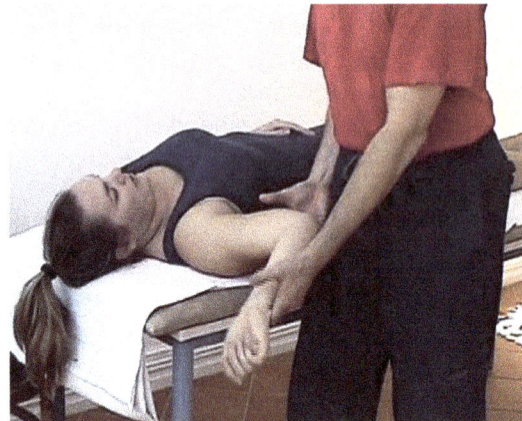

Picture 54.14

Technique 54.11 Deltoid

- Patient seated for middle deltoid, supine for anterior deltoid, prone for posterior deltoid.
- Lift the patient's arm.
- Ask the patient to relax their arm and allow their arm to drop.
- Assess the patient's ability to relax at 45 degrees, 90 degrees, 135 degrees abduction.

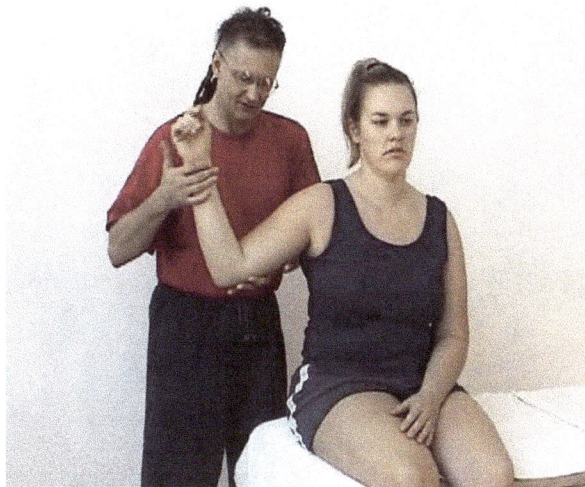

Picture 54.15

Technique 54.12 Biceps

- Patient supine or seated.
- Ask the patient to relax their biceps and allow their forearm to fall to a straightened (extended) position.
- Assess the patient's ability to relax at 90 degrees, 135 degrees flexion and just prior to full extension.

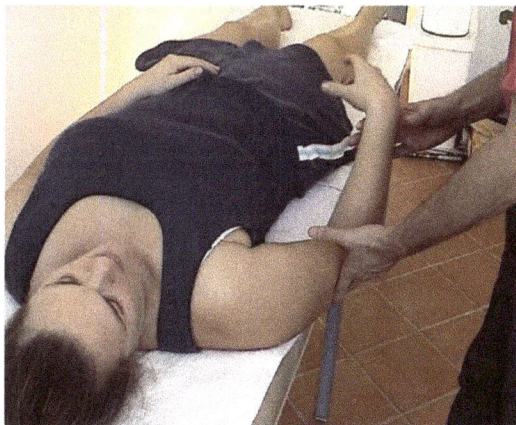

Picture 54.16

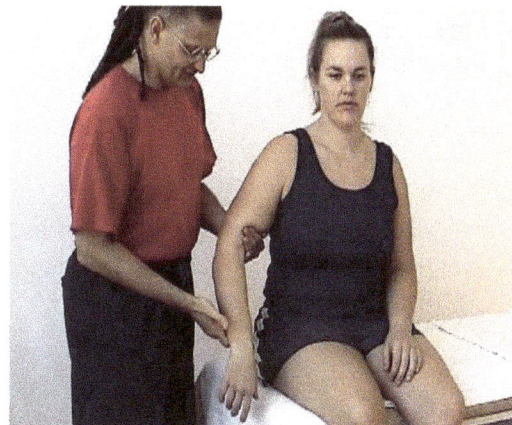

Picture 54.17

Technique 54.13 Triceps

- Patient seated.
- Pull back (extend) the patient's arm so the forearm is hanging vertically.
- Ask the patient to relax their triceps (and biceps) and allow their forearm to swing.
- Assess the patient's ability to relax at 45 degrees and 135 degrees flexion.

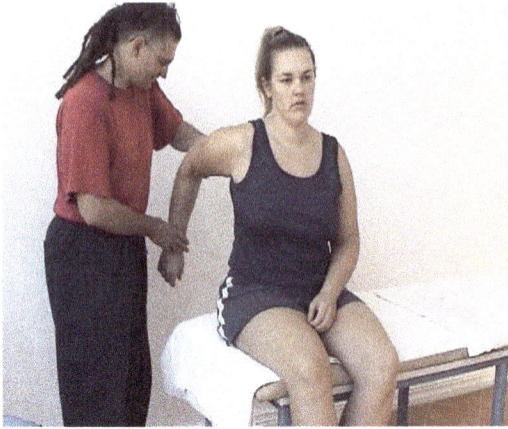

Picture 54.18

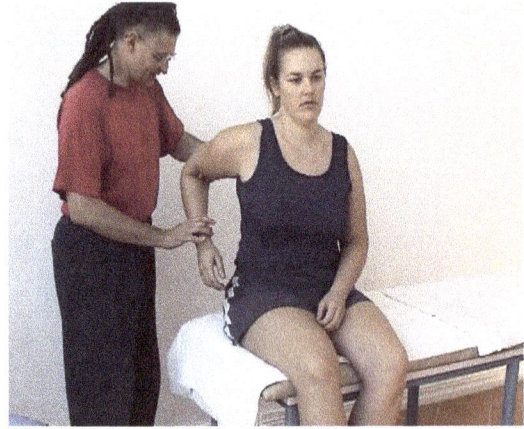

Picture 54.19

Technique 54.14 Medial forearm muscles (flexor carpi radialis, flexor carpi ulnaris, palmaris longus, flexor digitorum profundus, flexor digitorum superficialis and flexor pollicis longus) and Lateral forearm muscles (extensor carpi radialis brevis, extensor carpi radialis longus, extensor carpi ulnaris and finger extensor tendons)

- Patient seated or supine.
- Support the patient's arm.
- Ask the patient to relax their forearm and hand completely.
- Push the patient's forearm or wrist into flexion and extension.
- Pass the patient's forearm or wrist between the your hands.
- Catch it as it falls under gravity.
- Assess the patient's ability to relax.

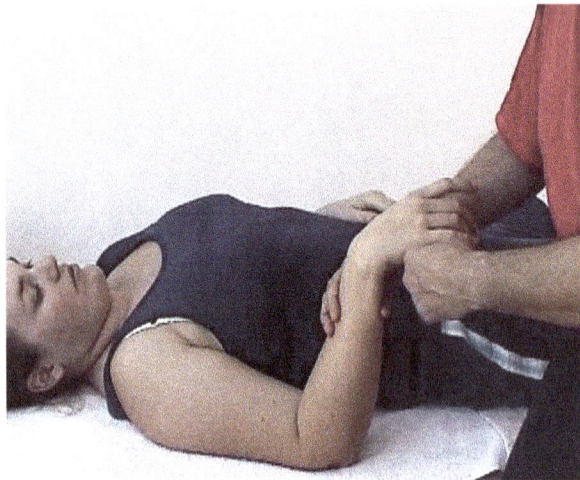

Picture 54.20

324

Technique 54.15 Iliopsoas

- Patient supine. The legs should remain extended.
- Lift up from under the patient's knees.
- Expect the knee to drop back (extend) down to the table when you let go.
- Assess the patient's ability to relax.

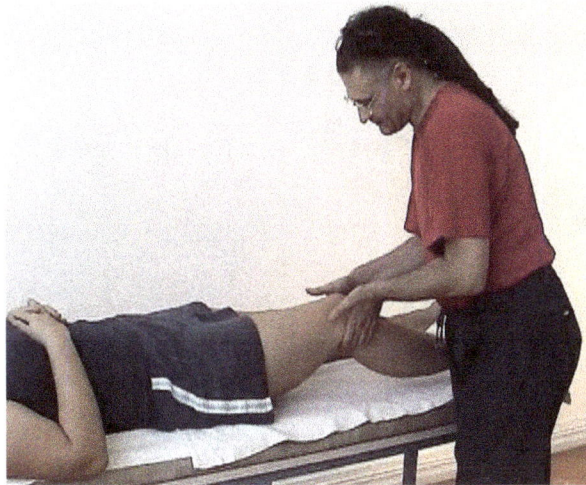

Picture 54.21

Technique 54.16 Quadriceps: (Rectus femoris, vastus lateralis, vastus medialis, and vastus intermedius)

- Patient supine or seated with legs hanging over the side of the table.
- Lift up one of the patient's legs.
- Ask the patient to relax their quadriceps and allow their leg to fall (flex).
- Assess the patient's ability to relax at 45 degrees flexion and full extension.

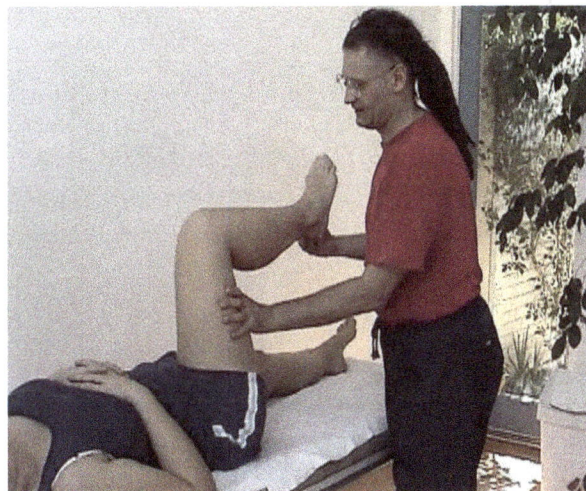

Picture 54.22

Technique 54.17 Hamstrings (Biceps femoris, semimembranosus and semitendinosus)

- Patient prone.
- Flex the patient's leg to 90 degrees.
- Grasp the patient's foot between both your hands.
- Ask the patient to relax their hip muscles and allow their leg to fall into flexion and extension.
- Assess the patient's ability to relax in both directions.

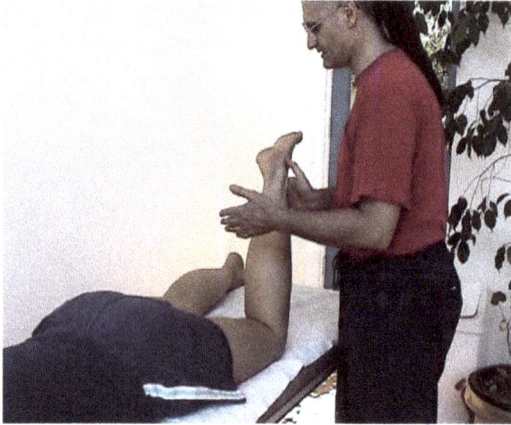

Picture 54.23

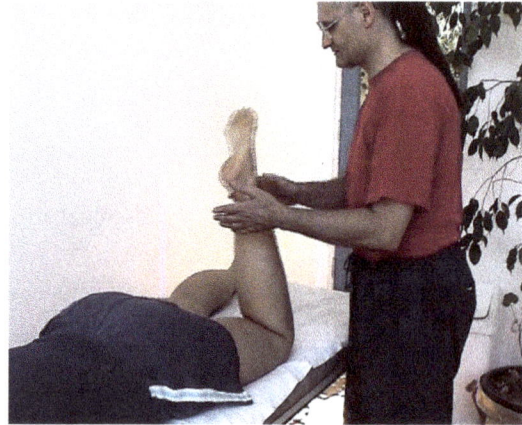

Picture 54.24

Technique 54.18 Hip internal rotators (gluteus medius and minimus) and hip external rotators (piriformis, obturator internus and externus, the gamelli and quadratus femoris)

- Patient prone.
- Flex the patient's leg to 90 degrees.
- Grasp the patient's foot between both your hands.
- Ask the patient to relax their hip muscles and allow their leg to fall into internal rotation and external rotation.
- Assess the patient's ability to relax in all directions.

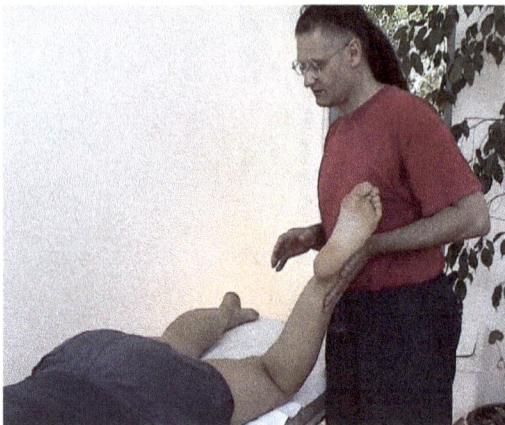

Picture 54.25

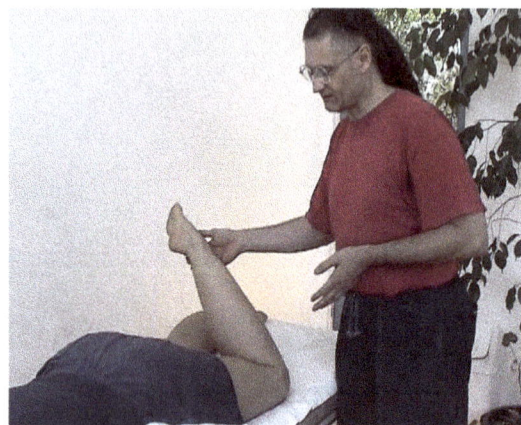

Picture 54.26

Technique 54.19 Hip abductors (Gluteus medius, gluteus minimus, tensor fascia lata and iliotibial tract)

- The patient is sidelying.
- Ask the patient to relax their leg from an abducted position.
- Assess the patient's ability to relax with the leg at full abduction and just prior to adduction.

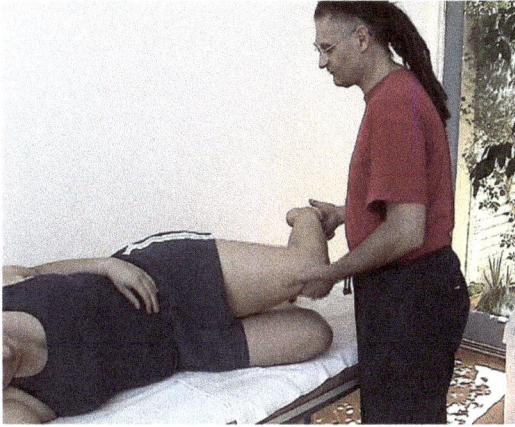

Picture 54.27

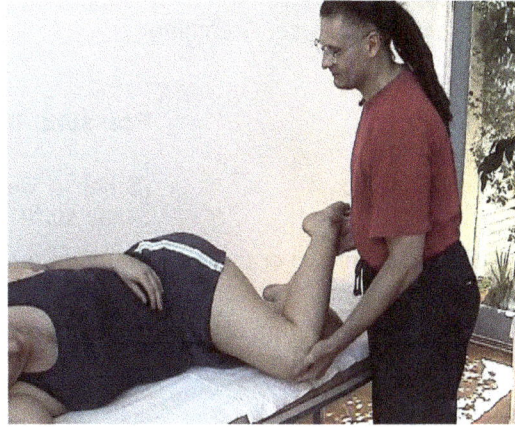

Picture 54.28

Technique 54.20 Hip adductors (Adductor magnus, longus, brevis, gracilis and pectineus)

- Patient sidelying with hips and knees flexed and on the table.
- Place a pillow between their legs
- Lift up the patient's legs. Lift up the patient's knee.
- Ask the patient to relax their adductor muscles and allow their knee to fall back to the table.
- Assess the patient's ability to relax.

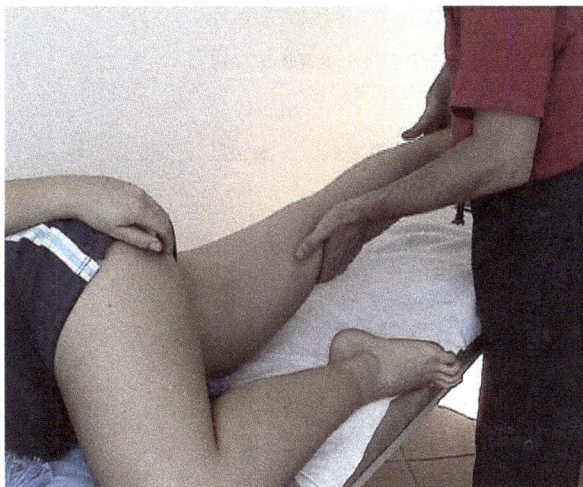

Picture 54.29

Key Components of Myofaction

Myofaction variables
6. Cross fibre force/ Transverse + Compression
7. Longitudinal force/ Stretch
8. Secondary force/ Torsion or Leverage
9. Internal contraction force/ Tension
10. Respiratory force/ Breathing

Applicators	Pressure/ Surface Area
1. One fingertip	(Small to Medium pressure Small surface area).
2. The heads of two or three distal phalanges (fingertips).	(Medium pressure Small to Medium surface area)
3. The heads of fingers of both hands, interdigitating	(Medium pressure Medium surface area)
4. The lateral side of thumb	(Medium pressure Medium surface area)
5. The thenar eminence	(Medium pressure Large surface area)
6. Opposition of fingers and thumb to grasp tissue and pull towards therapist	(Medium pressure Medium surface area)
7. The articular surface of the proximal row of IP joints (one knuckle or a row of knuckles)	(Medium to Large pressure Small to Medium surface area)
8. The pad of the thumb	(Medium to Large pressure Medium surface area)
9. The tip of the thumb	(Large pressure Small surface area)
10. The tip of the olecranon process	(Large pressure Small surface area)
11. The pisiform bone	(Large pressure Small surface area).
12. The tubercle of the scaphoid and the tubercle of the trapezium (heel of hand)	(Large pressure Medium surface area)
13. The proximal border of the shaft of the ulnar from the olecranon process	(Large pressure Medium to Large surface area)
14. The dorsal surface of the four proximal phalanges of fingers. (flat part on back of fingers of fist)	(Large pressure Large surface area)

Arrows

White arrow   The general direction of the muscle fibres and their attachments.

Blue arrow   The primary direction of tissue lockup. This is a transverse force, at right angles to the direction of the muscle fibre and always involves some compression The amount of compression required depends on how deep the tissue is, on the amount of initial tissue slack and on how much tension is taken up by the secondary and longitudinal forces.

Green arrow   The secondary direction of tissue lockup. The force may be in any direction other than the primary direction of tissue lockup, but it is usually a torsional (rotational) force. The secondary force may use a bone as a lever. The lever acts in a counter direction to the primary force to amplify that force.

Red arrow   The stretch direction of tissue lockup. This is usually along the line of contraction of the muscle and in the same direction as the muscle fibre. This is a longitudinal force. It is also the direction for assessing the ability of the muscle to relax and for correcting the passive component.

Yellow arrow   The contraction tissue lockup. This is along the line of the muscle fibres. It is a force produced by the muscle and acting on it from within it.

Hypothetical tissue lockup
(The more tension taken up by one the less tension is available for another)

Compression takes up	20%
Transverse force takes up	20%
Secondary force takes up	20%
Longitudinal force takes up	20%
Contraction force takes up	20%
Total tissue lockup is	100%

Bibliography

Daniels and Worthingham: *Muscle Testing* 4th Edition 1980 Published by W.B. Saunders Company.

Hartman, Laurie S DO, MRO. *Handbook of Osteopathic Technique* 2nd Edition 1985. Published by Hutchinson.

Hoppenfeld, Stanley M.D: *Physical Examination of the Spine and Extremities*. 1976 Published by Appleton-Century-Crofts.

Kapandji, I.A. *The Physiology of the Joints* 1974 Published by Churchill Livingstone.

Pansky, Ben PhD.,M.D *Review of Gross Anatomy* 4th Edition 1980. Published by Macmillan Co., Inc.

Wells, Katherine F. PhD: *Kinesiology* 5th Edition. 1971 Published by W.B. Saunders Company.

Williams and Warwick (Edited): *Grays Anatomy* 36th Edition. Published by Churchill Livingstone.

Index